Drug Dependence

To the memory of

FRANCIS E. CAMPS

Late Professor of Forensic Medicine, the London Hospital Medical College;
Ex-President, Society for the Study of Addiction;
First Chairman, Medical Council on Alcoholism;
First President, Association for the Prevention of Addiction

A source of inspiration and a pioneer of scientific research
in the field of dependency as well as in legal medicine

Drug Dependence

Current Problems and Issues

Edited by M. M. Glatt

Consultant Psychiatrist and Member of WHO Expert
Advisory Panel, Drug Dependence

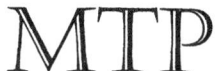

Published in the UK by
MTP Press Limited,
St. Leonard's House,
Lancaster, England

ISBN-13: 978-94-011-6149-7   e-ISBN-13: 978-94-011-6147-3
DOI: 10.1007/978-94-011-6147-3

Contents

Contents

List of Contributors

R. Battegay, MD
Professor Ordinarius of Psychiatry of the Medical Faculty at the University of Basel, Psychiatric University Out-Patient Clinic Petersgraben 1, CH-4051 Basel, Switzerland

Nils Bejerot
Socialmedicinska Institutionen, Karolinska Institutet, Industrivägen 13, Stockholm 60, Sweden

Peter G. Bourne
Special Assistant to the President for Health Issues, The White House, Washington, D.C. 20500, USA.

W. K. van Dijk, MD
Professor of Psychiatry, Psychiatrische Kliniek; State University of Groningen, Oostersingel 59, Groningen, The Netherlands

Stanley Einstein
Executive Director, Institute for the Study of Drug Addiction, 680 West End Avenue, New York, NY 10025, USA; Director, Jerusalem Centre for Drug Misuse Intervention, Jerusalem; Associate Professor, Department of Criminology, Barilan University, Ramat Gan, Israel.

Denys E. Fry, DE, BSc
Epsom Hospital Laboratories at West Park Hospital, Horton Lane, Epsom, Surrey, England

Max M. Glatt, MD, FRCP, FRC Psych, DPM
Consultant-in-Charge, Alcoholism and Drug Dependence Unit, St. Bernard's Hospital, Southall, Middlesex, England; Hon. Consultant, Department of Psychological Medicine, University College Hospital; Hon. Senior Lecturer, Medical School, University College Hospital, London.

John H. Langer, PhB, MA, EdD
Chief, Preventive Programs Section, Office of Public Affairs, Drug Enforcement Administration, US Department of Justice, Washington DC, USA

Donald B. Louria, MD
Professor and Chairman, Department of Preventive Medicine and Community Health, New Jersey Medical School, College of Medicine and Dentistry of New Jersey, 100 Bergen Street, Newark, New Jersey 07102, USA

Vincent Marks MA, DM, FRCP
Professor of Clinical Biochemistry, Department of Biochemistry, University of Surrey, Guildford, Surrey, England

Martin A. Plant, BSc, MA, PhD
MRC Unit of Epidemiological Studies in Psychiatry, University Department of Psychiatry, Royal Edinburgh Hospital, Morningside Hospital, Edinburgh, Scotland

E. Bruce Ritson, MD MRC Psych
Consultant Psychiatrist, Department of Psychiatry, University Department of Psychiatry, Royal Edinburgh Hospital, Edinburgh, Scotland

Reginald G. Smart, MA, PhD
Associate Research Director, Department of Evaluation Studies, Addiction Research Foundation, 33 Russell Street, Toronto 4, Ontario, Canada

Introduction

Drug dependence—according to the 1969 World Health Organization definition—is 'A state, psychic and sometimes also physical, resulting from the interaction between a living organism and a drug, characterized by behavioural and other responses that always include a compulsion to take the drug on a continuous or periodic basis in order to experience its psychic effects, and sometimes to avoid the discomfort of its absence. Tolerance may or may not be present. A person may be dependent on more than one drug'.

The substitution of the term 'Drug Dependence' in place of the previously employed terms 'Drug Addiction' and 'Drug Habituation' was recommended by a WHO Expert Committee in 1964. It was felt that there had been ongoing confusion in the use of the terms addiction and habituation and in particular, misuse of the term addiction. In 1965 the WHO Expert Committee 'was pleased to note the generally favourable reaction to the recommendations' made in the previous year and the gradual acceptance of the new term. In general, in subsequent years the term 'Drug Dependence' has gained increasing acceptance. Yet it would seem that difficulties may arise whatever term and definition may be used (Glatt, 1974), and although by and large the newer term seems more appropriate than the older definitions, one still often comes across the term 'Addiction', and this not only when discussing the matter with laymen or drug misusers themselves. The British Home Office, for example, when publishing annual statistics about the numbers of 'known' drug misusers, still talks of 'Addicts', referring in this connection in the main to opiates but also the stimulant cocaine. The latter produces a strong psychological dependence but no physical dependence, and if 'Addiction' were to imply essentially physical dependence, cocaine is certainly not a physical addiction-producing drug. In the present volume the term 'addiction' is still used occasionally (Dr N. Bejerot, for example, proposes a socio-medical classification of 'drug addiction'). Under the circumstances it may be of interest to remind readers that according to the (revised) old WHO definition (1957) 'Drug Addiction is a state of periodic or chronic intoxication produced by the repeated consumption of a drug (natural or synthetic). Its characteristics include: (1) an overpowering desire or need (compulsion) to continue taking the drug and to obtain it by any means; (2) a tendency to increase the dose; (3) a psychic (psychological) and generally a physical dependence on the effects of the drug; (4) detrimental effect on the individual and on society'. Incidentally, it might be opportune to mention here that the term 'overpowering' used in this definition (and similarly the term 'overwhelming' so often employed by drug misusers and uncontrolled drinkers) merely denotes a relative and not an absolute state. What is experienced as absolutely overpowering and overwhelming by one individual in a given situation and under certain circumstances, can be tolerated with a major or minor effort by another individual possibly under a somewhat different set of circumstances. In all aspects of drug dependance not only the 'agent' (the pharmacological nature of the drug concerned) but also the psychological-biological make-up of the individual ('host') and social and other environmental factors have always to be considered (Glatt, 1974). This applies to aetiology, the pace of developmental progress of the dependence-progress, treatment, rehabilitation, prevention, prognosis, etc. and is reflected in all contributions to this volume. All too often in the past attention was mainly directed to the nature of the drug without considering the drug user's personality and his social environment. Neglecting the importance of psychosocial factors was, for example, a prime factor in proving wrong the claims so often put forward in the 1950s and early 1960s that the (wrongly so-called) 'British System' of drug control helped to prevent drug misuse and drug epidemics. In fact, it seemed very effective as long as the users of opiates in the U.K. were relatively stable, middle-aged people with a good working record, i.e., 'therapeutic' or 'professional addicts'. The 'system' broke down as soon as there emerged, in the early 1960s, a new type of drug misuser, young, emotionally immature, socially and occupationally unstable individuals who started to take drugs 'non-therapeutically' and without 'professional' access (Glatt *et al.*, 1967).

Dependence can be psychological ('a condition in which a drug produces a feeling of satisfaction and a psychic drive that require periodic or continuous administration of the drug to produce pleasure or to avoid discomfort'—Eddy *et al.*, 1965) or/and physical ('. . . an adaptive state that manifests itself by intense physical disturbances when the administration of the drug is suspended . . . These disturbances, i.e. the withdrawal or abstinence syndromes, are made up of specific arrays of symptoms and signs of psychic and physical nature that are characteristic for each drug type'—Eddy *et al.*, 1965). Contrary to popular belief it is psychological dependence and not physical dependence which in the long run constitutes the main problem. Certainly, the physical abstinence symptoms which supervene on sudden cessation or very rapid reduction of the amount of the drug, can sometimes be very distressing and even life-threatening. But with skilled supervision, as a rule, this acute withdrawal syndrome can be handled relatively easily. What makes drug dependence so difficult to deal with in the long run, and is responsible for the unfortunate fact that, essentially, states of drug dependence are relapsing disorders, is psychological dependence, the user's recurrent desire to re-experience the instantaneous relief from emotional pain, the detachment from reality and escape 'from it all', or the euphoric 'high' or the 'buzz'. Social factors, too, such as 'subcultures', peer pressure, conditioning, etc. may play a big role in precipitating a relapse, after the individual had experienced a period of freedom from drug use (van Dijk). Physical dependence may be largely concerned in inducing the user not to discontinue his drug taking within a given 'bout', for example, for fear of the 'cold turkey' symptoms supervening on sudden withdrawal of narcotic drugs. Paradoxically, the barbiturate withdrawal syndrome (and similarly in rarer cases also the alcohol withdrawal syndrome) may often be much more dangerous than the much more widely feared opiate abstinence syndrome. Incidentally, the relative importance of psychological and physical dependence can possibly be illustrated by the example of compulsive gambling. Here of course there is no physical—and 'merely' psychological dependence. Nevertheless, compulsive gambling shows most of the characteristic features of compulsive drug-taking and drinking (Glatt, 1974).

In their initial recommendation of the term 'drug dependence' Eddy *et al.* (1965) emphasized that such a state would vary a great deal with the type of drug involved, and that therefore it was always necessary to designate the particular type of drug dependence in each specific case. Accordingly their paper described characteristics of drug dependence of morphine type, barbiturate-alcohol type, cocaine type, cannabis type, amphetamine type, Khat type, and of hallucinogen (LSD) type (given here in the order listed by Eddy *et al.*). To these seven types a later WHO Committee (1973) added a volatile solvent (inhalant) type.

This classification obviously includes both legally used and often widely socially accepted (and 'domesticated'—Jellinek, 1960) drugs, such as alcohol and tobacco, as well as illicit drugs. Relatively little concern was expressed in the past about the dangers of drug misuse as long as it was limited to alcohol, tobacco and (the usually ignored though widespread habitual excess intake by middle-aged women of medically prescribed) barbiturates (Glatt, 1962). It was the illicit use of drugs by the young which in the early 1960s aroused widespread concern. Clearly the fact that some drugs are legal and others illicit does not in itself not tell us anything about the risks or otherwise attached to their misuse. This of course is not fully appreciated by the public, as illustrated, for example by the so often heard pronouncement made by the parent who is so relieved to find that 'my daughter merely drinks quite a bit—but at least she does not take drugs'. A dependence-producing drug ('A drug having the capacity to interact with a living organism to produce a state of psychic or physical dependence—WHO, 1974') may rarely frequently or commonly '. . . be used medically or non-medically without necessarily producing such a state' (WHO, 1974), whether it is a legal or an illicit drug. But likewise the fact that such a drug or substance has been traditionally accepted by society—whether it is alcohol, tobacco (nicotine) or even coffee and tea (with the mild stimulant caffeine) or prescribed by the doctor (such as hypnotics, stimulants, or tranquillizers)—does not provide a guarantee or an immunity against the development of a state of more or less dangerous dependency. In most countries the problems caused by misuse of, and dependence upon, legal drugs—in particular alcohol—are much more widespread than those posed by illicit drugs; and in the UK—as in many other countries—the misuse of the (misleadingly so called 'soft' drugs) amphetamines, barbiturates, etc. and the vast overprescribing and overconsumption of tranquillizers, constitute much more prevalent problems that the consumption of 'hard' narcotics such, as heroin and methadone. All these problems will be touched upon in this volume by various contributors; in the main however it is the use of illicit drugs which is the main subject discussed in its multiple ramifications.

The 1964 WHO Expert Committee on 'Addiction-Producing

Drugs' arrived at its recommendation of the substitute term 'Drug Dependence' when '. . . attempting to find a term that could be applied to drug abuse generally'. Drug abuse was defined (WHO, 1965) as 'the consumption of a drug apart from medical need or in unnecessary quantities'. Drug dependence is of course only one of many possible harmful consequences of drug abuse (the term 'misuse' seems less pejorative than 'abuse'): consequences of acute intoxication, traffic accidents and other accidents, social and antisocial actions, etc. may all arise in occasional misusers although the likelihood of such occurrences will be considerably enhanced after occasional misuse has progressed to a state of dependence. In the past, the risks arising from dependence have perhaps been overemphasized if compared to the often ignored dangers arising from drug misuse; alcoholics for example are masters in sidetracking the therapist into largely irrelevant and difficult discussions as to whom he would call an alcoholic. Obviously excessive drinking in itself can have serious social, psychological domestic, and medical complications (Dr Smart's contribution p.263) whether or not it may fall under one or the other current definitions as to what is alcoholism; and the medical complications of drug abuse described by Dr Louria (p. 149) whilst of course more commonly seen in habitual and dependent drug takers may also occur in occasional drug users. One therefore should perhaps in the future lay much more stress on the risks of misuses of alcohol and 'other drugs' even though the type, frequency or dosage of such misuse may not yet qualify the user for the definition of 'Drug Dependent'. It is possibly for considerations such as these that so many of our contributors (eight out of twelve) have included the term 'Drug Abuse' in their chapter headings and this wider scope of the discussion is surely highly welcome. All the same, as regards the above-quoted WHO definition, doctors often strongly disagree as to what constitutes 'medical need', and what is an 'unnecessary quantity' for one individual may not be so for another; and moreover 'what constitutes use and abuse, or what is defined as such, may depend not only on pharmacological factors or the interaction between man and drug, or between man and society, but also on the prevalent view which happens to be taken at a given time by a given society' (Glatt, 1974).

The greatly varying views taken by different societies and different countries with their often conflicting but long-standing fashions as to the type of drug which is accepted makes international co-operation in an area such as drug misuse even more important—the more so under modern conditions of social mobility and international trade and travel. The drug scene in one country is bound sooner or later to closely affect neighbouring countries. It is interesting but an exceptional occurrence that the Swedish phenmetrazine epidemic (Dr Bejerot p. 69) or the misuse of non-narcotic analgines in Switzerland (Prof. Battegay p. 169) never really seemed to take an equally firm foothold elsewhere. The change in the drug scene described in the case of Scotland by Drs Ritson and Plant (p. 119) in the 1960s gradually involving younger people with their use of hallucinogens, amphetamines, barbiturates—apart from a minority who also took narcotics—and leading to the contemporary polydrug misuser, seems to have affected quite a number of countries simultaneously or successively in often very similar ways. Controlling the 'agent'—the dependency-producing drug—is of course not the only nor even the main approach in prevention; social, economic measures, mental hygiene, education—steps aiming at improving 'society' and 'host' are in the long run probably even more important (Dr Einstein p. 33, Dr Smart p. 263, Dr Langer p. 281) although this is clearly not an either—or question; prevention requires a comprehensive approach considering society, host and agent (Glatt, 1974). The recognition of the need for close co-operation among nations led to the international control measures and treaties starting in 1909. In spite of international co-operation in this field, international agreements still left the individual countries much leeway for the wildly different implementation of the recommendations of treaties. This is reflected, for example, in the differences between the 1914 Harrison Act (or at least in the way the act has been integrated) in the USA and the much more liberal recommendation of the Rolleston Committee in Britain in 1926. These differences were reflected in the widely varying approaches to control of illicit drugs between the USA and the much more permissive 'British System' which unlike American practices, largely left control in the hands of the medical profession. For many years, until the 1960s, the numbers of 'addicts' to the illicit drugs remained fairly steady, varying between 400 and 600 and an Interdepartmental Committee Report on Drug Addiction stated in 1961 that by and large the situation in the UK was well in hand—thereby confirming the views of many well meaning American observers that the permissive British System of drug control was greatly superior to the punitive American approach. But already at the time of the 1961 Report a number of changes foreshadowed the gradual deterioration in the British drug scene which has already been touched upon. The previously predominating middle-aged stable, therapeutic or professional morphine addict who kept to himself was replaced by the younger unstable non-therapeutic heroin and cocaine addict who usually initially bought his supplies from addicts who had received their drugs legally on a doctor's prescription and soon there emerged addict subcultures (Glatt *et al.*, 1967). Apart from the gradual rise in the numbers of addicts to narcotic drugs many youngsters began to misuse other drugs (amphetamines, cannabis, LSD) though at the time they generally kept away from barbiturates and often also from alcohol. The hastily reconvened Interdepartmental Committee in its Second Report in 1965 contained a far reaching reversal of its former views and proposals. Consequently since 1968 only specially licensed doctors—mainly those working in the newly established out-patient treatment centres have been allowed to prescribe heroin and cocaine to 'addicts'. In contrast to the often very generous overprescribing in the early and mid 1960s by a handful of London 'Junkie Doctors', the doctors at the treatment centres prescribed much smaller doses and started to replace heroin by methadone prescriptions; urine analysis for detection of drugs taken before accepting new applicants prior to acceptance at the Centre soon became routine (Prof. Marks and Dr Fry p. 295) The gradual rise in the numbers of known heroin and cocaine addicts seen prior to 1968 (when their number was 2782) began to level off and the general impression now seems to be that by and large the illicit drug problem has been contained—even though the numbers of illicit users are unknown. At the same time however considerable black market activity involved, apart from the previously peddled cannabis, LSD and amphetamines, also methadone (ampoules as prescribed in the Treatment Centres—unlike the oral methadone prescribed in the American Methadone Maintenance Clinics) 'Chinese Heroin' (mainly coming from the 'Golden Triangle' in the Far East, via Hong Kong) and barbiturates. Unlike the middle-aged woman who since the 1950s had been taking barbiturate tablets by mouth these youngsters dissolved the tablets and injected them intravenously, a highly dangerous practice often leading to the complications described by Dr Louria (p. 149) mainly in the case of narcotic drug misusers.

At present no one knows the extent of illicit drug use. Alcohol seems once again to have become the most popular drug of misuse also among the young; if it comes to 'other drug' most drug-using youngsters nowadays seem to be polydrug users adopting an 'anything goes method'. Drug dependence which made daily headlines in the 1960s seems nowadays to attract much less interest, and warning voices have rightly been raised against it becoming a forgotten issue. Some grounds for concern in this respect were recently summarised in the 1975/6 Annual Report by Scoda, the Standing Conference on Drug Abuse, which co-ordinates the work of several organizations nowadays active in this field. It has been estimated that 25 to 64% of narcotic addicts remain undetected. But also among 'known' addicts there has been a gradual increase from 1462 in 1962 to 1980 in 1974 (of whom incidentally the great majority—1557—were prescribed methadone as against 393 who received heroin prescriptions. Concern is aroused by the relatively large numbers of new addicts who come to the fore each year, for example 926 in 1975. This would indicate ready availability of illicit supplies (which is something that drug misusers speak of freely when discussing problems with their therapist) with the risk of involvement of organized crime*. The prevalence of (often drug related) criminal activities among 'addicts' is reflected in the finding that during 1975 483 were removed to penal institutions. This of course highlights the role of law enforcement officers in this field (Langer p. 281). Sixty-nine addicts had died in 1975. This reflects the need for

---

* A report in the *Sunday Times*—2 Jan., 1977—which came to hand after the above had been written—describes the activities of heroin dealers in London, . . . part of . . . secret Chinese societies that have recently set themselves up in Britain. . .' The organisation set up . . . is described by the Paper as '. . . sophisticated enough to replace one dealer with another as soon as he or she is caught; bureaucratic enough to keep accounts of the millions of pounds worth of heroin sold and held in stock; wealthy enough to keep empty flats as 'warehouses' for the heroin; and willing enough to engage in gangland violence in the manner of Chicago 'hoods'. The *Sunday Times* comments that 'Heroin is now such big, organised business here that Britain may have become a transhipment post for the much bigger profits available in North America'. This is why—so the Paper claims—'the U.S. Drug Enforcement Agency is setting up its own network of informers in Britain. . .' Incidentally, the lady mainly involved in the court case referred to in the paper had also tried to deal in heroin in Amsterdam, a city which in recent years had frequently been said to have become a main centre for the spread of drug misuse, because of its permissive approach. At any rate, reports such as these clearly highlight the implications of developments in one country for other countries, and the need for the closest cooperation. The prevention, as far as possible, of setting up big syndicates organising large-scale dealing in narcotics was of course one of the prime motives for the relative permissiveness of the 'British approach' that allows medical practitioners (though since 1968 only the relatively few who are 'licensed') to prescribe narcotic drugs to addicts.

medical supervision in view of the common medical complications (Louria p. 149). Many young drug misusers are rootless and homeless, indiscriminately using any drug they get hold of, and quite a few are admitted (sometimes repeatedly) to casualty wards for overdose (Louira p. 505) often of barbiturates. As regards treatment of polydrug users, this is not the province of the Treatment Centres which were set up 9 years ago to cope with the rising problem of narcotic drug dependence. But narcotic drug dependence has never been the main drug problem in the UK. The Alcohol and Drug Dependence Unit at St Bernard's Hospital, for example, has for over 15 years also accepted young dependents on drugs such as cannabis, amphetamines, barbiturates, as well as narcotics and has treated them by a community therapy approach and group psychotherapy, alongside alcohol patients (similar to the approach described by Battegay p. 169 and the one in a London prison described by Glatt p. 223). There is a great need for trying to detect, and to provide help for, young drug misusers in the community and quite a number of voluntary organizations are now trying to 'outreach' into the community.

However as stated above and described by Ritson and Plant (p. 119) in the case of Scotland, so also in England, it is alcohol that is the drug problem number one. This is confirmed by several other contributors to this volume in regard to other countries and it applies for example, also to the German Federal Republic where recent estimates have given the numbers of 'hard drug' consumers as 40 000 of whom 12 000 may be drug dependent, in comparison with an estimated 1.5 million German alcoholics (ICAA News, 1976). Moreover one million or more Germans are estimated to misuse pharmaceuticals. In the UK, medicinal drugs that may lead to dependence are tightly controlled under the Misuse of Drugs Act 1971 (except barbiturates which must rank amongst the most dangerous) that has taken the place of the former Dangerous Drugs Acts. As treatment of established drug dependents is difficult and often unsuccessful (Enstein p. 33, Battegay p. 169, Bourne p. 195) and as the many proposed new treatment procedures are as yet of doubtful and unproven value (Bourne p. 195), the task of prevention (Enstein p. 33, Smart p. 263, Langer p. 281) becomes even more vital. Education of the general public should aim at making people aware not only of the risks of the legal drugs alcohol and tobacco but also of prescribed drugs and of not expecting the doctor to have a miracle pill available for minor illnesses. In his turn, the doctor should try to ensure not to augment the number of drug misusers by unnecessary, or needlessly high or frequent prescribing. This must of course not lead to withholding narcotic analgesics in very painful or incurable conditions. Education, research, the role of doctors in avoiding the trap of inducing iatrogenic dependence (Bejerot p. 69), continuing attempts to reduce as far as possible such social determinants of drug misuse and crime as poverty, ignorance, insecurity, hopelessness, frustration, etc. (Langer p. 281), legal and fiscal measures (Smart p. 263) these and other approaches all have a part to play in the task of minimising the incidence of drug misuse. Collaboration between many agencies is necessary in the task of prevention as it is in the multidisciplinary team work required throughout the treatment and rehabilitation phases. Individuals with a very different psychological and constitutional make-up take drugs of widely differing composition under vastly different social conditions. There is no such person as 'the' addict and no such thing as 'the best' treatment. In each case the factors of importance in the given individual against his total social background requires evaluation followed by a choice of the combination of therapies best suited to his case.

Drug misuse is a complex phenomenon that as we have seen may vary in its manifestations according to social environment, local fashion and subculture, regional or national characteristics, etc. Acceptance of a given drug or otherwise may even affect symptomatology and the type of personality that may be predominant among drug misusers. In a culture for example that accepts heavy drinking as the norm—such as the French—even the average person, though he may be emotionally stable and mature, may become a heavy drinker, and in time develop alcoholism; in a different (for example Anglo-American) culture that frowns on heavy drinking, it will be in the main emotionally more unstable and 'vulnerable' individuals who will run the risk of social censure and ostracization by excessive drinking (Jellinek's 'acceptance-vulnerability' hypothesis, 1960). Because of the great importance of social factors in the genesis of alcoholism in France many French observers may consider alcoholism in the main a sociogenic disorder whereas in Britain and the USA many may consider alcoholism predominantly a psychogenic condition, because of the higher proportion of emotional problems in the pre-alcoholic personality. Similarly in a subculture that accepts cannabis smoking as the norm, even stable and mature personalities may become regular smokers without any guilt feelings. Likewise French alcoholics may not experience feelings of guilt, remorse, resentment, etc. (as their drinking pattern is after all not so different from the heavy drinking among their friends and neighbours) which are common features among British and American alcoholics.

Because of such differences affecting types, patterns and even manifestations of drug misuse in different countries, a great deal may be learned by comparing and contrasting experiences gained by expert observers in different parts of the world. The present volume contains reports written by experts from two continents and seven countries, all nationally and internationally well known, with special personal experience in the theme they themselves chose as their topic. Different viewpoints may also arise from the different perspective from which members of the various professional disciplines view the subject matter—although ideally sociologists should also take note of psychological and pharmacological factors, and psychiatrists of sociological conditions. Our contributors, though in the main psychiatrists, represent quite a number of professional disciplines concerned with drug misuse and dependence. Much of what is described in this volume by its various contributors holds in fact good anywhere and applies not only to the author's country and his professional discipline and viewpoint (for example van Dyck's 'vicious circles' of the development of drug dependence, p. 97, Louria's account of the medical complications p. 147, Marks and Fry's description of laboratory techniques and indications, p. 295, and Ritson and Plant's remarks on the applicability of their findings in Scotland to other industrialized countries p. 119). Other points touched upon may perhaps be more controversial although differences of opinion are more likely to arise between representatives of various professional disciplines or between individuals within the same country rather than originating from nationally different perspectives. Possibly more controversial issues touched upon in the present volume concern, for example, the infectious model of drug addiction (Bejerot p. 69 and also touched upon briefly by Louria p. 105), the place and the future of recently recommended innovative techniques (Bourne p. 195), the place of prison in the overall treatment programme (Glatt, p. 223) the mixing within the same community of alcoholics, other drug dependents (Battegay p. 169, Glatt

p. 223) and possibly also gamblers (Glatt) the social policy approach to prevention by reducing per capita drug consumption (Smart p. 263) Langer's (p. 281) plea for a definite though not predominant role of law enforcement in treatment and prevention programmes, and his statement that in fact most 'addicts' are somehow 'coerced' into treatment—with the implication that initially lacking motivation can indeed be often induced in an alcohol or drug dependent individual—a proposition with which incidentally the present writer wholeheartedly concurs, and Einstein's p. 33 critical analysis of theories explaining the non-medical use of drugs, of the consequences of the various definitions for intervention and treatment, and of suggested drug misuser-typologies.

Whilst touching on many aspects of the subject of drug misuse and dependence the present volume does not attempt to cover the whole subject comprehensively and systematically. Rather does it aim at discussing in greater depth than is frequently the case such aspects of the subject which for some reason or other are often not given the attention they deserve. Unlike the Editor's 'Guide to Addiction and its Treatment' (published by MTP in 1974) which aimed at providing a brief basic introduction to the whole field of dependence, the present text is directed rather at those professional readers with some postgraduate professional experience or interest in the subject matter. Whilst not a comprehensive textbook, the present volume contains a great deal of material on nature, causation, developmental progress, physical complications (though little on the much more common socio-domestic complications which are covered by many other texts on drug dependence), treatment, rehabilitation and prevention of drug misuse and dependence (or of its casualties). The finding that not all the experts contributing to this volume see eye to eye on all issues and problems touched upon only serves to underline the fact that so much in this field still awaits further 'elucidation—and that much further observation, research and interdisciplinary and international co-operation are required. At the same time—as for example pointed out by Bourne (p. 195)—with the all intriguing and highly necessary search for new and potentially more effective approaches, what may often be more important is the better and wider application of what is already known—and this is where authorative reviews and critical analyses and discussions of pros-and-cons written by observers with first-hand active experience in the particular field and with a wide knowledge not only of their own national scene but also of the international background may be of special value.

$$\star \quad \star \quad \star \quad \star \quad \star$$

Editor's summary and comments on the Chapters

1. EINSTEIN: ALCOHOL AND DRUG MISUSE TREATMENT: PROBLEMS AND ISSUES

Treatment of the drug misuser in order to be effective has to be understood in the light of various theories that have been put forward in an attempt to explain drug use, definitions of drugs, the treatment process and issues connected with non-medical drug use.

Four theories attempt to explain the non-medical use of drugs: biochemical, psychological, learning, and environmental theories. None of these theories can explain non-medical drug use satisfactorily: 'we do not know why people turn to drugs...'.

There are four traditional drug definitions: socio-religious, medical, legal, and scientific. Each of these has specific consequences for intervention and treatment processes.

A major factor bearing on treatment as an intervention technique is the question as to who is defined as a drug abuser. Analysis of the criteria employed to develop typologies of drug misusers indicates that they do not have sufficient empirical data to substantiate them. They can therefore not be used as a basis for predicting the course of drug misuse.

Einstein then discusses the questions why and how drug abusers should be treated. Formerly, the drug abuser was perceived as being an immoral or criminal deviant, nowadays he is commonly seen as a sick person. However, one has to decide carefully what kind of people (among drug misusers) need (what kinds of) treatment. The author proceeds to a critical analysis of the treatment process, the selection of the treatment site, screening systems, treatment goals and modalities, the need for treatment evaluation, follow-up, early case finding and prevention. He ends up with a discussion of the need to see 'treatment in context': treatment is only one of the many possible types of intervention and is not a panacea. One needs to understand why a given drug abuser treatment is chosen in preference to other forms of intervention; and it has to be carefully selected in order to have better results than in the past.

2. N. BEJEROT: THE NATURE OF ADDICTION

The Swedish psychiatrist Dr Niels Bejerot, pointing out that formerly addiction was considered to be a single entity, describes a socio-medical theory of addiction which he first put forward in 1965. According to the way dependence has been acquired, this classification divides addicts into three main groups: therapeutic, epidemic and endemic cases of addiction. To a certain extent Bejerot's 'therapeutic' and 'epidemic' types of dependence correspond to what in the U.K. has been called 'therapeutic' and 'non-therapeutic' addicts respectively; but Bejerot includes among his therapeutic types not only individuals originally introduced to the drug by their doctors during very painful illnesses for legitimate indications, but also 'addiction inadvertently caused by medical treatment', such as the nowadays common cases of dependence on hypnotics and tranquillizers subsequent to long-continued over-prescribing of these drugs by doctors (cf. Glatt, 1974: 'Iatrogenic Dependence'). Everyone would agree surely that the 'explosion' in prescribing these psychotropic drugs in the western world cannot be attributed to medical need. In the UK, incidentally, the formerly so popular prescribing of the more addictive barbiturates has decreased in recent years, and been replaced to a certain extent by the somewhat less dangerous tranquillizers. A third type among Bejerot's 'therapeutic group' ('self-established addictions') corresponds to the term 'professional addicts' in the UK, such as doctors and nurses.

Most of Bejerot's article deals with 'epidemic addictions' which, since the 1960s, have become common in western industrial countries. 'Epidemic addiction' requires for its initiation 'direct personal contagion between an established abuser and a novice'. The only major difference between the classical infectious disease model of illness and drug dependence as a communicable disorder is, as has been pointed out before, that unlike patients suffering from infectious diseases, in drug dependence the host wants and seeks out the agent. (Occasionally, however, one meets addicts who claim that their initial contact with drugs happened at parties where more or less well-meaning casual visitors virtually seduced and encouraged them to take such drugs or injected them into the newcomers' veins—though probably this is a rare occurrence).

Epidemic addictions, Bejerot points out, have occasionally been brought to an end by administrative measures. Additionally to examples he gives is a fairly recent experience in the UK in the late 60s. In 1967/8 the most striking development in the British drug scene had been the emergence of intravenous methylamphetamine as possibly the most widely misused drug among the young. This habit had arisen as the consequence of gross indiscriminate overprescribing by a very few GPs (another example of 'iatrogenic dependence'). In 1968 it was un-usual to meet a young drug misuser who did not also 'mainline' methylamphetamine. Despite many calls to do something about this new menace no steps were effective until in October an agreement was reached between the Ministry of Health, the General Services Committee of the British Medical Association, and the manufacturers of the drug, prohibiting further prescribing of the drug (except in hospitals). Within a short time the methyamphetamine epidemic had come to an end, and has not re-emerged since on the British scene. (Glatt *et al.*, 1969).

Another interesting point stressed by Bejerot that whilst in epidemic addictions men usually numerically predominate, among women this predominance becomes gradually less, the more such a drug becomes socially accepted and endemic within a population—a phenomenon also observed in the case of the accepted endemic drugs alcohol and tobacco. Another change taking place is that whilst maladjusted youths form the core of most drug epidemics, personality predisposition and social difficulties become less important the more widespread drug misuse becomes within a population. This of course is one further example reflecting the vulnerability-acceptance theory put forward by E. M. Jellinek in the 1950s in regard to alcoholism: the more accepted alcohol in a given population, the greater the likelihood that also ordinary, emotionally not vulnerable personalities can come to misuse it and in time become dependent (Jellinek, 1960).

One interesting point as regards the drug misuse in Sweden is the great popularity in the past of intravenous phenmetrazine—a form of drug abuse that never really caught on among British youngsters, in spite of the fact that way beck in the 50s phenmetrazine tablets were often taken habitually to excess by many women. Initially they had started them in order to slim only in time to become psychologically dependent and to continue with them quite independently from their original symptomatic purpose—an experience of interest in view of later points made by Bejerot.

'Endemic addiction', Bejerot's third group, means addictions that are constantly present in a country. Whereas epidemic-type addicts misuse many different drugs (in the UK, for example, for some years the polydrug misuser has been the most prevalent type), endemic-type addicts stay faithful to their habitual, socially sanctioned drug. Nonetheless, as Bejerot points out, alcoholics may under certain conditions take to sleeping drugs; and the misuse of barbiturates (and other hypnotics nowadays) was formerly very common among alcoholics in Britain (Glatt, 1961). Bejerot stresses that epidemic and therapeutic addiction constitute two different diseases, and he discusses the 'fundamentally different' groups who are at risk in regard to therapeutic, epidemic and endemic addiction. The middle-aged therapeutic addicts who are distressed by their dependence are usually quite different from epidemic, younger addicts (among whom character and personality disorders may be common), who take drugs for pleasure rather than for relief. These differences between the therapeutic and non-therapeutic (street) addicts in Britain—prevalent in the 50s and 60s respectively, probably explain the failure of the so-called 'British System' to prevent the emergence of the 1960 drug epidemic among the young. Bejerot stresses, however, the great differences in individual susceptibility to drug misuse, and to the development of drug dependence.

Bejerot stresses that susceptibility apart, exposure to, and massivity of contagion are factors in the development of drug dependence.

Bejerot finally discusses some theories put forward to explain addiction. Disturbed personality and social difficulties, he maintains, are not necessary for an individual to develop drug dependence: anyone can develop it '...if certain substances are administered in certain quantities during a certain period of time', although there are certain individual differences in dose and time necessary for the process to take place. Drug dependence—the compulsive phase—is in principle a condition essentially different from the preceding phase of (voluntary) drug abuse:

it 'assumes the character of a basic drive ... the addiction now dominating the individual and his way of life ... although even then the addict has not lost all voluntary control over his dependence. Bejerot sees the development of dependence as a short-circuiting of the pleasure-pain principle, addiction arising as an artificial drive ... as strong or even stronger than sexual drives'.

Results in epidemic-type addicts are poor, and Bejerot closes with the urgent plea to try to prevent such epidemics from arising in the first place, a task he regards as possible provided society—supported by public opinion—would be prepared to take the necessary measures.

3. W. K. VAN DIJK: VICIOUS CIRCLES IN ALCOHOLISM AND DRUG DEPENDENCE

Professor van Dijk, Professor of Psychiatry at the University of Groningen, attempts to obtain insight into the nature of alcohol and drug dependence by means of a multilevel concept of a series of vicious circles. The central feature of addiction is the addict's loss of freedom (and it is interesting in this connection to recall that years ago a Scottish worker has called the alcoholic's 'loss of control' the loss of freedom); van Dijk regards all other characteristics of dependence as special forms or effects of, or as additions to loss of freedom. Van Dijk distinguishes four vicious circles: pharmacological, cerebral, psychological, and social. Drug or alcohol use may cause metabolic changes (reflected in phenomena such as tolerance and withdrawal syndromes') which in turn lead to a need to take the drug again (pharmacological circle). Drugs taken to excess may damage cerebral tissues and thereby weaken the ego's resistance against further drug-taking (cerebral vicious circle). Unpleasant feelings and reactions that result from drug-taking are often quickly forgotten by further drug-taking (psychological vicious circle). Finally, drug-taking may have highly unpleasant social repercussions (for example, serious reproach by the spouse, rejection and ostracization by society), which produces the drug user's counter-reaction of further drug-taking (social vicious circle). Obviously these vicious circles reinforce each other's harmful operations, an important situation which would serve to explain their obstinate resistance to a 'cure'.

4. D. LOURIA: THE EPIDEMIOLOGY OF DRUG ABUSE AND DRUG ABUSE REHABILITATION

The American physician Donald Louria starts by briefly sketching the change in the type of the typical drug abuser seen in the USA in the mid-sixties: the newly emerging young, educated, well-off LSD and cannabis users were quite different from the economically deprived, often black heroin users. In the late 1960s and early 1970s the differences between these two groups became less distinct: cannabis, depressants and stimulants came now to be used by both groups, the well-off and the poor, with opium being more popular in the poorer areas, LSD among the affluent young sections of the community.

Previously few epidemiological studies had been carried out on the subject of illicit drug use but in the late 1960s a number of such investigations were undertaken in North America and Canada. Essentially they gave very similar results, which Louria illustrates by the obtained by the study of the New Jersey Medical School with which he has been prominently associated for years. Among the most interesting findings of this study was that students gave peer pressure, pleasure, and curiosity as the main reasons for their illicit drug use; peer pressure was by far the most important risk factor associated with drug use; there was a clear relationship between parental use of tranquillizers or tobacco (but not of moderate use of alcohol) and their children's illicit drug use. Louria considers risk factor analysis a very important technique in prevention campaigns.

Turning his attention to the sequential patterns of individual and community drug abuse, Louria found that the majority of suburban young marijuana smokers do not go on to more dangerous drugs; but those who do so, usually start with LSD, then continue with injecting stimulants and finally heroin. A change in individual cases from the sequential drug use pattern that is the usual one in the community, may be of significance as pointing to the presence of certain problems in that individual. In the inner city the sequence of drug use is quite different; here hallucinogens are often avoided by those who progress from tobacco, marijuana and pills directly to opiates.

The communicable infectious disease model of heroin abuse (discussed at length by Bejerot), 'whilst rejected by many'—has in

Louria's view the major advantage of serving as an intervention model. At the same time one must not forget that sudden changes in incidence of drug misusers may result from the natural course of the epidemic, rather than from treatment.

Louria continues by discussing patterns of drug abuse amongst students (epidemiological data obtained in 1974/5 showing that the legal drugs alcohol and tobacco once more constitute society's major drug problems, if compared to the more spectacular illicit drugs), and the relationship, 'if any', between marijuana use and the experimentation with more dangerous drugs such as LSD and heroin. Louria's studies indicate a possible connection between the frequency of marijuana smoking and the subsequent use of more dangerous drugs, such as LSD. Finally, a plea is made to apply epidemiological principles and analysis not only to the understanding of causation and nature of the drug abuse problem but also to rehabilitation programmes.

5. E. B. RITSON AND M. A. PLANT: THE INTERACTION BETWEEN ALCOHOL AND OTHER FORMS OF DRUG TAKING

Jointly written by a psychiatrist and a sociologist, this chapter describes problems of illicit drug use in Scottish culture where alcohol has always been the most widely enjoyed—and misused—drug. As the historical introduction outlines, opium, too, was popular in Scotland, as it was in England, during the nineteenth century, but there was little evidence of opium abuse in the first half of the twentieth century. In the early 1960s drug misuse suddenly 'emerged' among the young, and the authors review the relatively few clinical studies on drug takers carried out in Scotland, the surveys of drug-taking, and the information derived from police statistics. The main official response to drug abuse in Scotland consisted in increased police activity, as reflected in rising conviction statistics. Tightening up of legal supplies was followed by an increasing black market in illicit drugs. As regards the clinical response to drug abuse in Scotland, maintenance treatment remained uncommon.

As regards alcoholism, Scotland's rates are considerably higher than those of the rest of Britain. As anywhere else in Britain, in Scotland too there has been a rise in teenage drinking problems. Some of the heaviest (illegal) drug users are also heavy drinkers, and a similar relationship seems to exist between tobacco smoking and the use of other drugs. Evidence is cited also from the USA which indicates that many youngsters have added the newer, illicit drugs to the older legal ones, tobacco and alcohol. Growing preoccupation with drugs and alcohol among the young is often symptomatic of underlying social and psychological malaise.

Turning to the subject of prevention, the authors find that in Scotland (as of course also elsewhere) '...far less is spent upon education (concerning alcohol and drug abuse) than upon advertising alcohol and tobacco'—a familiar complaint throughout the western world. As the authors point out, many other trends found in Scotland are evident also in other industrialized countries. Moderate opinion supports the extension of licensing hours and increased availability of alcohol, whilst rejecting any enhanced availability of illicit drugs; and the authors reflect on the paradox that enables society to treat drugs with quite similar effects completely different because of national customs and the social meaning ascribed to their use. Young drug and alcohol abusers may not be fundamentally different from each other 'and yet society's reaction may be worlds apart'.

6. D. LOURIA: THE MEDICAL COMPLICATIONS OF DRUG ABUSE

By and large, psychological, psychiatric and social complications of drug misuse have been discussed in the literature much more frequently than its medical complications, partly perhaps because for some reason or other the recent worldwide epidemics of illicit drug use have attracted the interest of psychiatrists and sociologists much more than that of physicians specializing in internal diseases. Dr. Louria has been specializing in the subject he discusses in this chapter for many years. On the basis of his experiences he presents a list for each major category of drugs abused at the present time. Complications of misuse include overdosage (which he divides into three groups: respiratory depression, acute pulmonary oedema, and acute caridac arrythmia), endocarditis, infectious hepatitis, tetanus, malaria, neurological complications, renal dysfunction, and a miscellaneous group (septic arthritis, ostemyelitis, purulent myosistis, embolic lung infections, and possibly bacterial pneumonia). Amphetamine misuse leads to cardiovascular complications, infections, and possible brain damage. As Louria limits his descriptions to physical complications, a well-known mental complication (a paranoid schizophrenia-like picture) is here not included. In the case of hallucinogen use the possibility of teratogenic aberrations and chromosomal defects is controversial; there is the risk of self-destructive actions, and rarely homicide. Cannabis use may be a risk in driving a car; certain alleged physical effects (liver damage, chromosomal abnormalities, teratogenic effects, cerebral atrophy, and an organic brain syndrome) remain subjects of controversy. A number of other psychotropic drugs discussed by Louria include some which have been misused in Europe much less frequently than in the USA (MDA, Phencyclidine, STP). Solvent sniffing, too, has been observed in the UK rather infrequently, although in the past year (1976) quite a number of cases of glue sniffing were seen amongst young teenagers. Barbiturate misuse, on the other hand, has been quite common in the UK for several decades, formerly mainly in the middle-aged (during the last decade also among the young with their dangerous pattern of intravenous injection). The barbiturate withdrawal syndrome includes, like the alcohol withdrawal syndrome, also the possibility of delirium tremens. Louria's account finishes with a brief discussion of the important subject of neonatal dependence on opiates and barbiturates. Incidentally, in recent years cases have also been described of a foetal alcohol syndrome seen in infants born to women who drank heavily during pregnancy.

7. R. BATTEGAY: PSYCHOTHERAPY OF DRUG DEPENDENTS AND ALCOHOLICS

Alcoholism and drug dependence originate not only in pharmacological effects of the drug but also in constitutional, psychological and sociological factors. There are of course also psychological and social consequences (as well as causes) of drug abuse. Childhood may lay the basis for alcohol and drug dependence, in particular when conditions favour the production of anxiety. Alcohol and drug dependence are not only symptoms of the individual but also of the social surroundings, for example, they may reflect social drinking habits, the general prejudice towards non-drinkers, etc. Therefore one has to make use not only of the individual approach but one must also reach patients within a social framework.

Professor Battegay discusses the necessity, which may arise for various reasons, to take some patients out of their usual surroundings, at least for a certain time—although in general patients should be left as long as possible in their natural surroundings. The author then presents a detailed review of therapeutic techniques (which he has been using successfully for many years among his patients at the psychiatric clinics at the University of Basel): individual psychotherapy (supportive, analytical, hypnosis, behaviour therapy), and psychotherapies in which the individual is seen in his social context (group psychotherapy, family therapy, therapeutic community and community therapy). When discontinuing drink or drugs, the addict's only (though treacherous) support is taken away; therapy has to provide the addict with something that helps him to abandon his distorted view and to experience a participating human relationship. Voluntary treatment is preferable but not always accepted; often patients will require preliminary 'prepsychotherapy' in order to prepare them for real psychotherapy and create confidence. Of course, 'psychotherapy does not necessarily mean psychoanalysis'. The need is stressed for the very important aftercare—the psychotherapeutic as well as that carried out by the social worker. In this context the author discusses in some detail the personality of alcoholics and drug misusers, and stresses the need for alcoholics to remain abstinent and, similarly also in general for drug dependents not to take drugs. A possible exception is methadone maintenance which, in Battegay's view, however, dangerously '. . . limits . . . human freedom'.

Professor Battegay (like the present writer) has found special advantages in treating alcoholics and drug misusers in groups. Family therapy is valuable because, as Balint expressed it, 'the individual who drinks is often only a symptom of an unbalanced family'. Battegay describes the therapeutic community approach in which 'all members contribute to the ward administration', and ends with a plea that society should recognize that prophylaxis of the symptom 'drug dependence' must begin with readiness for confrontation with the problems of youth.

8. P. G. BOURNE: NEW AND INNOVATIVE TECHNIQUES IN THE TREATMENT OF DRUG ABUSE

Whereas the other contributors to this volume mainly dealt with familiar therapeutic techniques, Dr Bourne in his chapter discusses new and as yet not fully evaluated and somewhat controversial techniques. The continuing search for new techniques could be attributed to a belief held in some quarters that drug abuse may be due to a single cause, and possibly be remediable by a single therapeutic technique (which of course runs counter to today's predominant view of drug misuse being of multifactorial origin requiring a multidimensional approach). It would also be due to widespread frustration with present approaches, and to recognition that drug abuse problems, far from being homogeneous, require a wide variety of modalities geared to highly specific needs of the individual.

Dr Bourne discusses a number of key requirements for any new treatment approach as to acceptability, success, etc. Some of these new techniques if found successful in drug abuse field might later on be found applicable to the whole social service field. Anyhow there are very few if any completely new techniques, and what is more important is to apply available knowledge and techniques.

The author then discusses the (often neglected) need for and the difficulties in evaluating new techniques. As to conceptualization of the new techniques, one could classify them into those relating specifically to physiological aspects of addiction and to social rehabilitation respectively.

There follows a critical discussion of the techniques acupuncture, biofeedback, hypnosis, meditation, and electrosleep (with its attractions of being inexpensive and of being compatible with many—particularly oriental—cultures), a constellation of techniques aiming at relief of anxiety and possibly leading to biochemical changes in the brain, especially in the hypothalamus. Among the new pharmacological substances suggested as possible alternatives to methadone and other traditional programmes are propoxyphene napsylate (Darvon-N), apomorphine (here the pioneer work of Dr J. Y. Dent in London way back in the 1930s and 1940s in the treatment of alcoholism must not be forgotten), the B-adrenergic blocking agent propanalol, 1-alpha acetyl methadol (Laam) and the antagonists (in particular Naltrexone)—which block the effects of heroin but, because of their lesser effectiveness in suppressing narcotic hunger, require greater motivation on the side of the patient than in the case of methadone. The author closes his review with the reminder that with all the pharmacological approaches, addiction being primarily a social phenomenon, social rehabilitation will remain the cornerstone of the long-term approach. At the same time, work with some of these newer techniques holds out the intriguing hope for developing a non-pharmacological treatment which may induce specific physiological and biochemical alterations in the brain.

9. M. M. GLATT: A THERAPEUTIC COMMUNITY FOR DEPENDENT INDIVIDUALS IN PRISON

This chapter describes the setting up and the functioning of a therapeutic community (comprising compulsive gamblers as well as drug addicts and alcoholics) within a London prison. The principles at work in a therapeutic community with an emphasis on group therapy were set out in detail in Battegay's contribution, and the experiences over a number of years described in the present chapter that it is quite feasible to establish such a community within the confines of a prison, given understanding and therapeutic oriented staff attitudes. The task of actual treatment (i.e. mainly group therapy) falls mainly to the prison hospital officers each of whom looks after his own group of prisoner-patients. The atmosphere is non-custodial, and continual stress is laid on encouraging these patients' own initiative, sense of responsibility and motivation. A surprising finding has been the marked degree of mutual understanding and cooperation that developed very soon between the staff and these previously often very difficult and morose inmates. Aggressive 'acting-out', often seen in prisons hardly ever occurred, and the great majority, under the impact of group discussions and the general constructive attitude of other patients, in time seemed to acquire a greatly altered outlook. Compulsive gamblers, within this community, seemed well able to 'identify' with the drug misusers and the alcoholics.

Whilst such preliminary experiences seem highly encouraging, as yet no reliable long-term evaluation of the outcome has been possible.

Anyhow, neither such a prison nor a hospital unit stand a real chance of long-term success with patients without a planned, long-term aftercare programme, which should include special hostels, community aftercare, close collaboration with probation and voluntary services, etc.

This paper is of course not a recommendation to send addicts to prison which in itself—i.e. without a specific therapeutic oriented programme—does nothing for them. At best, prison treatment is only a side issue within the overall comprehensive approach needed for rehabilitation of addicts, and there is an obvious, urgent need to establish constructive alternatives to prison. On the other hand, there will always be alcohol and drug misusers or gamblers in prison for offences connected with their compulsive behaviour, and for a certain proportion among them the therapeutic community approach followed by a planned aftercare and rehabilitation programme certainly seems to hold out some hope. This type of approach therefore seems to deserve further large-scale study and evaluation.

10. G. SMART: SOCIAL POLICY AND THE PREVENTION OF THE UNIMODAL APPROACH

Concern with prevention should stem from lack of treatment acumen and the knowledge that, apart possibly from tuberculosis, all large-scale public health problems have been conquered with the help of primary prevention and not by treating individuals already affected. No major approach to prevention has been adequately tested. The choice therefore is arbitrary but Dr Smart's approach is based on the belief that a reduction of the frequency of alcohol and other drugs use will in time also reduce alcoholism and drug problems. The unimodal model of prevention has been studied mainly in regard to alcoholism. French and Canadian studies have indicated the lack of any clear difference in alcohol consumption between social, heavy and problem drinkers—in contrast to the more usually held view of a bimodal curve of alcohol consumption with a clear difference between normal and problem drinkers. Socio-cultural models—accepting the importance of social and cultural factors—suggest the establishment of proscriptive and prescriptive norms allowing controlled, integrated drinking. Adherents to this model ignore the importance of per capita consumption in preventing alcohol problems. As regards drug problems, the unimodal model and its implications are less well understood than in the case of alcohol, but, in Smart's view data available so far suggests that in order to reduce heavy drug use it may be necessary to reduce per capita consumption of drugs by the population at large.

The author then discusses the place of social policy in the prevention of drug problems. Social policy in regard to alcohol can easily be made by governments but not as regards illicit drugs. At present 'we appear not to know how to prevent illicit drug use'. As regards education on drugs, Dr. Smart believes that such programmes may indeed 'educate' but apparently without reducing drug use. There is need for experimental trials as regards social policy concerning alcohol and drug abuse.

11. J. H. LANGER: AN ENFORCEMENT PREVENTION PERSPECTIVE ON DRUG ABUSE

Social and political institutions operate the social mechanisms which control or try to regulate consumption of potentially harmful substances. Dr. Langer's paper stresses the need for a coherent strategy and the definition of the roles of institutions. He emphasizes in this connection the role played by law enforcement and the criminal justice system, without contending that these are the most effective means of handling drug abuse. Family, peer group, and socio-cultural controls may be the most effective type. The drug problem, however, is influenced by many agents of control and education, and society has to recognize the inter-relationships that exist between the roles of all these agents.

The 1974 Federal Response to drug abuse stressed that a balance had to be struck between, on the one hand, treatment, rehabilitation and education, and the criminal justice system on the other hand. The latter is nowadays the major source of drug abusers under treatment, and recent times have frequently witnessed better cooperation between enforcement and treatment programmes. In America as in European countries penalties for drug users (as different from dealers) have been reduced. Both the criminal justice system and the community require more education in the process of communication with each other.

Controversy has arisen in the past by the mode of application (too severe or too lenient, etc.) of the drug laws although the public, in general, regards these laws to be necessary. Of addicts in treatment, the majority were identified by enforcement and 'coerced' into treatment.

A basic difficulty for law enforcement agencies arises from laws which society does not wish to be consistently enforced without clearly saying so. Effective law enforcement depends on support by the public as well as on efficient enforcement techniques and judicial consistency, underlining the need for regular close collaboration with community groups, professional organizations etc.

For a variety of reasons drug abuse will remain with us in the near future, though it may perhaps decline if the public and special interest groups were to agree on basic preventative, educational and control measures; and if school and parents continue to teach very young children about drugs, their dangers, and constructive alternatives. Ultimately self-control rather than control from outside will see the solution to a drug crisis.

12. V. MARKS & D. E. FRY: DETECTION AND MEASUREMENT OF DRUGS IN BIOLOGICAL FLUIDS: THEIR RELEVANCE TO THE PROBLEMS OF DRUG ABUSE

Often clinicians may suspect that certain patients may use certain drugs although the patient denies it indignantly; or alternatively a doctor, for example when working in a prescribing drug treatment centre, may fear that the 'addict' does not take the drugs prescribed and sells them on the black market. Professor Marks and Dr Fry describe in this chapter certain laboratory methods which serve the purpose of detecting drugs in biological fluids under routine clinical conditions. A drug screening programme must adjust the methods used to the prevailing circumstances and to the type of locally popular drug, and must consider sensitivity and accuracy of procedures, as well as various other factors, such as time and available instrumentation (eg. rapid qualitative screening by thin-layer chromatography). Quantitative drug measurements are of doubtful value in the management of drug addiction.

The authors describe the methods in common use for the

extraction of drugs from urine and their detection by use of thin-layer chromatography—the technique commonly employed in screening programmes. This is followed by a discussion of the commonly used drugs and the methods employed for their identification and measurements.

In their 'general analytical considerations' the authors describe the techniques of extraction of drugs from urine by organic solvents; ion exchange procedures; non-ionic resin; the identification of drugs by thin-layer chromatographic techniques—which because of their non-specificity serve the purpose of screening procedures only, whilst positive identification of a specific drug requires the use of independent analytical methods; gas-liquid chromatography (used to confirm drugs detected by TLC); immunochemical measures (useful if only very small amounts of drugs are present); and finally, high-pressure liquid chromatography.

Next the authors consider in detail the use of the various techniques in the case of 'individual drugs', such as Diamorphine (excreted in the urine mainly as morphine and its derivatives) and Morphine (best detected in addicts' urine by TLC); Amphetamines; Methadone (extensively used in the treatment of heroin addicts both in the USA and the UK); barbiturates (detectable and measurable in blood and urine by means of many methods); Methaqualone (like barbiturates, commonly misused by young polydrug users in England); cannabis (where no satisfactory method for detection in blood and urine was available until simple and fairly sensitive radioimmunoassay techniques were introduced for this purpose in 1974); and LSD (whose detection and measurement in biological fluid is made very difficult because of its very low concentration). In their description the authors pay attention to such problems as multiple drug use, the sensitivity of the methods, and the dangers of, and methods of eliminating, misleading false positive results.

The usefulness of the methods outlined in clinical and forensic practice is discussed next—a subject matter which is described by the authors as '... one of virtual ignorance, surmise and speculation'. Limitations set by lack of available time and money rather than of suitable methods, reduce the ability of laboratories to detect and measure common drugs of abuse. Moreover, many factors (such as sensitivity and specificity of the analytical method used) affect interpretation of the obtained results. The clinician's question as to the quantity of a drug taken and to the frequency of its use, by a given drug user, cannot be satisfactorily answered by urine analysis. Factors affecting interpretation of results are discussed from both a technical and a clinical point of view. In discussing the 'clinical value of urine analysis' the authors emphasize the importance of specificity of method used when considering the significance of a positive urine test for drugs: for example, for positive identification of a drug thin-layer chromatography alone is unsatisfactory and has to be confirmed by other methods, because of the risk of false positive results ('Clinical Application of Drug Detection Methods and Interpretation of Results').

In diagnosis and treatment of addicts, urine analysis has not been used a great deal, although it could in the authors' view be an essential first step in the diagnosis of heroin and morphine addiction, especially as so often addicts are unreliable witnesses who often try to mislead the clinician. For example, they may confess to (or falsely claim) the use of heroin (in order to obtain legal supplies at the treatment centres), whilst denying the use of barbiturates etc.

The present writer's experience in a Drug Treatment Centre (at U.C.H.) and a large residential unit (at St. Bernard's Hospital) over the past ten years certainly bears out these views of Marks and Fry. On the other hand, drug addicts or people claiming to be addicts, nowadays know of course that their urine will be screened before being prescribed a drug such as methadone; they therefore make sure that before presenting themselves for the first time at a treatment centre they have bought and injected heroin and/or methadone for a while so as to ensure a positive urine result. But clearly, as the contribution by Marks and Fry shows, the laboratory can be of the greatest help to the clinician in this difficult field. Their extremely informative (though necessarily at times very technical) contribution, the last one in this volume, suitably rounds off and complements the observations, impressions and conclusions of the clinical and social field workers given in preceeding chapters; in particular their final paragraphs which underline the necessity of close collaboration of laboratory and clinical workers—one more indication for the need for integration of efforts and good communication between workers in many different disciplines if the best results are to be obtained in this fascinating but often baffling and frustrating subject of drug misuse and dependence.

And whilst in this last chapter of the present volume the authors are

primarily concerned with the drug—the 'agent', they make quite clear
that the 'agent's' importance in this connection can only be understood
against the background of the 'host'—the personality and intentions of
the user, and of the total social environment.

REFERENCES

Eddy, N. B., Halbach, H., Isbell, H. and Seevers, M. H. (1965). Drug
  Dependence: its Significance and Characteristics. *Bull. WHO*, **32**, 721
Glatt, M. M. (1972). The Abuse of Barbiturates in the United Kingdom. (U.N.)
  Bull. Narcot., **14**, 19
Glatt, M. M. (1974) *A Guide to Addiction and its Treatment: Drugs, Society and
  Man.* (Lancaster: Med. & Techn. Publ.)
Glatt, M. M., Pittman, D. J., Gillespie, D. G. and Hills, D. R. (1967). *The Drug
  Scene in Great Britain.* (London: Edward Arnold)
ICAA News (1976). *6th Drug Institute-Hamburg* Sept.–Dec., p. 8
Interdepartmental Committee Report (1961). *Drug Addiction.* (London:
  HMSO)
Interdepartmental Committee Second Report (1965). *Drug Addiction.* (London: HMSO)
Jellinek, E. M. (1960). *The Disease Concept of Alcoholism.* (Connect: Hillhouse
  Press)
SCODA (*Standing Conference on Drug Abuse*) (1975/6): Annual Report.
  London.
WHO Expert Committee on Addiction-Producing Drugs (1957). Seventh
  Report. *WHO Techn. Rep. Ser.*, **116**, 9
WHO Expert Committee on Addiction-Producing Drugs (1964). Thirteenth
  Report. *WHO Techn. Rep. Ser.*, **273**, 9
WHO Expert Committee on Dependence-Producing Drugs (1965). Four-
  teenth Report. *WHO Techn. Rep. Ser.*, **312**, 7
WHO Expert Committee on Dependence (1969). Sixteenth Report. *WHO
  Techn. Rep. Ser.*, **407**, 6
WHO Expert Committee on Drug Dependence (1973). Nineteenth Report.
  WHO Techn. Rep. Ser., **516**, 8
WHO Expert Committee on Drug Dependence (1974). Twentieth Report.
  WHO Techn. Rep. Ser., **551**, 14

ACKNOWLEDGEMENTS

It is a pleasure to express my thanks to a number of people—to the
authors of the various chapters in this volume for their valuable and
searching contributions, and to Mr David Bloomer, Managing Director
of MTP, his staff and my Personal Assistant, Mrs Phyllis P. Buffam, for
their unfailing assistance throughout all stages in the preparation of this
book.

PART I
Nature, Aetiology, Epidemiology

CHAPTER 1

Alcohol and drug misuse treatment: Problems and issues

S. EINSTEIN

Treatment of the 'alcoholic' and the 'drug misuser', if it is to be an effective tool, must be understood in the light of theories posited to explain drug use, definitions of drugs and their associated consequences, the process of treatment and its all too often politicalization, as well as the various critical issues associated with the contemporary non-medical use of drugs.

THEORIES

Four general theories have been posited to explain the non-medical use of drugs. There are of course, variations on each one. The basic common denominator for all of these theories is that they have little empirical and predictable data to substantiate them. The following account is designed not only to abstract these theories but to point out consequences each one may have on determining who the treatment agent(s) should be; it is summarized in Table 1.

BIOCHEMICAL–PHYSIOLOGICAL THEORIES

These theories assume that either drug users have a predisposition to drug use, or once they have begun drug use they suffer from a condition analogous to a biochemical deficit that requires drugs (specifically narcotics) for relief. The analogy of the diabetic is often used by proponents of this theory.

There are three major objections to this type of theory:

1. There should be few if any abstinent drug users who function

Table 1 Etiology of the non-medical use of drugs and some derived consequences

I Model	II Process for drug adaptation	III Theoretical assumptions about types of drug users	IV Activity level for non-drug adaptation	V Preferred treatment agent	VI Successful treatment outcome
Bio-chemical-physiological, genetic	Biochemical deficit genetic pre-disposition	Homogeneity	Minimal to nil	Bio-chemists Ex-addicts Recovered alcoholics Geneticists	An arrested bio-chemical disorder
Psychoanalytic development of personality	Regressed or fixated psychosexual development (oral addict personality)	Homogeneity	Moderate to maximally active	Psycho-analysts	Sublimated oral personalities or more mature psycho-sexual personality development
Learning	Conditioning (Classical, operant)	Homogeneity	Minimal to maximally active	Behavior therapists	New non-drug overt behavioral adaptations (conditioned ex-addicts)
Environmental	Retreating from external milieu via drugs	Homogeneity	Minimal to nil	Builders, urban planners, etc.	Drug users or non-users in better environment
Psycho-sociological ('Burning Out')	Not given	Homogeneity	Moderate to minimally active	None, self change	Tired ex-addicts and/or socially acceptable drug substitutors
Altered states of consciousness	Normative need naturally determined	Heterogeneous	Moderately to maximally active	None specific self change possible	Substituted altered states of consciousness (drug or non-drug related)

reasonably well without chemical substitution. This is obviously not the case, notwithstanding the gloom that colours present treatment outcomes. There are obviously many drug users who have changed their styles of life away from the non-medical use of drugs.

2. If an addict is put on an appropriate dose of methadone, his biochemical deficit should be taken care of and he should not be involved in using other narcotics simultaneously. This is also obviously not the case, as many methadone treatment centers can testify to.

3. The model contemporary non-medical user of drugs is most often a multiple drug user. This raises the issue of whether there are multiple biochemical deficit systems, paralleling each other, or even interacting with one another. These would have to account for drug families as divergent as central nervous system depressants and stimulants, psychedelics as well as the various fadist substances that are tried (e.g., bananas, peanut butter, etc.)

While the biochemical-physiological theories may leave much to question they may be useful if understood as a social message. The drug user, irrespective of his aetiology, may be telling us to stop looking at him as both the cause of his drug use as well as the answer to his drug abstinence. In simplistic terms he may be telling us that if he were born with most other physical conditions, and perhaps some psychiatric ones, we would not be blaming him. Indeed we might be offering help without moralization. Indeed society may perceive the drug user as having a monkey on his back which he is to rid himself of with little help from us. The drug user may feel that he has the monkey plus society on his back which a theory based on predisposition may partially alleviate.

The major consequence of this theory for treatment agents would be to emphasize the roles of the biochemists, and perhaps geneticists, and to minimize the role of traditional therapists as well as ex-addicts.

PSYCHOLOGICAL THEORIES

These theories are primarily related to the theorists notions of normal and abnormal psychological development. The theory to be presented is the psycho-analytic one developed by Dr. Freud and furthered by his disciples. To understand it we must recognize that it was developed to explain drug use at a time when barbiturates, amphetamines, and psychedelics such as LSD were not known by him or his colleagues either as medicants or as hedonistic substances. Indeed alcohol was the major drug of use and misuse during Freud's times, as it remains at present.

The central thesis in this theory is that individuals either become fixated or regress to an oral level of psychosexual development and that this leads to an addict personality.

This theory suffers from two major difficulties:

1. Freudian theory assumes that for each level of psychosexual development, there are associated only certain diagnoses. Yet a standardized mental status on any large group of drug users, even single substance ones, will result in the entire spectrum of diagnoses.

2. Being an oral personality, whatever that means, does not necessarily mean turning to the non-medical use of drugs. Of the various other alternatives there is eating, love making, talking, playing the clarinet, etc. Obviously, retrospective tagging is not equivalent to empirically based predictability.

The major consequence of this theory for treatment agents is that we would only use psycho-analytically oriented treatment agents. A second consequence would be asking the government to take on the expensive and long-term individual treatment of drug users. It would appear that the group who would immediately benefit from this theory are the couch makers in every community.

LEARNING THEORIES

These theories are primarily concerned with the learning processes that underlie adaptation. Conditioning theories have been posited to explain the non-medical use of drugs.

At first glance these theories seem eminently correct. They suggest that there are internal and external stimuli that serve to reinforce drug related behaviour, and that interfering with them will result in inhibitary processes which ultimately should result in the cessation of the non-medical use of drugs.

The conditioning thesis is either based on theories of classical (Pavlovian), or of instrumental (Skinnerian) conditioning. In classical conditioning, the relationship of the unconditioned stimulus to the conditioned stimulus is crucial. In instrumental conditioning the ratio of reinforcement is crucial. In addition, the instrumental thesis differs from classical concepts in that it posits that the behaviour that is conditionable is normal for the species, and that the ratio of reinforcement simply calls out the particular behaviour. Thus, drug orientated behaviour would have to be assumed to be normative for the human species. There may be obviously some questions to this, particularly in terms of non-medical drug use.

Of perhaps greatest import is that neither of these theories can adequately handle the multitude of stimuli that are necessary to explain drug use. They can only adequately handle a minimal number of stimuli at any given time. And the non-medical use of drugs assumes stimuli for the drug of first choice, route of administration, the drug experience (which is often a negative one which should lead to inhibition and not to reinforcement), the meaning of the drug experience, whether drug use takes place in isolation or in a social group, multiple drug use or single drug use; types of detoxification (medical or cold turkey, in the streets, jail or medical facility), etc. The point is that there are too many stimuli, singly or in combination for the two conditioning theories to adequately handle.

The major consequence of conditioning theory for treatment agents is that we would use behavioural therapists rather than other types.

ENVIRONMENTAL THEORIES

The environmental theories are in a relative sense the most recent and in many ways the most simple. They are based on the assumption that specific environments either induce drug orientated behaviour or interfere with it. The most commonly known variation of this theory is Retreatism. This theory, developed by analyzing the drug behaviour of Negroes in Harlem, assumes that youngsters retreat into drug use, which they witness all around them, when they recognize that there is little likelihood of their actually escaping from the negative impact of their environment.

The major difficulty with this theory is that it assumes that the impact of economic or social poverty, given drug availability, will lead more often than not to drug use.

The spread of the non-medical use of drugs to all segments of society, all over the world raises serious questions for this thesis. As does the fact that all people who experience the impact of societal pressures, with limited options for escape, do not turn to drugs. Related to this is that many of those who cease the non-medical use of drugs, and never return to it, do not return to a community that is less personally traumatic.

The major consequence of environmental theories for treatment agents is that we would not really need any—rather we would need bulldozer operators, architects, builders and urban planners. If indeed we took this route we should remind ourselves that a house is not a home and that a geographically planned area is not a community.

In summary we are left with the reality that none of these four theories adequately explain the non-medical use of drugs; none can be used in a predictable sense. Indeed we do not know why people turn to drugs or why some who do, stop, and of these some subsequently return to them again, whilst many others never do. This need not be too depressing a state. There is much that we do not understand about human functioning, and yet we are often called upon to intervene in as effective a way as possible.

DRUG DEFINITIONS

Altering a person's drug use style, via treatment, implicitly makes assumptions about drugs themselves. A viable treatment plan must come to terms with how it defines drugs and the meaning and value it imputes to them. This is necessary because if we do not have a working definition of drugs, then we would obviously not have any drug misuse, or non-medical use of drugs. It is drug misuse that has resulted in the contemporary decision to treat or incarcerate drug users.

There are four traditional sources of drug definitions. Each is associated with specific consequences.

SOCIO-RELIGIOUS DEFINITION

The socio-religious definition is based on the ritualization and social use of drugs. Within this context drugs are condoned or condemned in terms of social, political, economic and religious factors. Medical and psychiatric issues play no major role in the determination of social pharmacology. And treatment has rarely been turned to as a preferred technique for changing a person's drug related behaviour. Rather social and/or religious stigmatization, isolation and various forms of political intervention have been used.

MEDICAL DEFINITION

Medical definitions are based on the thesis that when chemicals are prescribed by medical representatives, solely for the purposes of relief from pain, return to a particular level of health, maintenance of a particular level of health, or treating and/or curing disease, that such use is legitimate. This legitimacy, which is a form of actual or imputed control by others than the drug user (i.e., the physician), results in the chemical being categorized as *medicines*. All other use (i.e., recreational drug use, expanding the mind, getting high, etc.) results in a designation of *drugs*. This distinction is important since most people feel that they use medicines while others use drugs. And it is the uncontrolled user, who is or has become, visible, that is the focus of the drug treatment efforts. Medical definitions also suggest that leadership in treatment intervention should be the primary province of physicians, notwithstanding that they are as well, or as ill-trained for this as any other professional.

LEGAL DEFINITION

The legal definitions are based on the simple notion that if a substance is dangerous to a person and/or his community, the substance and the person should be controlled. Thus we control growth, manufacture, distribution, sale, possession, importation, etc., via licensing, incarceration, fines and death. We control the visible drug user who comes to our attention by removing him from the mainstream of his community. Treatment as a process is rarely used in the legal arena. At best, it is a facade for removing a person. Legal definitions also have resulted in faulty drug classifications. Two widely used classifications are *hard and soft* drugs, and the notion of *dangerous* drugs. Obviously drugs are just drugs and there are no undangerous ones. Lastly, legal definitions may result in the notion that the preferred intervention agent is a law enforcement representative. Three consequences derive from this. Empirically, none of man's appetites have yet to be adequately controlled by laws. Secondly law enforcement agents are in no better position via training, skills, status, etc., than any other group to intervene effectively. And lastly, the focus of the law enforcement agent, in terms of what his community asks him to do, more often than not runs counter to the logic, goals and process of treatment.

SCIENTIFIC DEFINITION

The scientific definition of a drug as any active, chemical substance which alters the structure of functioning of a living organism, has the virtue of not being judgemental but has the distinct limitation of being irrelevant to the contemporary use and misuse of drugs. The general public, community leaders, policy planners and makers are not concerned about scientific issues in terms of drug use. They are concerned about certain people, using certain drugs, in certain ways, for certain reasons, in their neighbourhoods. It becomes quite clear then that treatment as a process is not related to drug definitions, but rather to defining who the drug addict, drug misuser, abuser, etc., is.

THE DRUG MISUSER

Continuing with the the premise that a major factor that determines the use of treatment as an intervention technique is who we define as the drug abuser, an analysis of the criteria for existing typologies is in order. Table 2 schematizes some of the factors that have been utilized in the development of drug misuser typologies.

All of these typologies suffer from face validity. They appear to be eminently logical. And indeed they are; and that is their greatest failing. They seduce the treatment planner into believing that these typologies are scientifically sound when indeed all of these typologies have one common denominator: they do not have sufficient empirical data to substantiate them. Because of this, they are useless in making predictions about the course and/or cessation of drug misuse. Indeed the greatest failing of these typologies is that we are unable to predict or plan the most efficacious type of treatment intervention for a specific type or individual at a given point in their treatment career. This is primarily so because we tend to forget that at best, the particular typology tells us something about *what* a person is doing in terms of drug related

Table 2 Factors involved in alcohol and drug misuser typologies

The Drug	*Typology*
Type of Drug Used	Cokie, A-head; Pot head; Wino.
Frequency of Use	Greezy Addict; Chippying; Weekend User.
Amount of Drugs Used	Coke Habit; Jones; Heavy Drinker; Tasters.
Status of Drug	Junky; Lush.
Drug Effects	Pain Prone Addicts.
Drug Pattern	Multiple Drug Abuser; Single Substance Users.
The Drug User	
Age of Initial Drug Misuse	Primary and Secondary Addict.
Visibility	Street (Junky); Hidden (Drug Abuser).
Psychiatric Classification	Addict Personality; Oral Personality.
Sociological Classification	Retreatists; Two Worlders; Hustlers.
Length of Drug Misuse	Burning Out; Acute or Chronic; Chronic Drinkers.
Manner of Drug Taking	Needle Addict; Greezy Addict.
Initiator of Drug Misuse	Iatrogenic; Self.
Source of Drug	Medical Addicts; Maintained Addicts.
Source of Drug Use Support	
Source of Categorization	Adjusted Addicts; Ex-Addicts; Recovered Alcoholics.
Meaning of Drug Use	Reactive Drinkers; Social Drinkers.
Consequences of Drug Use	Physically and Psychologically Degenerated Alcoholics.
Moral Classifications	Dope Fiend; Decadent Drinkers; Immature; Gratifiers.

behaviour rather than *who* he is. And it is the *who* that is crucial in treatment planning and not the *what*. These typologies and their associated profiles of characteristics which are generally stereotypes, lead us to view the drug misuser as falling somewhere along a criminal–sick gradient. The acceptance of this assumption more often than not precludes evaluation of the intervention between the drug user, his drugs of choice and his environment. In doing this it leads the lay and professional public to generally focus only on the user himself as the centre of the problem and to demand of him that he solve his own problems.

WHY TREAT THE DRUG MISUSER?

The third issue that must be raised is whether the drug abuser's present status (life style adaptation) is such that he should be treated and/or what treatment will be of help to him and to those he affects.

For a long time it was felt that excessive drinkers and other kinds of drug abusers were immoral individuals. One just assumed that they were unable to handle events which most of the world could and thus turned to drugs out of personal weakness and for illicit pleasure.

The obvious intervention for a moral condition is theologically or philosophically based. But these interventions have had little effect on changing man's appetite behaviour.

The 'immoral' perception soon changed into the criminal-deviant notion of drug abuse. This type of analysis often led to discussion about whether drug users were involved in crime prior to their drug involvement; the crimes were against property or against people; or whether drug use reinforced a core criminal condition.

The obvious treatment for criminals is punishment. Being modern, we call the process of removing the drug abuser from his mainstream of living 'rehabilitation'. The judicial system determines the length of and geographical locus of the 'rehabilitation' that is needed, other penal system representatives determine the focus of the 'rehabilitation', and the general community responsible for funding this process, sees to it that only minimal funds are spent. After all, the drug abuser got himself into this mess, and surely part of his treatment is that he learn how to get himself out of it.

In recent years, professionals, nonprofessionals, and groups best designated as unprofessionals, have taken to viewing drug abuse as a symptom of psychopathology, necessitating verbal and/or chemotherapeutic intervention. The evidence is clear:

1. Who but a sick person would stick a needle into his arm?
2. Who but a sick person would buy drugs illicitly without really knowing their contents?

3. Who but a sick person would take drugs whose consequences are unpredictable?

Each of us can add more such questions. The trap—and there is one inherent in such rhetorical questions—is that many kinds of people are involved in all types of bizarre, irrational, illogical behaviour, and may not necessarily be psychologically or socially sick, given the agreed upon mores and rituals of the time. For example, consider discussing the perils of drug use while smoking in a hallway which is improperly ventilated, after having consumed an excessively rich meal, washed down by alcohol—which is typical of a drug abuse conference scene.

The main point is that once we view the drug abuser as being sick, we automatically fall into the trap of assuming and recommending 'treatment' for him. The choice between using traditional or avant garde modalities is but a minor one once our initial perception is set of the person and his 'problem'.

Given a heterogeneous population of drug abusers, with a homogeneous goal system, using techniques whose effectiveness for a given person is not predictable, the treatment outcome is most often abysmal.

In order to protect our own images we have foisted upon our colleagues and the general community the notion that treating the drug abuser is difficult and their prognosis is guarded. The general approach is that if the drug abuser gets better—translated, that means he gives up his drugs of choice—he was a good and motivated patient and was able to profit from our professional expertise and skill. We cured him. If the patient continues his drug use, this is manifest evidence that he was unmotivated, and a poor treatment risk who could not profit from our skill. Strangely enough, no one ever assesses the level and kind of motivation present in a given treatment agent, let alone what his therapeutic skill really is.

The crucial issue obviously is not that treating the drug abuser is difficult, rather it must be: what are the sources of difficulty in working out a tailored treatment plan for a person who needs to be treated?

Confronting this issue means that we must be cognizant of what kinds of people need and can use what kinds of treatment. Perhaps a major source of difficulty is that we continue to view the drug abuser as a homogeneous entity whose actions and needs are quite distinct from most others. He is an 'addict personality', a 'passive aggressive', a 'drug dependent personality', a 'retreatist', etc. One could spend hours listing the categories that we self-righteously lump the drug abuser into. That is, until he turns out to be a friend or relative.

THE TREATMENT PROCESS

There are presently four major treatment modalities used to change man's appetites: the verbal, conditioning-aversive, chemotherapeutic, and altering states of consciousness. The use of any of these modalities for drug users suffer from two continuing problems. Firstly the drug user may not meet the minimal criteria for effectively utilizing one, or any one of the four during a particular point in his treatment career. Secondly, and perhaps of greater importance, these modalities are often confused with treatment—which they are not. Treatment is an entire process, whereas therapy is the use of a particular technique or modality. Thus whereas it is possible for a person to be in therapy, and not in treatment, the opposite is not possible.

The treatment process is schematized in Table 3. It is initiated with understanding why we choose treatment for a given drug user rather than other forms of intervention, and goes on to issues of selection of treatment site, to screening systems, goal selection, role determination, modality determination, ongoing evaluation, follow up and includes early case finding and prevention. Therapy is only one factor in this process.

It is within this context for example that we must come to understand whether the use of methadone, either for detoxification or maintenance, or behaviour therapy, or meditation, or hypnosis, or alpha waves, or verbal techniques are treatment or therapy. The outcomes for either choice may not, and in all likelihood cannot be the same. Similarly the roles of treatment agents, drug users and the community at large cannot be the same. The difficulties associated with treating any drug misuser becomes manageable when we set forth a complete treatment procedure, pinpointing all of its facets, and when we remember that treatment is not equal to therapy.

Table 3 Treating the drug abuser—a schema

Process	Drug abuser	Purposes and issues	
		Intervention agent	Community at large
I. Standardized screening —evaluation	Relationship to evaluation site Assess person's present strengths Assess person's present weaknesses Assess person's use of community resources Possible registration Baseline data for future evaluation	Selection of evaluation site Assess attitudes (specific to drug user, drug abuse, social pharmacology) Assess knowledge of resources Assess use of resources Criteria for screening in and out	Selection of evaluation site Assess attitudes (specific drug user, drug abuser, social pharmacology) Assess knowledge of available resources Assess utilization of resources Assess gaps in resources Assess priorities for intervention Assess consequences of registration Criteria for screening and their consequences
II. Goal setting	Meaningful for person Achievable by person Acceptable to person Flexible for person	Acceptable to treatment agent Flexible for treatment agent Referral to resources	Acceptable to community Flexible for community Availability of needed resources

45

Table 3 (continued)

Process	Purposes and issues		
	Drug abuser	Intervention agent	Community at large
III. Role definitions	Person's role defined	Treatment agents Role defined	Community's role defined
	Implicit and explicit rights, responsibilities and obligations	Implicit and explicit rights, responsibilities and obligations	Implicit and explicit rights, responsibilities and obligations
IV. Treatment modalities	Appropriate for person	Appropriate for treatment agent's training	Appropriate relevance other priorities
	Determine relationship to conjunctive and ancillary services	Appropriate to treatment agent's availability	Appropriate relevance fiscal consideration
	Assess effect of treatment site	Tone of treatment	Criteria for treatment programmes
		Determine relationships to conjunctive and ancillary services	Delivery of care system
		Continuity of care	Delivery of intervention system
		Continuity of responsibility	Selection of treatment site
		Central case manager	
		Effect of treatment site	

V. Re-evaluation

Assess status of
functioning
Goal re-assessment

Assess attitudes
and motivations
Criteria for evaluating
drug users functioning
Goal system assessment

Treatment modality
assessment

Assessment of other
services' effectiveness
Referral and/or
termination
Assessment for
ongoing training

System for feedback

Assess attitudes

Assess community
Life style functioning
Criteria for
evaluating drug users
Community
involvement and
functioning
Goal system
assessment
Treatment modality
assessment
Assessment of
availability and
utilization
of other services
Reassessment of
criteria for
treatment programmes
Assess consequences
of termination
Goals, funding and
criteria for training
programmes
System for feedback

47

Table 3 (continued)

Process	Drug abuser	Purposes and issues	
		Intervention agent	Community at large
VI. Follow-up	Status of functioning	Assess attitudes and motivation	Assess attitudes
	Referred to needed resources	Assess drug users functioning	Assess drug users functioning
	Role definition as potential intervention agent	Assess treatment efforts	Assess community life style functioning
		Assess criteria for termination	Assess treatment effort
		Assess referral system	Assess delivery of care system
		Assess effects of other services	Assess effects of termination
		Assess gaps in needed other services	Assess effects of site treatment
		Develop drug user typology	System for feedback
		Assess effects of site of treatment	
		System for feedback	

48

VII. Early case findings	Signs and symptoms	Criteria for signs and symptoms	Criteria for signs and symptoms
	Possible registration	Registration issues (i.e., jeopardy)	Registration issues (i.e., contagion)
	Pre-treatment orientation	Pre-treatment orientation skills	Pre-treatment orientation consequences
	Role definitions	Role definitions	Role definitions
	Consequences	Consequences	Consequences
VIII. Prevention	Non-drug alternatives	Delivery of hope	Delivery of hope
	Going beyond drugs	Systems of alternatives	Systems of alternatives
		Develop adaptiveness typology	Social vs. legal control
		Going beyond drugs	Culture and media intervention
			Going beyond drugs

SELECTION OF TREATMENT SITE

The actual site of and for treatment is a crucial issue which is most often overlooked. The most common decision in terms of a treatment site is for it to be away from where we live. The patient, treatment agent and the public at large tend to agree on this. Rarely do we ever ask the about-to-be-patient unless a constituency model of treatment is used. The reason for the geographical distance is self evident: We are offering treatment to stereotypes whom we fear, rather than to humans who we don't know.

The general rule in planning where a program is to be situated must be related to treatment goals. If the goal is to return the drug misuser to an active, heterogeneous community life, the program should not be isolated from the community.

The content of the treatment will also determine the site of treatment. If a methadone maintenance program utilizes a daily pick up system, then the people it serves should not be made to travel for an inordinate amount of time. This is particularly so if it will interfere with such conventional behaviour as school, work or family activities. If a single-substance narcotic addict is to be detoxified, and he manifests no serious medical or psychiatric problems, his detoxification should be tried on an out-patient basis, rather than automatically in a hospital. Another consideration in choosing a treatment site is the actual length of treatment. If it is the live-in, self-help or halfway house variety, the site should be in an active community and not too distant from other necessary adjunctive or ancillary services. If it is an out-patient facility and if one wants to respect the need and desire for confidentiality of treatment, the site should be one which casual observers can not easily categorize as the 'drug addict place'.

Not to take these factors into consideration when choosing a treatment site can only result in emphasizing the uniqueness of the drug misusers behaviour and characteristics and his treatment needs. This will tend to reinforce the stereotype of him that is held by both the community at large and treatment agents. It can also facilitate the drug misusers identification with this stereotype.

Thus, the actual site of treatment is a crucial factor in accentuating or minimizing the drug misuser stereotype. It obviously will also effect delivery of services, treatment outcome and the kinds of early case finding and prevention programs that are carried out.

SCREENING SYSTEMS

This is the first step in a projected procedure, which must include assessment of the strengths and weaknesses of the individual, past, present and anticipated future; in conventional, deviant, and drug oriented areas of adaptation. One should also assess whether the individual prior to drug use has had a history of turning to community and private resources. This will permit a realistic determination of types of referrals to be used. If the person has never used resources, just giving him a name and address is not a referral, it is 'dumping'. For this type of person, programme staff should accompany him the first few times to the referral source. Combined with information derived from significant others, evaluation should help determine the following issues:

1. The type of intervention, including treatment, that is necessary if any.
2. Treatment goals
3. Areas to be focused on
4. The roles and responsibilities of the treater and the treated.
5. The roles and responsibilities of ancillary and conjunctive services.

One might also utilize initial screening as the opportunity for registration for a central registry if this has a health-services function rather than a police function. If treatment is needed, the next obvious step in planning is the selection of appropriate goals.

TREATMENT GOALS

Abstinence is a legitimate goal only if there are medical or psychiatric reasons which contraindicate continued drug use. Otherwise, abstinence is but one of a number of techniques through which treatment goals may be achieved. The logic of this, and its reality, is quite simple: one can rarely change a person's drug behaviour without changing other parts of his behaviour. The evaluation procedure permits the determination of which behaviour can be or should be changed. Since the drug misuser is the focus of the treatment, he should have an active role in goal setting.

Various goal systems may be developed in order to meet the immediate and future needs of the different types of drug abusers being

Table 4   A proposed goal system for the treatment of drug abusers

Palliation	Evaluation indicates that behaviour changes are unlikely because the physical, mental or social condition is too deteriorated. Palliation will permit minimizing of the pain the person is experiencing.
Disability limitation	Evaluation indicates that level of functioning has become increasingly inadequate through time. The goal is stopping the dysfunctional behaviour or deterioration before it gets worse.
Rehabilitation	Evaluation indicates that the person has functioned on a healthier level at other times in his life and the strength to do so again are present. Rehabilitation will permit the person to return to a previous level of satisfactory functioning.
Maintenance plus	Evaluation indicates the person is generally functioning on a satisfactory level but that he needs help in one or two areas. Maintenance plus will permit the individual to reinforce his present satisfactory functioning and will either limit his present dysfunctions or teach him viable alternatives to them.
Promotion	Evaluation indicates unutilized strengths and skills. Promotion will permit the individual to function on a level he has never functioned on before.

treated. A given goal must, however, be selected to meet four criteria: meaningfulness, achievability, acceptability and flexibility.

The logic underlying this for the patient is once again quite simple. If the goal is not meaningful or acceptable why should the patient aspire to it. If it is not achievable, at that point in time, it simply becomes another frustrating barrier in the person's treatment attempt, and indeed may lose him to any future, viable treatment. If it is not flexible then the treatment process is not hand tailored to the person. If this is so we are maintaining empty rituals rather than a treatment process.

The goal criteria need only be acceptable and flexible for the treatment agent and the community at large. If the goals are not acceptable one can anticipate attempts by treatment agents and for the community to undermine the treatment efforts. The clearest contemporary examples of this in the USA are heroin maintenance for the addict or controlled social drinking for the alcoholic.

Goal determination is distinctly associated with the model of delivery of services that is to be utilized. There are different consequences for patient, treatment agent and the community at large when a medical model or a constitutency model is used. The activity level, rights and responsibilities change in each model for all concerned. The issue is not which system is better, but what are the consequences.

Achievement of a goal is obviously related to the choice of treatment modalities, the availability of these modalities and other resources that may be needed, the comprehensiveness of the care offered, the coordination of the treatment effort, and the post-treatment follow-up. A proposed goal system for the treatment of drug abusers is given in Table 4.

TREATMENT MODALITIES

The correct choice can only be based upon whether or not the specific technique relates favourably to the achievement of the selected goal. At this point in time it is impossible to predetermine which goals are best achieved with particular treatment modalities. Although this remains a key difficulty in treating the drug misuser, to blame this difficulty on the patient is, at the very least, self-defeating for everyone.

Choice of a specific modality obviously should depend on whether the person has the ability to benefit from it, let alone partake of it. Too little consideration is given to the availability of staff who have the expertise with a particular technique to implement and utilize it effectively. Professional schools rarely if ever prepare the future therapist or treatment agent to work with drug abusers. Most often such training is obtained, most inadequately, on the job, making it difficult to devise and study what adequate treatment is.

Hope, a necessary ingredient for taking a chance on changing one's way of adapting, is not one of the core courses taught to adult professionals in schools. Without the communication of hope, the treatment process becomes a series of technical movements which may lead to playing at life, not living or learning from it.

Another consideration regarding treatment modalities is the meaning imputed to them by both the professional and lay public. Many believe that if the drug misuser has been in some form of verbal therapy and gained insights, significant changes should be forthcoming, particularly drug abstinence. But gaining insights does not necessarily lead to their productive use, as many of us who have been in therapy so well remember. Similarly many treatment agents have tended to negatively assess the variety of drug and non-drug related mind altering techniques (i.e., bio-feedback, hypnosis, yoga, meditation, psycholitic, etc.) without really understanding their appropriate utilization.

Underlying the chemotherapeutic treatment of the drug abuser is the unrealistic notion that there are chemical solutions to maladaptive socio-psychological functioning. First, there are no magic drugs. Second, a major task in treating the treatable drug misuser is to help him to turn to others, to people rather than things or drugs, in meeting his everyday needs. A therapeutic drug will not place a person in the mainstream of conventional living, particularly if he never lived there before. A medicine will not decrease deviant behaviour if conventional behaviour has little meaning for the drug abuser. The use of chemotherapy when the person has legitimately been evaluated as being untreatable at a given point in time, as a holding operation, or as a last resort will be communicated in just this fashion to the client. This can surely lead to increased frustration, and a reinforcement of hopelessness. Something—a chemical—is not better than nothing. Nothing is equal to nothing. Obviously, treatment modalities have, as do the human beings being treated by them, distinct limitations. Success with both the techniques and the persons being treated depends upon our knowing the specifics of these limitations.

Verbal therapies demand that a person be word-oriented rather than action-oriented, and that he be able to tolerate anxiety as he seeks insights into his behaviour. When the person cannot tolerate and respect his anxiety, and self-medication is available to allay a variety of discomforting feelings, the therapeutic process becomes endangered.

When the patient is action oriented and the therapist is word oriented, they are often unable to reach a common understanding. The difficulties of arranging a viable therapeutic relationship often outweigh any projected accomplishments. Verbal therapies are also predicated on the person not only being able to achieve insights but to effectively use them. As a species man has demonstrated some difficulties with the former criteria, and great difficulty with the latter.

Another critical issue is that without continuous delivery of appropriate services, as they are needed, and without someone taking full responsibility for the delivery of care, a central case manager, fragmentation is sure to arise, and the drug abuser is bound to be blamed for the inefficiency and ineffectiveness of the treatment system.

The necessary components for successful treatment are not always present, but when they are, treatment is obviously as possible for the drug misuser as it is for others.

TREATMENT RE-EVALUATION

Constant evaluation and re-evaluation is necessary in order for the most appropriate choice of goals and treatment modalities, as well as treatment agents and ancillary and conjunctive services for particular patients.

From a goal perspective, treatment should be terminated once goals have been achieved, unless new goals are set. From a modalities perspective, techniques should be changed, given changes in goals and skills of the patient at a given point in time. From a treatment agents and community resources perspective new treatment agents should be brought in when other specific modalities are needed. Likewise new community resources should be developed when re-evaluation points the need for this.

FOLLOW-UP EVALUATIONS

At some point in time after termination from treatment, that dreaded drug misusing patient with the infamous poor prognosis must be revisited. He must give an accounting of his daily behaviour so that we can decide if the whole treatment process was worth it. For most conditions, the process of follow-up attempts to determine if the person is in some way healthier than he was prior to therapeutic intervention, and perhaps feeling a bit more comfortable. If the person's level of functioning is in spite of treatment then we are all in trouble.

Notwithstanding the fact that follow-up is generally an act of lip service in the treatment of drug misusers, when it is done at all, three areas are most often focused on: present use of specific drugs; present vocational and/or school status; and present involvement with the law.

This triad is in part a piece of drug use stereotype. Obviously a real *bona fide* drug mususer uses illicit or licit drugs for the wrong reasons, does not work, and therefore has a criminal status. If he's cured—through our efforts—he may drink and smoke, be unemployed or employed in a job he may be ill suited for, or which is only minimally productive for his community, and hopefully his criminal acts will fit into blue or white collar categories (crimes with class).

At best the 'cured' drug misuser can achieve the status of being an ex-addict or a recovered alcoholic. The underlying assumption is that: 'Once an addict or alcoholic then always an addict or alcoholic'. The social crime that the drug user has commited is that he has permitted himself to be tagged as a visible uncontrolled loser in cultures which respect controlled winners.

Follow-up, if it is to have meaning, should have little to do with verifying stereotypes. Rather it should result in learning what a person's present functioning is like, given his present strengths and weaknesses against a background of available resources. From the patient's perspective it should help pick up clues as to whether further intervention is necessary and if so, what kind, with what goals, and which treatment agents. From the treater's perspective it should permit a clear assessment of whether the treatment process was effective and what it was about the entire process that reinforced or inhibited a positive treatment outcome. It should also serve as a guide for learning new techniques. From the community's point of view, a key question to be answered is: was it all worth it? Communities have the right to determine fiscal spending on the basis of facts and not anecdotes.

The fact that a person has given up his use of particular drugs and illegal behaviour to support his drug appetites may be a considerable attainment for the individual, but if he remains a burden to his society, if his abilities remain unchannelled for the good of his community, the general public may legitimately ask whether all of the treatment efforts were worthwhile.

Obviously, this type of analysis pinpoints yet another difficulty in assessing treatment of the drug abuser. Whose criteria and what criteria are to be used for assessment? The value that one places upon human life, functioning, productivity, and community participation will vary given different perspectives. The point to remember however is that similar dilemmas are present in the treatment of other physical, psychological and social conditions. Drug abuse is not unique.

Another source of difficulty experienced by many who treat the drug misuser is that they themselves often feel a lack of hopefulness in their own lives, that they may be bogged down in personal and professional adversities which they cannot turn into successful outcomes, and for whom the boundaries of their life space are so constricted that only minimal alternatives for daily functioning are available and/or experienced.

Perhaps what we need, if we are to retard the increase in the use and misuse of drugs, is to develop new professions, such as hope communicators, adversity-to-success specialists and alternative analysts.

EARLY CASE FINDING

Early case finding, which has developed from the field of contagious diseases should be an integral part of a treatment process. There are some distinct limitations to this technique when it is simply extrapolated into the area of drug misuse intervention.

Implicit in the use of early case finding is the notion that if we intervene early in a persons non-medical drug use career that the treatment outcome is more positive as well as predictable. There is little empirical evidence to substantiate this, since we don't fully understand why people do or do not turn to drugs, cease or return to drugs.

Secondly is the implicit promise that if we interfere in the persons life and remove him from his present life space that our techniques will be of some help to him. Once again we must acknowledge that there are no techniques or processes which have predictive value for the drug misuser.

Lastly is the implicit promise that should early case finding jeopardize the person in any way it will only be for a limited time. The reality is that the jeopardizing consequences of early case finding may last a life time for the individual and may significantly interfere with such conventional areas of functioning as school, work, residence, etc.

From the treatment planners and communities perspective, early case finding may serve to empirically plan for necessary resources and treatment agents.

From the novice drug misusers perspective, early case finding may serve to sensitize him to what treatment is all about, to orient him to available community resources, to initiate contact with a treatment process and to train and/or educate him in the non-drug alternatives which are available for achievement of his goals.

PREVENTION

Preventing the misuse of drugs, and reinforcing their appropriate or socially–medically approved use has become an area of increasing concern and importance for all segments of society, particularly in industrialized nations. The logic of the concern and the associated efforts is quite simple. Increasingly we have given up on drug misusers, involving them in what euphemistically passes for treatment and, instead, the effort is to save the non-drug user and more specifically non-users from populations at risk.

In the process we have mixed up prevention, education and training, as if they were equivalent. The reality is that prevention is a process which is meant not only to inhibit certain behaviour but to facilitate and reinforce other behaviour. Education is a process in which a hetero-geneous group becomes the focus of certain goals and techniques and terminates this process as a heterogeneous group, particularly in terms of decision making. Training on the other hand is a process or technique by which a heterogeneous group is aided in becoming a homogeneous one for specific skills, values, abilities, attitudes, etc.

These distinctions are not minor ones as programmes attempt to reinforce certain patterns of drug use and inhibit others. Do we need or want heterogeneous or homogeneous groups of citizens in regard to the use and misuse of all drugs? Do we need drug aware and sensitized citizens or simply maximally functioning friends, neighbours and family? What criteria should be developed, if any, to screen in and screen out individuals from drug related prevention–education programs of any type? These are just some of the issues that must be confronted when we begin to consider the development of drug prevention programmes.

Prevention, if it is to be viable, should be based on the non–drug alternatives to experiencing and adapting to life, rather than the drug oriented ones. The major reason certain drugs cannot be used is not related to their danger. There are no undangerous drugs. Every society has always, and no doubt will continue to decide which drugs are in and which are out as a function of arbitrary social decisions.

Meaningful prevention means that we go beyond drugs, rather than remaining fixated on them.

TREATMENT IN CONTEXT

Treatment of the drug misuser can only be understood against a background of immense and rapid change in daily living as well as the multiplicity of factors that affect the contemporary non–medical use of drugs. Table 5 schematizes these factors.

Since the industrial revolution and its concomitant technological advances, we have more people, attempting to meet their increased needs in less space, being bombarded by more noise, living longer, with more free time that they don't know what to do with, and threats to national and personal identity and existence have significantly increased. Institutions such as the family, the school, and the church, which in previous times instructed people in the rituals of the good life and how best to live life and not play at it, are increasingly ineffective in their efforts. At the same time there is an increasing number of chemicals available to more and more people of all ages against a background of progress through chemistry.

Techniques and rituals are needed to help people—drug abusers as well as abstainers, and those in between—to take a chance on non–drug options for experiencing life. Treatment is only one of the options.

Unfortunately many treatment agents and policy makers don't view treatment as being only one of the options open to us.

Table 5   Factors affecting the non-medical use of drugs

Drugs	Characteristics of users	Behaviour of user
Type Frequency Amount Manner Pattern Meaning	Age Vocational status Sex Mental status Race Physical status Ethnicity Economic status Religion Social class Marital status I.Q.	Physical and psycho-social functions and dysfunctions; conventional and deviant life styles
Scientific knowledge	*Attitudes: Intervention agents*	*Attitudes: General communication*

Theories
  Treatment
  Drug use
  Drug action
  Altered state of
    consciousness
Classification
  Drug use
  Drug users
  Non-drug users
  Drugs
Research
  Role
  Techniques
  Relevance
	Drugs
	Drug use
	Drug misuse
	Drug users
	Stereotypes
		Drugs
		Drug use
		Drug misuse
		Drug users
		Stereotypes

Treatment	*Public policy:* *local and national*	*Politics*
Types of programmes	Laws	Service related delivery
Site of treatment	Policies	Non-service related delivery
Evaluation methods and procedures	Procedures	
Goal setting systems		
Roles		
Treatment modalities		*Economics*
Policies and procedures		Legal facets
Ongoing evaluation		Illegal facets
Follow-up systems		
Early case finding		

Education–prevention	*Mass media*	*Philosophy–religion*
Drug related alternatives	People oriented patterns of living	Drug related rituals
Non-drug related alternatives	Drug oriented patterns of living	Non-drug related rituals
Decision making		
Respect for people		
Respect for feelings		*Culture*
Respect for drugs		Drug related
Built in inequities of living		Non-drug related
Role definitions, associated rights, responsibilities, obligations and consequences		

Much of the hopelessness and breast-beating arises from our confusion about treatment, what it can and can't accomplish, and from our less than clear interpretation of what drug abuse or misuse means.

There are at least three kinds or sources of drug abuse. These are:

1. Abusing drug laws: the breaking of drug related laws, mores and rituals by using particular drugs in particular ways and for particular reasons.
2. Self abuse: the direct or indirect consequences, resulting from the use of drugs for other than medically approved reasons, to the person taking the drug(s).
3. Abuse of others: the direct or indirect consequences of the use of drugs for other than medically approved reasons to people other than drug misusers.

Developing alternatives to the non-medical use of drugs does not necessarily mean treatment. Other viable alternatives begin to be possible if we can determine the type of drug misuse we are considering at a given point in time. Having decided that, the next step is to decide what the focus of intervention is to be. We have the choice of focusing our efforts on:

1. the drugs themselves;
2. abstainers–individuals who have never used drugs or those who have ceased their drug misuse;
3. active drug misusers;
4. intervention agents–teachers, clergy, treatment agents, parents, peers, etc.; and
5. the general community.

Having decided upon the type of drug misuse we wish to affect, and what the focus is to be we can then decide the area of possible intervention.

Treatment is only one of the possible types of intervention (see Table 6). Choosing it is as arbitrary a decision as any other that we might make. But once we have chosen it, based on careful thought rather than as a panacea, we should have better results with it than was our general experience when treatment was a euphemism for isolating us, the good people from them, the bad drug users.

Obviously, this decade will be one of more drugs, and surely more

Table 6 Types of intervention in drug misuse

Areas of intervention (I–X)	Focus of intervention (a–c)	Sources of drug misuse		
		Drug related Laws, mores rituals (A)	Self abuse (B)	Abuse of others (C)
I. Treatment (Including Early Case Finding and Prevention)	a. Drugs b. Abstainers c. Drug Users d. Intervention Agents e. General Community			
II. Education	a. Drugs b. Abstainers c. Drug Users d. Intervention Agents c. General Community			
III. Attitudes	a. Drugs b. Abstainers c. Drug Users d. Intervention Agents e. General Community			

Table 6 *(continued)*

		Sources of drug misuse		
Areas of intervention (I–X)	Focus of intervention (a–c)	Drug related laws, mores rituals (A)	Self abuse (B)	Abuse of others (C)
IV. Media	a. Drugs b. Abstainers c. Drug Users d. Intervention Agents e. General Community			
V. Culture	a. Drugs b. Abstainers c. Drug Users d. Intervention Agents e. General Community			
VI. Religion	a. Drugs b. Abstainers c. Drug Users d. Intervention Agents e. General Community			

VII. Laws, Policies Procedures

    a. Drugs
    b. Abstainers
    c. Drug Users
    d. Intervention Agents
    e. General Community

VIII. Politics

    a. Drugs
    b. Abstainers
    c. Drug Users
    d. Intervention Agents
    e. General Community

IX. Economics

    a. Drugs
    b. Abstainers
    c. Drug Users
    d. Intervention Agents
    e. General Community

X. Research

    a. Drugs
    b. Abstainers
    c. Drug Users
    d. Intervention Agents
    e. General Community

people. But whether more people will be using and misusing more drugs will have little to do with the difficulties of treating the drug misuser. Rather it will have to do with understanding in a real way the difficulties and pleasure of life and how best to experience both.

REFERENCES

Barber, B. (1967). Drugs & Society. (Russell Sage Foundation: New York)
Barton, H. H. (1971). Brief Therapies. (Behavioral Publications: New York)
Brecher, E. M. (1972). Licit and Illicit Drugs. (Little Brown and Co: Boston)
Brotman, R. and Freedman, A. (1968). A Community Mental Health Approach to Drug Addiction. (US Government Printing Office: Washington, DC)
Brown, C. (1970). Manchild in the Promised Land. (New American Library: New York)
Burroughs, W. (1900). Junkie. (Ace Publishing Corp: New York)
Burris, D. S. (1969). The Right to Treatment. (Springer Publishing Co: New York)
Burton, A. (ed.) (1969). Encounter. (Jossey Bass: San Francisco)
Caldwell, V. W. (1900). LSD Psychotherapy. (Grove: New York)
Casriel, D. (1971). (Daytop, Hill and Wang, New York)
Cohen, C. (1972). Multiple drug use considered in the light of the stepping stone hypothesis, *Intern. J. Add.* **7**, 27–56
Cohen, A. Y. (1971). The journey beyond trips: alternative to drugs. *J. Psychodelic Drugs* **3**, 16–21.
Coles, R., *et al.* (1970). Drugs and Youth (Liveright, New York)
Cross, J. N. (1968). Guide to the Community Control of Alcoholism (American Public Health Association: Washington, DC)
Crowley, R. (1939). Psychoanalytic literature on drug addiction and alcoholism, *Psychoan. Rev.* **26**, 39–54
DeRopp, R. S. (1968). Master Game: Pathways to Higher Consciousness Beyond the Drug Experience. (Dell, New York)
Dole, V. P. and Nyswander, M. (1965). Medical treatment for diacetylmorphine (heroin) addiction, *J. Amer. med. Ass.* **193**, 646–650
Dole, V. P. and Nyswander, M. (1968). Methadone maintenance and its implications for theories of narcotic addiction. *Res. Publ. Ass. Res. Nerv. Ment. Dis.*, **46**, 359–366
Duncan, T. L. (1965). Understanding and Helping the Narcotic Addict. (Fortress Press, Philadelphia)
Ebin, D. (ed.) (1961). The Drug Experience. (Orion Press: New York)
Edwards, G. (1972). Reaching Out: the Prevention of Drug Abuse Through Increased Human Interaction. (Holt, Rhinehart, Winston: New York)

Einstein, S. and Jones, F. (1965). Group therapy with adolescent addicts: use of a heterogeneous group approach. *In* 'Drug Addiction in Youth' Harmes, E. (ed.) (Pergamon Press: Oxford)

Einstein, S. (ed.) (1971). Methadone Maintenance. (Marcel Dekker: New York)

Einstein, S. (ed.) (1972). The Non-Medical Use of Drugs: Clinical Issuès. (Institute for the Study of Drug Addiction: New York)

Final Report (1963). President's Advisory Commission on Narcotic and Drug Abuse. (US Government Printing Office: Washington, DC)

Franks, C. M. (1966). Conditioning & conditioned aversion therapies in the treatment of the alcoholic, *Intern. J. Add.* 1, 61–98

Ford Foundation (1972). Dealing with Drug Abuse. (Praeger Publishers: New York)

Frykman, J. (1971). A New Connection. (Scrimshaw Press: San Francisco)

Hess, A. (1971). Deviance theory and the history of opiates, *Intern. J. Add.* 6, 585–599

Jaffe, J. H. and Brill, L. (1966). Cyclazocine, a long acting narcotic antagonist: Its voluntary acceptance as a treatment modality by narcotic abusers. *Intern. J. Add.* 1, 99–123

Hoffman, H. von. (1900). We are the People our Parents Warned us Against. (Fawcett-World: New York)

Keniston, K. (1968). Heads and seekers: Drugs on Campus, counter culture and American Society. *Amer. Schol.* 38, 97–112

King, R. (1972). The Drug Hang Up. (Norton Publishers: New York)

Kramer, J. (1971). Controlling Narcotics in America, Part I. *Drug Forum,* 1, No. 1, 51–70

Kramer, J. (1972). Controlling Narcotics in America, Part II. *Drug Forum* 1, No. 2, 153–168

Laing, R. D. (1969). The Divided Self. (Penguin Books, Inc: Middlesex, UK)

Lennard and Associates (1971). Mystification and Drug Misuse. (Jossey Bass: San Francisco)

Marin, P. and Cohen, Y. (1971). Understanding Drug Use. (Harper and Row: New York)

Menninger, K. (1963). The Vital Balance. (Viking Press: New York)

Metzner, R. (1968). The Ecstatic Adventure. (MacMillan: New York)

Meyer, R. (1972). Guide to Drug Rehabilitation: A Public Health Response. (Beacon Press: Boston)

Michener, J. A. (1971). The Drifters. (Random House: New York)

Nyswander, M. (1956). The Drug Addict as a Patient. (Grune and Stratton: New York)

Proceedings. (1971). Third National Conference on Methadone Treatment. (US Government Printing Office: Washington, DC)

Proceedings. (1972). Fourth National Conference on Methadone Treatment. (National Association for the Prevention of Addiction to Narcotics: New York)

Rachman, S. and Teasdale, J. (1969). Aversion Therapy and Behavior Disorders. (University of Miami Press)

Report of the Commission of Inquiry into the Non-Medical Use of Drugs, Treatment, Information, Canada, Ottawa. (1972)

Robins, L. N. and Murphy, G. E. (1967). Drug Use in a normal population of young Negro men. *Amer. J. Pub. Health*, **57**, 1580

Roszak, T. (1900). Making of a Counter Culture. (Doubleday: New York)

Slater, P. (1970). The Pursuit of Loneliness. (Beacon Press: Barton)

Szasz, T. S. (1972). The ethics of addiction. (Harpers)

Szasz, T. S. (1900). Law, Liberty and Psychiatry: An Inquiry into the Social Uses of Mental Health Practices. (MacMillan: New York)

Task Force Report (1967). Narcotics and Drug Abuse. (US Government Printing Office: Washington, DC)

Terry, C. E. and Pellens, M. (1971). The Opium Problem. (Patterson and Smith: Montclair, New Jersey)

Watts, A. (1962). The Joyous Cosmology-Adventures in the Chemistry of Consciousness. (Panthean Books: New York)

Weil, A. (1972). The Natural Hind. (Houghton, Mifflin: New York)

Weisman, T. (1972). Drug Abuse and Drug Counseling. (The Press of Case Western Reserve University: Cleveland)

Wikler, A. (1965). Conditioning factors in opiate addiction and relapse. *In* 'Narcotics' Wilner, D. M. and Kassebaum, G. C. (eds.) (McGraw Hill: New York)

Yablonsky, L. (1965). Synanon: The Tunnel Back. (MacMillan: New York)

Zborowski, M. (1969). People in Pain. (Jossey Bass: San Francisco).

Zinberg, N. E. and Robertson, J. S. (1972). Drugs and the Public. (Simon and Schuster, New York)

CHAPTER 2

The nature of addiction

N. BEJEROT

INTRODUCTION

Until recent years drug addiction has been considered as a single entity, and any division of the condition has been along pharmacological lines, with addictions divided into morphinism, cocainism, and so on. With the mass spread of addiction among the youth, particularly since World War II, a growing number of observers have realized that addiction is not one condition, and most of them have discerned two different types. Kolb (1924) referred to various personality disorders and medically induced addictions; Lindesmith (1965) described them as the old and new types of addiction; Brill (1966, 1968) differentiated therapeutic and street addicts; James (1967) described the new type of addicts by their own term, 'junkies' and Ball (1970) made a division into metropolitan heroin abuse and middle class white addiction where the drugs are obtained by legal or semi-legal means.

A SOCIO-MEDICAL CLASSIFICATION OF ADDICTION

In 1965 I put forward a socio-medical classification of addictions based upon the way in which the addiction has been acquired. This classification divides addiction into three main groups: therapeutic cases, epidemic and endemic cases (Bejerot 1965, 1969).

THERAPEUTIC CASES

These are characterized by the fact that they have not been introduced into their abuse by an established addict. They may be subdivided into three groups.

(1) Addiction arising as a result of a consciously accepted risk during medical treatment

This is mainly a matter of the relief of pain in incurable and dying patients, and a complicating addiction in these cases has to be accepted. Generally there is no great problem with regard to these addictions

(2) Addiction inadvertently caused by medical treatment

Earlier morphinism sometimes started in this way, but nowadays the risk of addiction is small in correct medical treatment of pain.

On the other hand it is not unusual for nervous and anxiety-ridden patients to become addicted through long over-consumption of tranquillizing drugs and sleeping tablets. The risk is particularly great if the patients wander from one physician to another, and receive drugs from several physicians simultaneously without any coordination of the medication. Many physicians also prescribe tranquillizing and sleeping tablets in an irresponsible way, and thereby initiate addiction in their unsuspecting patients.

The therapeutic cases have in recent years been completely over-shadowed by the epidemic addictions. However, even the therapeutic addictions are probably rising rapidly in number parallel with the great increase in the prescribing of psychotropic drugs during the last 10 years. Freyhan (1971) reported that production of tranquillizers has doubled in the USA in the last 4 years. During 1970 5000 million doses of tranquillizing drugs, 3000 million doses of amphetamines and 5000 million doses of barbiturates were produced in the USA. A third of all Americans between 18 and 74 are reckoned to have taken psycho-active drugs of some kind during 1970. 'We must face up to the fact that we cannot account scientifically for this consumption rate of therapeutic drugs. There is no evidence of an increase in the incidence of drug-treatable psychiatric disorders to match the astronomic increase of prescriptions.'

(3) Self-established addictions

These are old and familiar phenomena. Through the ease with which they can obtain drugs, medical staff have always run a risk through self-administration of dangerous drugs in conditions of pain, depression or stress.

In none of these three groups of therapeutic cases is there any marked tendency to draw others into drug abuse. The individual cases are often very severe, but they are not contagious, with some reservation for addicted physicians, some of whom draw their wives into addiction. They also have a marked tendency to be careless in prescribing dangerous drugs to patients. Already in 1915 Brown declared that 'certain physicians unhappily leave behind them a sad trail of addicts. In most instances these physicians are themselves addicts.'

EPIDEMIC ADDICTIONS

It is often considered that some kind of microbe is involved if we talk of epidemics. Other forms of contagion occur, however. We had, for instance, bizarre mass phenomena during the Middle Ages, such as epidemics of dancing (Hecker, 1833). Local outbreaks of suicide and arson occur now and then.

The literature abounds in descriptions of small, local, mental epidemics, and I will quote a recent report from Britain (Benaim *et al.*, 1971): 'An epidemic of falling, confined to one single class of a large comprehensive school in a London suburb, is described. There were 24 adolescent girls in the class, all in the 16–17 age group, and the class was involved in examinations. The school authorities decided to close down the class one week before the end of term, when eight girls and a young locum teacher lay unconscious on the floor. Most of the girls affected belonged to the 'in-group': the very bright, the Greek, the Jewish and the one coloured girl were unaffected.'

One of the protagonists of the epidemic was admitted to hospital for observation, and there she started a hysterical 'pregnancy epidemic' in her ward.

The epidemic addictions have a number of characteristics which differentiate them radically from addictions of the therapeutic type.

Contagion

The type of epidemic addiction which now afflicts most Western industrial countries has, as a prerequisite, direct, personal contagion between an established abuser and a novice. No one can learn to inject drugs into the veins unless he has been taught by an experienced person. It is perhaps less widely known that you cannot even learn to smoke hashish properly without being taught the technique.

As early as 1968, Cameron, Chief of the Drug Dependence Unit of WHO, pointed out that there is only one major difference between the classical infectious-disease model of illness and drug dependence as a communicable disorder. With infectious diseases, the host does not seek the agent of infection. At worst the host may be indifferent to the agents of such disesases as cholera or malaria. But with drug dependence, the host wants and seeks out the agent.'

The contagious element in youth addictions has been observed by a number of research workers (Brown, 1915, Hill, 1962, Bewley 1965, Chapple and Marks 1965, Glatt 1965, MacDonald 1965, Ausubel 1966, Brill 1966, Scher 1966, Teigen 1966, Evang 1967, Cameron 1968, Blum et al. 1969, Cohen 1969, James 1969, Kleber 1969, Lindberg, B. 1969, Ball and Chambers 1970, Blachly 1970, Eddy 1970, Retterstøl 1970, Alström 1971, Brown et al. 1971, Cockett 1971, Jaffe and Hughes 1971, Glasscote et al. 1972, Hughes et al. 1972 *a, b*, Hughes and Crawford 1972, Jonas 1972, Rathod 1972, Tec 1972, Johnson 1973, Levengood et al. 1973, Nahas 1973, Bourne 1974, DuPont 1974).

De Alarcón (1969) has traced in detail the paths of infection in a heroin epidemic in Crawley, a new town outside London (Figure 1).

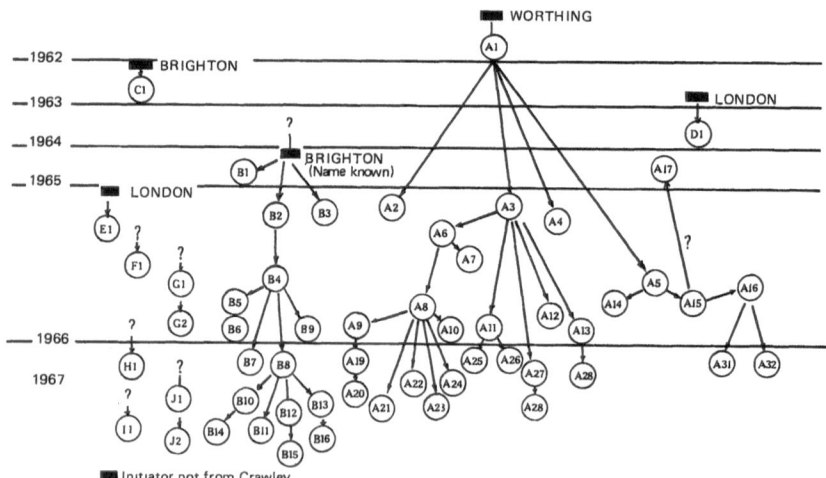

Figure 1 The spread of heroin abuse in Crawley 1962–67 (from De Alarcón, 1969). The sociogram illustrates the chain of transmission from one subject to another for young people living in Crawley in 1967 Only three cases were known to have given up heroin spontaneously after the first few injections

Contagion in epidemic addiction occurs almost exclusively through close personal contact. Earlier it was believed that pushers initiate people into abuse of this type. Pushers come into the picture at a later stage, and then they play a pernicious role as suppliers and reinforcers.

Rapid spread

The number of therapeutic cases in a society is usually fairly stable, while drug epidemics seem to develop by geometric progression as long as potential risk groups remain and drug policy remain unchanged. The heroin epidemic in Britain doubled every sixteenth month between 1959 and 1967 (Bewley *et al.*, 1968). The Swedish amphetamine epidemic doubled about every thirtieth month between 1948 and 1968 (Bejerot, 1970).

Historic boundaries

The epidemic addictions always start suddenly, as when a spark lights a forest fire. On the other hand, it may smoulder in the undergrowth a long while before the flames break out in full force.

Drug epidemics may be brought to an end, as was the great amphetamine epidemic in Japan after the World War II (Tatetsu, 1963; Brill and Hirose, 1969) or the Chinese opium smoking, which was checked by drastic action after the revolution in 1949 (Blaustein, 1962). The cocaine epidemics in England and Germany in the 1920s were also checked by administrative measures (Spear, 1969).

Geographic boundaries

The drug epidemic may be limited to a school, a district in a city, a region, or a country. Epidemic addictions are always checked for some period of time by political and geographic boundaries even if communications across the borders are lively.

The injection of amphetamines, which started in Stockholm in the forties, was practised by about 400 individuals before the first known cases appeared outside Stockholm in 1954, when one of my addicted patients moved to Gothenburg. Before 1966 the Danish authorities did not know of any intravenous addicts. Swedish peddlers had made energetic attempts to sell central stimulants in Copenhagen, but failed completely until 1967. In the early months of 1968, there was already a daughter epidemic of a few hundred cases of intravenous abuse in

Copenhagen, and one year later there were an estimated 500 cases. In 1972 there were about 3500 intravenous drug abusers in Denmark, mainly teenagers, and most of them were using opiates (morphine base).

Ethnic boundaries

For a long time, alien citizenship in Sweden gave almost complete protection from being drawn into intravenous drug abuse, even for people living in Stockholm—the centre of the Swedish epidemic of amphetamine abuse. In 1965 there was a breakthrough into the large Finnish population in the Stockholm area and, in 1966, a daughter epidemic broke out in Helsinki. The first cases of intravenous abuse in Norway were reported in 1967; all of them had lived for some time in Sweden. Some other aliens had also learnt the injection technique in Sweden and then returned to their home countries with this experience.

Even in the little epidemic of falling girls described above, the ethnic boundaries were strong enough to protect the non-Anglian girls although they attended the same school class.

The ethnic barriers for the spread of drug epidemics are weak if the epidemic has its centre in groups with a wealth of international contacts and considerable international mobility. The cannabis epidemic among jazz and pop musicians and students illustrates this point.

Age distribution

The epidemics first affect narrow age groups. Thinner sniffing usually occurs in young teenagers (Litt and Cohen, 1970), hashish smoking in the upper teens and the early twenties; intravenous drug abuse originally spread among 20–30 year olds.

The more a drug epidemic spreads, the broader the age distribution becomes. In the spring of 1965 there were very few persons under 20 or over 40 who took drugs intravenously in the Stockholm arrest population. Yet at that time 39 per cent of the arrestees between 25 and 30 were injecting drugs (Figure 2).

The rates for this advanced form of abuse in the youngest (15–19) and oldest (40–44) age groups in the arrest population increased tenfold from 3 to 30 per cent between spring 1965 and spring 1967 (Bejerot, 1972). The mean age of Swedish amphetaminists is about 26, which is the same as for American heronists (Brill, 1968).

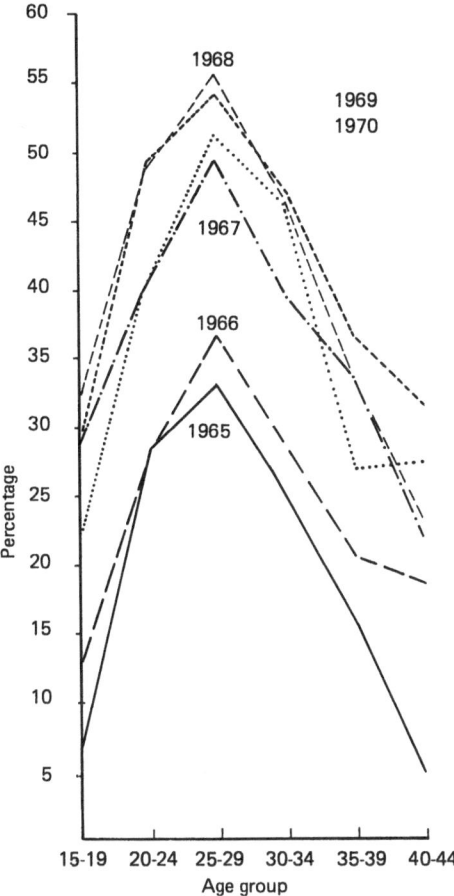

Figure 2 Percentage of drug abuse of intravenous type in different age groups among male Swedes arrested under the criminal code in Stockholm, April 1965 to June 1970.

Sex ratios

While the ratio of men to women is usually about 1 : 1 in addiction of therapeutic origin, and women may even be over-represented in this group (Brill, 1968), men are always over-represented in epidemic addiction. The male excess tends, however, to diminish the more widely spread the epidemic becomes and the older it grows.

In the beginning of a drug epidemic there are often six or seven men to every woman involved, but the difference falls successively to three or four men to every woman. The sex ratios in various drug epidemics are discussed by Ball and Chambers (1970) for the USA, Brill and Hirose (1969) for Japan, Bejerot (1970) for Sweden, and Glatt *et al.*, (1967) for England.

In drug epidemics which have finally become a socially accepted and endemic phenomenon, the proportion of women increased successively (as, for instance, in the use of tobacco and alcohol in industrial countries), but has still not reached the ratio 1:1.

Group boundaries

Hashish smoking was brought to Scandinavia by American jazz musicians in the late 1940s. For a long time hashish was confined to just these circles in Scandinavia.

In 1965 it was estimated that there were only a few hundred hashish smokers in Sweden, nearly all in Stockholm, and centered around one jazz restaurant. Four years later there were tens of thousands of students and school children all over the country who had tried hashish, and it is now difficult to estimate the number who are severely addicted.

Intravenous drug abuse, on the other hand, represents quite another epidemic and affects different groups; in Sweden until 1965 mainly bohemians and criminals.

Massivity

Drug abuse, as opposed to addiction, is often a symptom of maladjustment of various kinds; this is particularly the case when the drugs of choice cannot be obtained legally. Then it is often deviating individuals who are prepared to break social norms and engage in criminal activity in order to obtain illegal drugs for which, in the beginning, they have no craving; it is the maladjusted youths who form the core of most new drug epidemics. It should be remembered, however, that many youths start on drugs during a critical phase in what might otherwise have been a normal course of development. Also, when addicts are asked why it was they had taken the first dose, the reason most commonly given was that it was out of curiosity or the desire to belong to an 'in-group' (Ball 1970, Cameron 1968, Brown *et al.*, 1971).

The more widespread abuse becomes, the more exposed to drugs the non-abuser will be, and the less predisposing personality disorders and social difficulties are required for an individual to be drawn in. This corresponds to the massivity phenomenon in epidemics spread by microbes: there is an *increased morbidity risk on increased concentration of pathogenic agents in the environment.*

This mechanism has been exemplified clearly in the present cannabis epidemic where, after a time, large groups of ordinary youth have been drawn in through the massivity effect in their environment. Walters *et al.*, (1972) express this phenomenon rather drastically, 'thus, not only in the college studied, but probably in most others like it, the non-user has become, in a *statistical* sense, deviant.'

Fashion in choice of drugs

The great Japanese epidemic of drug abuse after World War II concerned exclusively methamphetamine (Brill and Hirose 1969). Abuse of central stimulants began in Sweden in the forties with amphetamine. During 1957–58 the new slimming drug phenmetrazine (Preludin) came into the picture and took the place of amphetamine. For a period methylphenidate (Ritalin) was very popular. When Preludin was taken off the legal market amphetamine, illicitly manufactured, came back into fashion.

Fashion for method of administration

For a long time, central stimulants were taken orally in addict circles in Sweden. In the mid-1940s addicts began to dissolve the drugs and inject them directly into the veins. At the end of the 1960s there were not many addicts who were content to take the drugs by mouth.

In America, subcutaneous injections of opiates was for a long period the usual method of administration. The intravenous technique was introduced in the early thirties (O'Donnell and Jones 1970, Baden 1972) and came to be the dominant method of administration.

In Hong Kong people still smoke opiates, although it is usually heroin they smoke these days (Hess 1965, Whisson 1965).

In comparison with therapeutic cases, the epidemic addictions constitute a different form of illness, even if the addicts are dependent upon the same drug. The most alarming factor in the situation is that *all addicts of epidemic type are potentially contagious.*

ENDEMIC ADDICTIONS

Endemic addictions are addictions which are constantly present in a country, and which have arisen as a result of a more or less socially accepted use of certain addicting substances for enjoyment, relaxation, or stimulation. Many endemic addictions in the distant past began as epidemics. It is possible that we today are witnessing the conversion of a marijuana epidemic into an endemic in the United States.

Among endemic addictions we can include opium smoking in the old China after the initial epidemic phase; hashish smoking in North Africa, coca chewing among South American Indians, alcoholism among the ancient Israelites (Keller, 1970) and in a large part of the world today. Alcoholism exists mainly in Christian areas, while Buddhist and Muhammadan countries up to the present have been spared this, thanks to their religious precepts. It appears that Muhammad not only eradicated alcoholism in North Africa and Asia Minor, but also the grape vine.

Since endemic forms of addiction arise on the basis of the drug being more or less socially tolerated within the country, these addictions affect a more average and 'normal' selection of the population than the epidemic addictions. Epidemic addictions mainly affect special population groups (youth, bohemians, criminals, etc.).

While abusers and addicts of epidemic type have a strong tendency to change from one type of intoxicant to another ('poly-drug-abusers', 'multiple addiction') (Bewley and Ben Arie 1968, Mitcheson *et al.*, 1970, Balter *et al.*, 1971, Birdwood 1971, Dodson *et al.*, 1971, Mirin *et al.*, 1971), addicts of endemic type—like those of therapeutic origin—have a strong tendency to keep to their habitual and socially sanctioned intoxicant (Brill, 1968). If morphinists of therapeutic type cannot obtain morphine they do not then go over to central stimulants or cannabis (but sometimes to the socially accepted alcohol or sleeping tablets); morphinists of epidemic type on the other hand, experiment willingly with other illegal drugs in an abstinence situation. The alcoholic, with his endemic form of abuse, does not begin to sniff thinner or smoke hashish if his source of supply is cut off, for instance through a strike (Bjerver *et al.*, 1965), but in some cases he may abuse sleeping tablets and other socially accepted preparations instead.

AT RISK GROUPS

The groups afflicted by addiction of therapeutic, self-established, epidemic and endemic type differ fundamentally from each other. The different personality patterns are thus intimately connected with the different paths into addiction, i.e., the reason why the addicting drug originally came to be used.

THERAPEUTIC ADDICTION

Here addiction has by definition occurred as a complication to medical treatment. The drugs were usually prescribed for continuous or repeated pain, anxiety and stress, or insomnia. Those affected by therapeutic addictions are mainly middle-aged people (Brill, 1968). Women and men are affected about equally, and women may even predominate.

Those who are afflicted by therapeutic addiction are often more ambitious than the average, but also more sensitive to criticism and set-backs. Various forms of neuroses, frustration and depression are common background factors in addiction of this type.

Criminality and antisocial conduct are rare in this group. These socially responsible, rather over-ambitious, anxious and sensitive people stand psychologically more removed from epidemic addicts than the average population.

Self-established addiction

It is mainly physicians and nurses who are affected by self-established addiction, and the condition is almost always therapeutic in origin, and due to self-medication for pain, stress, frustration or depression.

Modlin and Montes (1964) refer to a number of investigations from the United States, England, Germany, Holland and France; these all show that physician-addicts comprised about 15 per cent of all known addicts in these countries. The group is 1 per cent of all American physicians (Winick, 1965), and there is much to suggest that it is of about the same proportion in Europe. This makes addiction 30–100 times as frequent among physicians as among the rest of the population—in countries without a great drug epidemic, we must add.

EPIDEMIC ADDICTION

We can easily show that drug abuse of epidemic type is over-represented during certain periods, in certain societies, in special age groups, subcultures and social classes. Those who are drawn into drug epidemics, particularly in the early stages of an epidemic, differ as a group in almost every variable from those who are afflicted by therapeutic addiction. In epidemic addictions it is mainly young, unstable, immature, adventurous and easily led individuals who experiment with drugs. There is also a risk for individuals with school or work problems, and those who for any reason have difficulty in being accepted in the ordinary gangs, and therefore are prepared to take drugs in order to be accepted at least by aberrant groups (James, 1969). Those youngsters who experiment with injections are a much more deviant group than those experimenting with hallucinogens (cannabis, LSD, etc.).

All epidemic addicts have in common that they are not seeking relief from pain, anxiety or insomnia, but instead are looking for enjoyment, intoxication, kicks. It is therefore not surprising that epidemic addicts have been found to show a greater tendency than the average towards other forms of pleasure-seeking behaviour before the development of drug abuse. As a group they have early experience of tobacco and alcohol, an early sexual debut (Backhouse and James, 1969, Johnson *et al.*, Riley *et al.*, 1971), have been more promiscuous (Cohen *et al.*, 1972), and even in other ways they have proved themselves more desirous of recreation and more 'advanced' than the average youths in their age and social strata (Kolb, 1962). As a group they have often had greater difficulty in tolerating frustration and in realizing long-term goals, which may have been expressed in truancy, absence from work, frequent change of job, vagrancy, etc., prior to initiation into drug abuse (Kolb, 1962). Many, particularly the nucleus of the epidemic group, have an early and extensive history of criminal activity (Bejerot, 1970).

It is important to remember that what has been said applies only statistically for the group of epidemic addicts as a whole. Individuals differ in their susceptibility to drug abuse and in their susceptibility to the development of severe dependence. The individual variations are very large, even in the most serious forms, such as intravenous abuse. Also the susceptibility of the individual changes, not only with age, but also with incidental crises and strain.

What has been described here represents the personality factors correlated with a high susceptibility to epidemic addiction. They represent minor variations in a relatively stable, normal distribution of character traits in the population. Susceptibility, however, represents only one of the components in the development of epidemic addiction. The other components are exposure to, and massivity of, contagion. It is principally the degree of exposure which determines who, and how many, will be drawn into the various addiction epidemics. The weakest are drawn in as soon as they are exposed to risk, but even average or 'strong' personalities can be drawn in when the massivity of contagion is high.

When an epidemic has become as widespread as marijuana smoking in USA, the personality factor declines in importance. Johnson (1973) showed that marijuana smoking could be predicted on the basis of four variables: sex, tobacco smoking, religious participation, and political sympathies. Of non-religious, left wing, cigarette-smoking males, 97 per cent had tried cannabis. Of very religious, right wing, non-cigarette-smoking females only 4 per cent had ever tried cannabis. If a fifth variable is added, the proportion of intimate friends who smoke marijuana, marijuana smoking can be predicted with almost 100 per cent accuracy; this last variable is the most important, particularly with regard to regular smoking of cannabis. Thus, the primary factor in understanding why a college student used marijuana is the proportion of his friends who use it. It is the non-religious, left wing, tobacco smoking males who will have the greatest proportion, 76 per cent of cannabis smoking friends, whilst only 2 per cent of the religious, right wing, non-smoking females will have a large proportion of friends smoking cannabis.

Epidemic and therapeutic addiction: two different diseases

The fundamental differences between the two main types of addiction, the epidemic and therapeutic, do not seem to have been observed before the mid-1960s (Bejerot, 1965).

From Table 1 it is apparent that epidemic and therapeutic addiction represent two different morbid conditions, not only with regard to the initiation mechanism and circumstances generally, but also the persons affected, their social and psychological characteristics and even their attitude to their disease: therapeutic addicts experience their dependence as a great tragedy, they feel shame and guilt because they are unable to resist the craving, and they try to hide their drug problem from others by every means they can. Epidemic addicts, on the other hand, tend to regard drug intoxication as the most desirable experience in the world,

Table 1   Some contrasts in two types of opiate dependence
(from Brill, 1968)

Characteristic	Non-medical (Street addict)	Medical
Usual age range of cases Male/female ratio	18 to 30 (avg. 27) 6 or 8 men to each woman	30 and beyond (avg. 40). Female incidence equals that of male
Locale	Cases tightly clustered in specific metropolitan areas.	Cases dispersed
Drugs used	Heroin is the drug of choice; multiple drug use is the rule, marijuana frequent	Morphine and demerol the prevailing drugs; heroin rare in U.S., infrequent abroad
Psychiatric classification	Character and person-ality disorders	Neuroses, depressions, and psychoses; psychosomatic disorders
Psychiatric history	Conduct disorder only	Long history of subjective symptoms, often psychosomatic
Severity of habit	Fluctuating but char-acteristically severe	Varies in severity; unknown proportion of cases thought to follow stable dosage
Degree of economic disability	Severe as a rule often to the point of vagabondage (periodic)	Serious but often not complete; many retain a degree of marginal productivity
Effect of maturation	A proportion of cases recover as they age (loss of capacity for euphoric reaction?)	Probably not a factor
Condition after drug withdrawal is com-pleted	Marked physical and mental improvement is the rule	An underlying psychiatric disturbance may be uncovered or existing one increase in severity

Characteristic	Non-medical (Street addict)	Medical
Delinquency	Frequent before, and during addiction; also seen after	Delinquency not a feature prior to addiction; tends to be limited to technical infractions during addiction
Way in which habit began	Usually 'on the street' under social pressure of a group and seeking pleasure	Under medical conditions. For treatment of a complaint
Social use of drugs	Frequent use in groups	Solitary use only
Psychic contagion	Primary mode of spread May assume epidemic proportions	Not a problem
Attitude toward drug use	Often seen as highly desirable	Guilt and anxiety

the climax in life; they can talk indefinitely about their drug experiences with other addicts, just as boys talk about girls and sex.

ENDEMIC ADDICTION

The endemic addictions are only represented in Europe by alcoholism, which in Sweden is the most important nation-wide disease since tuberculosis was brought under control.

It is well-known that alcoholism affects people from all classes of society, in all occupations and all environments (Lisansky, 1967). In spite of extensive research it has not been possible to prove that there are any special personality types who are particularly predisposed to the development alcoholism, nor any special types who are free from risk.

The low rates of alcoholism among Jews (Glatt, 1970) and Chinese in Western societies strongly suggests that cultural factors and social values with respect to the use and abuse of alcohol are of greater significance than individual personality deviations for the development of alcoholism.

A hereditary factor has also been demonstrated in a study of persons adopted during the first month of life (Goodwin *et al.*, 1973). When one of the biological parents had been treated in hospital for alcoholism, the children had a far higher rate of alcoholism than other adoptees.

Choice of career is also important. The free professions, musicians, actors, authors, journalists, artists, physicians, etc. have a high rate of alcoholism, as have commercial travellers. There is some self-selection to all occupations, but hardly enough to explain the high rates of alcoholism associated with 'interesting' jobs. It is possible that the requirement to get up early in the morning, and be in a fit state to work, prevents persons with routine working hours from indulging in excessive drinking during the week.

THE BIOLOGICAL NATURE OF ADDICTION

Regardless of the type of addiction, the compulsive nature of the condition is common to all cases, and is expressed in most of the definitions. Thus in the WHO definition of 1950 there is mentioned 'an overpowering desire or need (compulsion) to continue taking the drug and to obtain it by any means.' Vogel *et al.*, (1958) declare 'drug addiction may be defined as a state in which a person has lost the power of self-control with reference to a drug and abuses the drug to such an extent that the person or society is harmed.'

THE SYMPTOM THEORY OF ADDICTION

There is a school of thought which has gained widespread support, particularly in the mass media, which looks upon addiction as only a *symptom* of psychological or social maladjustment. It follows from this theory, as its protagonists repeatedly point out, that nothing can be done about the addiction until the underlying individual or social causes of the condition have been cured.

We all agree that *abuse* of alcohol and drugs, like, for instance, criminality and prostitution, may be—and often is—a symptom of individual and social disturbances, but, once established, alcoholism and other addictions are no longer symptoms, they are themselves deeply rooted morbid conditions which are characterized by their own dynamics of development.

This argument can be illustrated with the simple, every-day example of nicotinism, which is one of the most banal of all drug dependencies, in spite of the marked excess morbidity and mortality connected with it (Haybittle, 1966, Bell and Laing, 1969). Most people who smoke tobacco started in the lower teens, or even earlier, usually to imitate their elders and to look grown-up. In the beginning it was often unpleasant, and the youngsters suffered from headache and vomitting, but they coughed their way through one packet of cigarettes after the other to prove to themselves and others how grown-up they were.

The ambition to look big may have been the underlying cause which induced the teenager to begin smoking, but this can hardly explain why the same person, 30 years later, may be smoking a packet of cigarettes a day. The cause—to look grown up—no longer exists, but the individual, as we know, still finds it very difficult to stop smoking? Why? It is because he has developed a nicotine dependence. Cigarette smoking is now no longer a symptom, and it has not been so since the teenage period of abuse. The craving for cigarettes has become *a condition of its own*, a disease if you like, and far more serious than our commonest illnesses, dandruff, warts and caries, and only nicotine either smoked, or in the form of tablets, etc. can satisfy this craving (Jarvik *et al.*, 1970, Glick, 1971). The same applies to morphinism when it has arisen as a complication to the treatment of pain. Even if the pain was temporary and later disappeared completely, the morphinism remains and develops according to its own dynamics.

These examples demonstrate that a disturbed personality and underlying social problems are not essential prerequisites for an individual to develop a drug dependence. In principle any individual and any animal will develop an addiction if certain substances are administered in certain quantities during a certain period of time, even if there are large individual differences in the dose and time required for the development of addiction. The more potent a dependence-producing substance, and the more pleasant its psychopharmacological effects, the quicker and stronger is the development of addiction.

ADDICTION AS A BASIC DRIVE

An established drug dependence thus becomes a force in itself and follows its own laws. It is the same, for instance, with a lung cancer which is directly caused by tobacco smoking. Even if the causal mechanism—smoking—is discontinued after the development of cancer, the tumour progresses nonetheless according to its own dynamics. We could agree with the German 19th century philosopher, Hegel, and say that in these processes a dialectic change occurs in the development. A certain quality (A) 'abuse' (e.g., 'experimental smoking') after successive quantitative increments (i.e., repeated experimental smoking) after a time changes to a new quality (B) 'dependence' (in this case nicotinism). Quality B may then through quantitative accumulation (prolonged smoking) give rise to a third quality (C) (cancer of the lung), which follows its own laws, increases quantitatively and finally leads to the last quality (D) which is death.

We should be in agreement now that drug dependence is in principle a condition essentially different from drug abuse. Even if there are intermediary stages that are difficult to classify, in most cases there is no great difficulty in differentiating abusers from those who have passed the abuse phase and have developed a well-defined addiction. At the abuse stage the individual can steer his consumption and intoxication through his own free will (precompulsive stage). In time, however, according to the addictive quality of the drug, the dosage, the intensity and duration of abuse and individual factors, abuse can change into dependence, and then it assumes the character of a *basic drive* (the compulsive stage). The individual now loses the power of mastering his craving for the drug, the addiction dominates the individual and his way of life. With regard to cocaine and heroin, this condition usually develops after only a few weeks of continual abuse, but it can occur much more quickly—in fact it can develop at the first contact with the drug. With barbiturates and amphetamines it usually takes months of intensive consumption of large doses before addiction arises. Alcoholism, on the other hand, usually takes years of abuse to develop: a couple of years in young people, far longer in the middle aged.

The addicting power of the drug thus varies greatly. Intravenous administration results in a quicker and stronger dependence than if the drug is taken orally. Monkeys develop alcoholism in a few weeks if they are given copious amounts of alcohol intravenously (Seevers, 1968).

When drug dependence has developed the character and strength of a natural drive, the addict has not necessarily lost all voluntary control over his drug consumption. The individual—at least in the case of humans—always retains some power of modifying his behaviour. For a long while the drug-dependent person tries to hide his drug consumption or to steer it into socially accepted forms. The alcoholic tries as long as possible to remain sober at work and perhaps also while driving. The intravenous addict attempts in the beginning to conceal from his relatives that he is taking drugs. The same applies to the average person in regard to sexual instincts; he postpones his sexual activity until the situation is suitable.

It should be observed that unreliability, manipulation and simulation, so characteristic of addicts (Kolb, 1962, Duncan, 1965), are in fact a defence for their craving for drugs, and this phenomenon—which might be called 'pseudopsychopathy', and which clinically is often erroneously considered to be a manifestation of primary character disturbances—is strongly marked even in those cases where the individual has not demonstrated any abnormal psychological tendencies before the inception of addiction. We recognize this behaviour from the defence of sexual behaviour in every-day life. For instance, we know that an individual who is usually honest and reliable in other respects, may lie when he has to protect some extramarital love affair which is vital to him. Natural drives make the unfaithful husband prevaricate about repeated committee meetings, business trips, scientific congresses or what ever smoke screen he uses to hide his instinctive behaviour.

Thus, even when a certain behaviour is an expression of a natural or acquired drive, an individual still has considerable freedom in forming the details in and around the desired experience, but he/she has little power to suppress it.

From clinical experience we know that drug effects are often valued above sexual satisfaction by addicted humans and animals, both quantitatively and qualitatively. Seevers (1969) writes 'all the evidence suggests that, following an initial experience, drug-seeking is probably as powerful a drive in human and animal behaviour as food and sex, and in susceptible individuals may supercede either or both.' This gives some idea of the difficulty of treating addiction. How many people suffering from sexual difficulties would accept castration as a solution of their problems? Practical experience from the prison services is instructive here. Before it was possible to treat dangerous sexual delinquents with hormones, these men were often interned for life or until they reached old age. They were usually offered castration and immediate release, but this was often refused. They preferred to remain locked up—but with the opportunity of masturbating—rather than be rid of their dangerous sexual drives, and return to society as free men.

Rado (1963) has described the addict's situation very tellingly in a single sentence, 'the patient does not suffer from his illness, he enjoys it'. On the other hand this does not mean that the addict is not burdened by many severe problems. The emotional debit and credit of addiction, however, speak for continued drug consumption, and that is the usual result.

Let us for one moment consider the commonest of our forms of addiction—alcoholism. We know that the alcoholic can drink away his money, family, work and social position, and lose everything that previously was important to him. The only explanation of how he can accept this slow psychological, economic and social deterioration is that the successive painful losses are outweighed by the immediate satisfaction which alcohol gives him.

Will power and craving often collide in every-day life, and we need not be psychologically disturbed or weak-willed individuals to be unable to master our desires. We need only think of all the fat people who so whole-heartedly desire to be thin. The desire to eat tempting food, however, is usually stronger, for which reason their curves increase with the years (Swanson and Dinello, 1970). Consider then that the craving for drugs in most kinds of addiction is far more insistent than the desire to eat excessively.

Obese patients provide many parallels with addicts: they are often quite incapable of steering developments in spite of strong medical support; they are unreliable in reporting what they consume, they often insist that they 'just haven't taken anything at all' although they continue to gain weight. If they are admitted to hospital for slimming ('weaning') they have a tendency to smuggle in unpermitted calories, and after discharge there is a very high risk of relapse.

Just as with addicts, overweight people want to get rid of the complications of their special enjoyment without being prepared to sacrifice the source of enjoyment itself. On the other hand they willingly undergo worthless 'treatment' (as massage for obesity or 'advice' for addiction) if it does not jeopardize the satisfaction of their craving. In the same way the alcoholic seeks assistance for his gastritis or ulcers, his insomnia or irritability, but he is not prepared to give up alcohol. Usually the heavy smoker will try all possible medicaments for his chronic bronchitis, but generally he rejects the only adequate measure—to stop smoking.

THE PLEASURE–PAIN PRINCIPLE

We have now reached the core of the problem. It is easiest to understand the process of addiction, the paradoxical symptomatology, its poor prognosis and chronic character if we see the development of dependence as a short-circuiting of the pleasure–pain principle, and addiction as an artificial drive that has arisen in this way, as strong or even stronger than sexual drives.

The pleasure–pain principle seems to be the primary biological steering mechanism for the whole animal world including humans, with optimal pleasure as the goal. To obtain pleasure—whether it is to eat and drink, to find warmth, security and friendship or to obtain sexual satisfaction—some kind of effort is required. In the same way effort is needed in order to avoid discomfort—irrespective of whether it is hunger, thirst, pain, cold, loneliness, sexual deprivation, etc. We can say that the pleasure–pain principle is the unconscious regulator in the animal world, and it furthers the adjustment of the individual and the survival of the species.

The pleasure-pain principle has internal barriers preventing or counteracting abuse of the normal biological pleasure mechanism which might hazard the individual's adjustment, or the ability of the species to survive. Even the strongest pleasurable sensation, the sexual orgasm, is followed by a quiescent period. This has as a result that even the most libidinous young male can spend time on other activities between his sexual activities, behaviour which may be essential to life, such as building a nest, hunting, etc.

Some people may object that we humans are not animals guided only by instincts, and perhaps they will point out that we daily force ourselves to do many unpleasant things: We get up early to go to work, where perhaps we have unpleasant and dull tasks to perform. It requires little further consideration, however, to understand that the unpleasantness would soon be still greater if we did not struggle through our daily measure of disagreeable tasks; we would lose our job, the respect of friends and relatives, and in time risk a process of social rejection. On the other hand if we struggle through our difficulties we receive various rewards for our pains—income, respect, security—sometimes perhaps only a good conscience but that is not a bad satisfaction either. The main difference in the way human and animal behaviour is guided by the pleasure-pain principle is that humans are more capable of following long-term goals, denying themselves satisfaction for the moment and enduring present discomfort in favour of future pleasure. This long-term socio-cultural satisfaction of pleasure requires a learned character moulding.

THE SHORT-CIRCUIT MECHANISM

What happens if we "short-circuit" the pleasure–pain mechanism and give the individual unlimited means of gratifying his desires? This has been demonstrated by the neurophysiologists Olds *et al.*, (1954). It was observed that when electrodes were implanted in the pleasure centre in the brain of rats, and these were given the opportunity to self-stimulation, there was a positive reinforcement with the characteristics of a primary reward. 'With electrodes correctly placed and with the current correctly set, it was possible to generate more motive force with a brain stimulus reward than with any other reward ordinarily used in animal experimentation' (Olds and Milner, 1954). These research workers also showed that the reinforcement of brain stimulation could be so strong as to lead to death from starvation or collapse from physical exhaustion under self-stimulation.

In Ann Arbor, Seevers (1969) and his coworkers have experimented with rhesus monkeys which, by means of an ingenious apparatus, were enabled to self-administer drugs intravenously. All the common drugs of dependence proved to be reinforcing in the monkeys, and the pattern of abuse in man and monkeys proved to be strikingly similar (Schuster *et al.*, 1969). When central stimulant drugs were administered the monkeys took the drug day and night for a period of about 6–9 days without sleep and with practically no food or fluids. Then they were exhausted, took some fluid, and slept or rested for a few days. After that they ate and drank and then started again on the next intensive injection period of about a week, and so on. This periodic abuse is completely governed by pharmacological and physiological factors, and is typical also for human addicts on stimulants when they have access to an ample supply of drugs. When an amphetaminist is asked why he stops his period of heavy abuse he often says it is because his mouth is so dry that it is difficult to swallow, 'it feels like a laryngitis'. At this stage the body and the mucous membranes are so dehydrated that the discomfort of continued drug administration exceeds the satisfaction obtained.

SPONTANEOUS ADDICTION IN THE ANIMAL WORLD

It is also of theoretical interest that addiction occurs spontaneously in the animal world, especially among social insects.

Among ants there are many species that have this special type of pleasure seeking behaviour. Hölldobler (1971) describes how one of these ant species, *Formica polyctena*, adopts beetles and larvae *Atemeles pubicollis*, whose secretions are greatly desired by the ants. Even filter paper soaked with the beetle secretion is carried into the nest by the ant hosts. He was able to demonstrate that not only did the ants feed the beetle larvae, but the presence of beetle larvae reduced the normal flow of food to ant larvae, while the presence of ant larvae did not affect the flow of food to the beetles. These and other ants, e.g. *Lasius flavus*, also harbour the beetle species *Lomechusa*, whose larvae feed on the ants' own larvae. When they are disturbed the ants will carry the beetles to safety before their own offspring (Lindroth and Nilsson, 1959). Thus for the delights of the beetle secretion the ants are prepared to offer their own offspring. This leads our thoughts to the opium smokers in old China; it was not unusual for them to sell their wives and children in order to buy more opium.

Seevers (1969) reports other types of spontaneous addiction in the animal world. 'Certain animals in their natural habitat behave much like man in seeking drugs. Stock-raisers in various countries have long suffered economic losses when their horses, cattle, or sheep discover the so-called "loco-weeds". Once having come under the influence of these toxic herbs, animals often will refuse other fodder and greedily seek them, and even influence other animals to eat them, often with fatal results.'

CONCLUDING REMARKS

It is important to understand these deeply rooted biological phenomena. Many behavioural scientists are unfamiliar with these natural forces in addiction, and they often interpret them as deprivation conditions (deprivation of love, acceptance, self-confidence, security, social and material assets, etc.) or as a result of unfortunate habit forming. Such aetiological factors are of great significance in the inception of abuse, but the fully developed addiction is in principle a condition of quite a different quality.

Nowadays pharmacologists are aware that certain substances give rise to severe dependence conditions regardless of who takes them; but it has not been pointed out previously that these conditions assume the character of basic drives. A generation ago even pharmacologists did not always realize that certain substances could cause serious dependence conditions if, for scientific reasons, the scientist tested them on himself for a time. The prominent pharmacologist Louis Lewin (1931) says in his classic ethnopharmacological work *Phantastica*, 'during recent years I have seen among men of science frightful symptoms due to the craving for cocaine. Those who believe they can enter the temple of happiness through this gate of pleasure purchase their momentary delights at the cost of body and soul.' But the addict is prepared to do this, and he finds a thousand reasons to avoid adequate treatment, and a thousand ways back to his drug experiences.

Considering the failure of the cocaine dependent scientists and countless physician–morphinists to rid themselves of an addiction, the average addict of epidemic type can have little chance of overcoming his drug craving by his own free will, handicapped as he often is by a personality disorder, a criminal record, low social status and lack of skills.

In all serious illnesses where the results of treatment are poor, it is of utmost importance to concentrate upon prevention; this applies all the more when the condition is also contagious. History shows that it is quite possible to stop even very widespread drug epidemics if society is prepared to take the measures necessary, and if the policy is supported by public opinion.

REFERENCES

Alarcón, R. de (1969). The spread of heroin abuse in a community. *Bull. Narcot.*, **21**, (3) 17

Alström, C. H. (1971). Some problems of society's struggle against contagious addictions. *Excerpta Medica Internat. Congress Series No. 274*, 215–218.

Ausubel, D. (1966). Drug addiction: Physiological, psychological, and sociological aspects. (Random House, New York)

Backhouse, C. I., James, I. P. (1969). The relationship and prevalence of smoking, drinking and drug taking in (delinquent) adolescent boys. *Brit. J. Addict.* **64**, 75

Baden, M. (1972). Narcotic Abuse: a medical examiner's view. *New York J. Med. April 1*, 834

Ball, J. (1970). Two patterns of opiate addiction. *In* 'The Epidemiology of Opiate Addiction in the United States' Ball and Chambers (eds.), p. 81. (Charles C. Thomas: Springfield, Ill.)

Ball, J. (1970). Onset of marihuana and heroin use among Puerto Rican addicts. *In* 'The Epidemiology of Opiate Addiction in the United States' Ball & Chambers (eds), p. 167. (Springfield, Ill.: Charles C. Thomas)

Ball, J. and Chambers, C. (1970). Overview of the problem. *In* 'The Epidemiology of Opiate Addiction in the United States'. Ball and Chambers (eds.), (Charles C. Thomas: Springfield, Ill.)

Balter, M. and Manheimer, D. (1971). Patterns of psychotherapeutic drug use among adults in San Francisco. *Arch. Gen. Psychiat.* **25**, 385

Bejerot, N. (1965). Aktuell toxikomaniproblematik. *Läkartidningen* **50**, 4231

Bejerot, N. (1969). Social medical classification of addictions. *Int. J. Addict.* **4**, 391

Bejerot, N. (1970). Addiction and Society. (Charles C. Thomas: Springfield, Ill.)

Bejerot, N. (1972). A theory of addiction as an artificially induced drive. *Amer. J. Psychiatry* **128**, 842

Bejerot, N. (1975). Drug Abuse and Drug Policy: An epidemiological and methodological study of drug abuse of intravenous type in the Stockholm police arrest population 1965–1970 in relation to changes in drug policy. *Acta Psychiatrica Scand.*, Suppl. 256, (Munksguant: Copenhagen)

Bell, J. A. E. and Laing, D. H. (1969). Statistical analysis of mortality rates of cigarette, pipe and cigar smokers. *Canad. med. Ass. J.* **100**, 806

Benaim, S., Horder, J. P. and Anderson, J. (1971). 'The falling girls'. Observations on the dynamics of a hysterical epidemic. *Proc. Vth World Congress of Psychiatry*, p. 201. La Prensa Médica Mexicana, Mexico City

Bewley, T. (1965). Heroin and cocaine addiction. *Lancet,* **i**, 808- 810
Bewley, T., Ben-Arie, O. and James, I. P. (1968). Morbidity and mortality from heroin dependence 1: Survey of heroin addicts known to the Home Office. *Brit. med. J.* March 23, 725
Bewley, T. and Ben-Arie, O. (1968). Morbidity and mortality from heroin dependence 2: Study of 100 consecutive inpatients. *Brit. med. J.* March 23, 727
Birdwood, G. (1969). The Willing Victim. (Secker and Warburg: London)
Bjerver, J. and Neri, A. (1965) Alkoholkonsumtionens förändringar våren 1963 hos måttliga alkoholförtärare och hos personer med alkoholproblem. *In* Alkoholkonflikten 1963. (Norstedt and Söner: Stockholm)
Blachly, P. H. (1970). Seduction: A conceptual model in the drug dependencies and other contagious ills. (Charles C. Thomas: Springfield, Ill.)
Blaustein, A. P. (ed.) (1962). 'Fundamental legal documents of Communist China.' p. 237. (South Hackensack, N. J.: Rothman)
Blum *et al.* (1969)
Bourne, P. (1974). Addiction. (Academic Press: New York)
Brill, H. (1966). Sociological aspects of drug dependence in the U.S.A. and Great Britain: Importance of the dimension of social contagion. *Excerpta Medica Internat. Congress* Series, No. 129, 267
Brill, H. (1968). Medical and delinquent addicts or drug abusers: a medical distinction of legal significance. *Hastings Law J.* **19** (3), 783
Brill, H., Hirose, T. (1969). The rise and fall of a methamphetamine epidemic: Japan 1945–55. *Seminars Psychiat.* **2**, 179
Brown, B., Gauvey, S., Meyers, M. and Stark, S. (1971). In their own words: addicts' reasons for initiating and withdrawing from heroin. *Internat. J. Addict.* **6**(4), 635
Brown, L. P. (1966). Enforcement of the Tennessee anti-narcotics law of 1915. *In* 'Narcotic Addiction' O'Donnell and Ball (eds.), p. 34. (Harper and Row: New York/London)
Cameron, D. (1968). Youth and Drugs. *J. Amer. med. Ass.* **206** (6) 1267
Chappel, P. A. and Marks, V. (1965). The addiction epidemic. *Lancet* **i**, 288–289
Cockett, R. (1971). Drug abuse and personality in young offenders. (Butterworths: London)
Cohen, S. (1969). The drug dilemma. (McGraw Hill: New York)
Cohen, M., Klein, D. and Oaks, G. (1972). Age of onset of drug abuse in psychiatric inpatients. *Arch. Gen. Psychiat.* **26**, 266
Dodson, E., Alexander, D., Wright, P. and Wunderlich, R. (1971). Patterns of multiple drug abuse among adolescents referred by a juvenile court. *Pediatrics* **6**, 1033
Duncan, T. (1965). Understanding and Helping the Narcotic Addict. (Prentice-Hall: New Jersey)
DuPont, R. L. (1974). "Epidemic". *J. Amer. med. Ass.* **227**, 1380
Eddy, N. B. (1970). Current trends in the treatment of drug dependence and drug abuse. *Bull. Narcot.* **22** (1), 1–10

Evang, K. (1967). Symposium om prevention av narkomani. *Soc. Med. Tidskr. skriftserie*, **34**, 21

Freyhan, F. A. (1971). Use and misuse of psychoactive drugs. Proc. Vth World Congress of Psychiatry, p. 12. La Prensa Médica Mexicana, Mexico City

Glasscote, R., Sussex, J., Jaffe, J., Ball, J. and Brill, L. (1972). The treatment of drug abuse. Joint Information Service, Washington, D.C.

Glatt, M. (1965). Reflections on heroin and cocaine addiction. *Lancet*, **ii**, 171–172

Glatt, M., Pittman, D., Gillespie, D. and Hills, D. (1967). The Drug Scene in Great Britain (Edward Arnold: London)

Glatt, M. (1970). Alcoholism and Drug Dependence among Jews. *Brit. J. Addict.* **64**, 197

Glick, S. D. (1971). Titration of oral nicotine intake with smoking behaviour in monkeys. *Nature* **233**, 207

Goodwin, D. W. (1973). Alcohol problems in adoptees raised apart from alcoholic biological parents. *Arch. Gen. Psychiatry* **28**, 238–243

Haybittle, J. L. (1966). Cigarette smoking and life expectancy. *Brit. J. prev. soc. Med.* **20**, 101

Hecker, J. F. C. (1833). Epidemics of the Middle ages. Translated in 1844 by Babington, B. G. (Woodfall and Son: London)

Hess, A. (1965). Chasing the Dragon. (Amsterdam: North-Holland Publishing Co.)

Hill, H. E. (1962). The social deviant and initial addiction to narcotics and alcohol. *Quart. J. Stud. Alcohol* **23**, 279

Hölldobler, B. (1971). Communication between ants and their guests. *Sci. Amer.* **3**, 86.

Hughes, P. H., Senay, E., Parker, R. (1972a). The medical management of a heroin epidemic. *Arch. gen. Psychiatry* **27**, 585–591

Hughes, P. H., Barker, N., Crawford, G. and Jerome, J. (1972b). The natural history of a heroin epidemic. *Amer. J. public Health* **62**, 995–1001

Hughes, P. H. and Crawford, G. A. (1972). A contagious disease model for researching and intervening in heroin epidemics. *Arch. Gen. Psychiatry* **27** (2), 149–155

Jaffe, J. and Hughes, P. H. (1971). Heroin epidemics in Chicago. Proc. Vth World Congress of Psychiatry, p. 22. La Prensa Médica Mexicana, Mexico City

James, I. P. (1967). Suicide and mortality amongst heroin addicts in Britain. *Brit. J. Addict.* **62**, 391

James, I. P. (1969). Delinquency and heroin addiction in Britain. *Brit. J. Criminology* **9**, 108–124

Jarvik, M. E., Glick, S. D. and Nakamura, R. K. (1970). Inhibition of cigarette smoking by orally administered nicotine. *Clin. Pharmacol. Therapeut.* **4**, 574.

Johnson, B. D. (1973). Marihuana users and drug subcultures. (John Wiley and Sons: New York)

Johnson, M. S., Abbey, H., Scheble, R. and Weitman, M. (1972). Survey of adolescent drug use. *Amer. J. public Health* **164**, 164

Jonas, S. (1972). Heroin utilization, a communicable disease? *N.Y. State J. Med.* **72**, 1292–1299

Keller, M. (1970). The great Jewish drink mystery. *Brit. J. Addict.* **64**, 287

Kleber, H. D. (1969). Narcotic addiction—the current problem and treatment approaches. *Connecticut Medicine* **33**, 113–116

Kolb, L. (1924). Types and characteristics of drug addicts. *Mental Hygiene* **9**, 300

Kolb, L. (1962). Drug Addiction. (Charles C. Thomas: Springfield, Ill.)

Retterstøl, N. (1970). Narkotikamissbruk. (Läromedelsförlagen: Stockholm)

Riley, D. N., Jamieson, B. D. and Russell, P. N. (1971). A survey of drug use at the university of Canterbury. *New Zealand med. J.* **74**, 475, 365

Scher, J. (1966). Patterns and profiles of addiction and drug abuse. *Arch. gen. Psychiatry* **15**, 539–551

Schuster, C. R., Woods, J. H. and Seevers, M. H. (1969). Self-administration of central stimulants by the monkey. *In* 'Abuse of Central Stimulants', Sjöqvisk and Tottie (eds.) p. 339. (Almqvist and Wiksell: Stockholm)

Seevers, M. (1968). Psychopharmacological elements of drug dependence *J. Amer. med. Ass.* **6**, 1263

Seevers, M. (1969). Drugs, monkeys and men. *Michigan Quart. Rev.* **1**, 3

Spear, H. B. (1969). The growth of heroin addiction in the United Kingdom. *Brit. J. Addict.* **64**, 245

Swanson, D. and Dinello, F. (1970). Severe obesity as a habituation syndrome. *gen. Psychiat.* **22**, 120

Tatetsu, S. (1963). Methamphetamine psychoses. *Folia Psychiat. Neurol.* Suppl. No. 7, p. 377, Tokyo

Tec, N. (1972). The peer group and marijuana use. *Crime and Delinquency* July, 298–309⁻

Teigen, A. (1966). Narkotikabehandling i sluten anstalt. Cited by Melldahl, I. E. (1966). *Psykisk Hälsa* **2**, 54–63

Vogel, V., Isbell, H. and Chapman, K. (1948). Present status of narcotic addiction with particular reference to medical indications and comparitive addiction liability of the newer and oldest analgesic drugs. *J. Amer. med. Ass.* **14**, 1019

Walters, P., Goethals, G. and Pope, Jr., H. (1972). Drug use and life-style. *Arch. gen. Psychiat.* **26**, 92

Whisson, M. (1965). Under the Rug. Council of Social Services: Hong Kong)

Winick, C. (1965). Epidemiology of narcotics use. *In* 'Narcotics', Wilner and Kassebaum (eds.), p. 3. (McGraw-Hill: New York)

CHAPTER 3

Vicious circles in alcoholism
and drug dependence

W. K. van Dijk

INTRODUCTION

Psychopathological processes and phenomena are complex by nature. By this we mean that they can be described and studied on several levels, e.g., the physical, chemical, biological, psychological, sociological, and others. For this reason two types of conceptual and terminological tools are used in psychopathological research and practice.

The tools belonging to the first group are characterized by the fact that they originate in a specific branch of science, their use making sense in that particular field only; so the 'pH of consciousness', or 'the projection of the turnover of catecholamines' or the 'role-expectance of the integration' are nonsensical expressions. Concepts and terms in the second class, however, are more generally encompassing; they can be applied meaningfully in several fields with fruitful results. One of these terms is 'vicious circle', other examples being: 'cause', 'integration', 'feed-back', 'information', and 'learning'.

It should be noted that both groups of concepts—namely the unilevel on the one hand and the multilevel on the other—are useful in their own way. The fruitfulness of unilevel concepts lies in their power to split up a complex phenomenon into several aspects and to analyse one isolated aspect. Their disadvantage, however, is the loss of view on the whole phenomenon in its multilevel complexity, or, still worse, the reduction of an intricate phenomenon to the single aspect studied— in the worst case denying the importance of other aspects. The multilevel concepts, on the other hand, are useful by virtue of their unifying property, their nearness to the real complexity of the phenomena and the avoidance of one-sidedness. The risk in their use, however, is that they may lead one to lose sight of the need for continuing abstraction and analysis, thus blocking further progress in research and practice.

In this chapter we shall try to clarify some vexed problems concerning alcoholism and drug dependence by means of the multilevel concept of a 'vicious circle'.

THE CONCEPT OF VICIOUS CIRCLE

A vicious circle is a process or state of affairs in which a cause or condition brings about or fosters an effect, which in its turn produces, maintains or reinforces the original cause or condition. For practical reasons the concept of vicious spiral with its features of progression and reinforcement—positive feed-back in cybernetical terms—is included in this definition. As opposed to simple causes which work in a direct, rectilinear way, so to speak, the causal factors in vicious circles have a circular mode of action.

In both the use and abuse of alcohol and other drugs linear as well as circular operating forces play a part. With a progression, however, of the mode of use from incidental or casual use to excessive use, the circular mechanisms become more and more important. Finally, in the stage of addiction, a certain limit is passed and the vicious circles are firmly established, forming a highly characteristic feature of this psychopathological state.

The shift from rectilinear to circular mechanisms is connected with a developing disequilibrium between the operating forces on the one hand, and the ability of the person in question to keep up with the forces or their effects on the other. The functions of mastering, canalizing, directing, controlling and maintaining an equilibrium between the various forces and processes which play a role in human life is, in the psychoanalytic view of psychopathology, generally attributed to the ego. From the point of view of ego-theory there are, broadly speaking, several possible ways of describing and clarifying the disequilibrium mentioned, namely: 1. the ego is relatively too weak (the weakness ensuing from the different etiological causes and conditions known in psychopathology); 2. the operating force is relatively too strong; 3. the effect is relatively too strong. The word "relatively" in the sentence above is not superfluous, because the three factors by which the disequilibrium is brought about are interdependent. It is, however, important to indicate them separately not only from the point of view of theoretical insight, but also for correct diagnosis and rational therapeutic strategy. As an example of the latter, compare psychotherapy aiming at a strengthening of the ego with measures which may be taken to lessen the social pressures which lead the dependent person to take the drug, and with the administration of chemicals to block the desired pleasurable effects of the drug.

VICIOUS CIRCLES IN ALCOHOLISM AND DRUG DEPENDENCE

The mechanism of vicious circles can most clearly be seen in the advanced states of dependence that we call addiction. It is not our intention to add to the great number of existing definitions by providing one more of our own. Some general remarks only will be made. First of all it should be noted that addiction is a broad clinical concept used to describe a more or less specific behavioural pattern in relation to the use of alcohol and other drugs. The pivotal characteristic of this pattern is the fact that the addict has lost his ability to decide of his own free will "to use or not to use" in every condition and at any time. That is not to say that he will be intoxicated every second of the day for the rest of his life. On the contrary, there may occur shorter or longer periods in which he can use the drug in a way more or less adapted to the standards of the culture he lives in. This mostly happens when there is an inhibiting restraint from outside, or when the psychological and social circumstances are favourable. But sooner or later the moment will occur when he will be unable adequately to direct his behaviour in relation to the drug concerned. In this sense the loss of freedom has to be regarded as the central feature of addiction and all other characteristics of dependence described by many authors in many different ways are either specific *forms* or *effects* or *additions* to this basic feature. They may be put together with the central characteristic in various ways so as to form different syndromes of addiction or dependence: all, however have in common the distinctive feature of loss of freedom.

Specific *forms* of the loss of freedom are exemplified by the loss of control against inability to abstain; *effects* of the loss of free will include being overwhelmed by the urge to take the drug in inappropriate places or occasions; *additions* to the basic feature may take the form of belonging to a particular (sub)group (hippies, junkies, skid row or middle class alcoholics), belonging to a certain age group (adolescent or middle-aged), or falling into certain diagnostic categories or possessing particular personality traits (psychopathic, neurotic, depressive, sexual inadequacy, etc.). Much confusion has arisen by the fact that some authors include one or more of the specifications, effects or additions into their definition of dependence or addiction, whereas others do not. The same fact may explain the contradictory outcomes of research in several aspects of dependence.

In this paper we will confine ourselves to the basic feature of dependent behaviour, taking for granted that the term 'loss of freedom' is clear in itself and leaving aside the practical difficulties which may arise when operationalization is needed for specific research purposes. Two points, however, should be added to the concept of dependence (addiction): firstly that the addictive syndromes have in common that they are "relatively autonomous"; and secondly that they are self-perpetuating.

By the first point we mean that, whatever combination of initial causes and conditions may have led to the addiction syndrome, once the critical point has been passed, a particular behavioural state comes into being, which is more or less independent of the primary generating forces. As for therapy, relative autonomy means that in most cases merely removing the initiating factors does not suffice; special measures must be taken, aimed at handling and treating the addiction syndrome as such.

The statement that the addiction state is self-perpetuating means that spontaneous recovery is exceptional; on the contrary, if no help is offered there is a tendency for the condition to worsen.

Both features are highly remarkable: why, for example, continue the use of a drug when the effects are so unpleasant and harmful? They cannot, in my opinion, simply be explained by a single rectilinear cause nor by a combination of such causes. Ample research on different aspects of dependence has so far failed to resolve the problem in this way. It is, however, possible to get more insight into the phenomenon of addiction by means of the concept of vicious circles.

In addiction we may, generally speaking, distinguish four vicious circles: the pharmacological, the cerebral, the psychological and the social one.

THE PHARMACOLOGICAL VICIOUS CIRCLE

The use of alcohol or drugs may cause metabolic changes if the single doses are large enough and the use is repeated several times over a certain period. Such changes have been demonstrated in experiments *in vitro* and they manifest themselves in the clinical phenomena of tolerance (an increase of the dose is needed to attain the same effect) and withdrawal syndromes (a sudden interruption of a drug's use brings about unpleasant or even serious physical and psychological signs and symptoms). In some types of dependence the persistent need for the drug and the inclination to increase the dose may to a high degree be explained by a change of metabolism. The continuing use of the drug however, maintains or intensifies the metabolic change, which in its turn is responsible for the need to take the drug again. Cause (use of drug) and effect (metabolic change) bring about and maintain each other in a circular way by mediating pharmacological mechanisms, and it is thus reasonable to speak of a pharmacological vicious circle.

THE CEREBRAL VICIOUS CIRCLE

In some cases the excessive use of a drug has a damaging influence on cerebral tissues, the functions of which form the basis for regulation and integration of behaviour. The outcome is, in terms of ego-theory, a weakening of the ego. This means a reduction of the mental powers for regulating and controlling the use of the drug, and this, in turn, implies that the motives for taking the drug have the opportunity to come into effect more easily. Because of the mutual relationship of cause (drug use) and effect (disorganisation of behaviour) linked by cerebral damage we may speak of the cerebral vicious circle.

THE PSYCHOLOGICAL VICIOUS CIRCLE

The psychological vicious circle refers to the mental concomitants of behavioural and cognitive dysfunction. Unpleasant somatic and mental feelings produced by the drug, feelings of guilt and shame, the fearful notion that decreasing the use or abstaining from the drug would be better, the gloomy aspects of reality, etc., play an important role. The easiest and most effective way to get rid of these annoying feelings is to take the drug, and in this way a vicious circle arises.

These aspects of the circular psychological process may be described in terms of learning theory, particularly operant conditioning. Moreover we may point to the infantomimetic effects of drug use, Levy, (1958). By this is meant a regression to a more infantile behaviour with an increase of the affective and instinctive components and a decrease in the rational, controlling and synthetic functions of the ego. From a psychoanalytical viewpoint we may see a shift from the reality-principle to the pleasure-unpleasure principle, as well as an increasing predominance of primary over secondary processes. Since in all aspects mentioned the causes and effects influence each other to and fro via psychic mechanisms, we speak of a psychological vicious circle.

THE SOCIAL VICIOUS CIRCLE

This circular process has to do with the fact that addiction has social consequences which in their turn maintain or reinforce the use of the drug, the term social being used here in a broad sense, including economical, judicial, spiritual and other aspects. The social sequel may be summarized as a dysfunction and, finally, a disintegration within the groups in which the addict is or was functioning. This process has harmful effects on the addict. We may only mention the reproaches of the spouse and other members of the family, the sometimes violent quarrels, the contempt and withdrawal of friends and acquaintances, the tensions and conflicts in the occupational sphere, the economic problems, criminality in some cases, etc.

At the micro-social level, as well as at the meso–and macro-social levels, mechanisms of stereotyping, stigmatization and isolation combined with rejection arise in most cases, finally resulting in a more or less complete dropping out by the addict from the several social groups and society at large.

The factors indicated above engender in the subject negative feelings, which foster an attitude of "let oneself go into the state of being an addict", often combined with attempts to find companionship in social groups which make less social and moral requirements and accept the drug using habits or even encourage them. All this means a fixation of the role-behaviour of a drug-addict or an alcoholic, which state reinforces the use of the original drug or even more harmful ones. As an instance of the latter we may point to the fact that social rejection or severe penal measures against marijuana users may in some uses tip the balance and change a not yet established but risky habit into a stable and harmful one.

The social processes described fit well into the concept of vicious circle.

CONCLUDING REMARKS

I hope that the foregoing discussion has demonstrated that, on the one hand, the wide-ranging, multilevel character of the concept of vicious circle enables us to apply it to several aspects of the complex phenomenon of dependence, whilst, on the other hand, in each of the different levels it is 'coloured' by the laws pertaining to that particular aspect. So the dynamism of the pharmacological vicious circle is, in a sense, 'stricter' than that of the psychological or sociological ones. What they share in common, however, is that generating forces and effects mutually influence each other.

After the short discussion of the operation of the four vicious circles in drug dependence some general remarks may be added.

1. The model of circular mechanisms is a general one; particular circular mechanisms should be specified in relation to the individual drug and stages of dependence. In alcoholism, for instance, first the psychological and social vicious circles seem to be preponderant, whilst later on the pharmacological one begins to play an important part, the cerebral vicious circle only coming into the picture after prolonged drug use over a period of several years. In marijuana, however, the pharmacological and the cerebral vicious circles are lacking, as far as we know at the present. Moreover, the model seems apt to throw some light on the puzzling problem of multiple drug use: here the social and psychic vicious circles are preponderant.

2. It is generally accepted that the origin of the process leading to dependence cannot be attributed to one single cause or condition. On the contrary, there is a network of causes and conditions. Broadly

speaking these comprise: (a) the psychopharmacological properties of the drug; (b) the social meaning and value of a drug and of drugtaking as such; (c) the personality structure of the person who takes the drug; (d) the environmental influences and circumstances. These factors, in close interaction give rise to the process which eventually leads to dependence. The same concept of a combined action of multiple etiological factors applies to the operation of the vicious circles. As a general rule the vicious circles complement and reinforce the harmful operation of each other, which fact may explain why addiction is so hard to cure. According to this, only a multilevel attack upon each type of vicious circle may produce a positive result. According to the theoretical considerations outlined above the most effective method to stop and remove a vicious circle adopts three approaches: (a) to reduce the original factor; (b) to strengthen the ego; and (c) to reduce the effect of the drug.

Theoretically this can only be done by taking combined somatic, psychological and social measures, however difficult this may be in practice in many cases of dependence.

REFERENCES

Levy, R. I. (1958). The psychodynamic functions of alcohol. *Quart. J. Stud. Alc.* **19**, 649.

CHAPTER 4

The epidemiology of drug abuse
and drug abuse rehabilitation

D. LOURIA

INTRODUCTION

During the first half of the 20th Century, there were surprisingly few
careful epidemiologic analyses relating to the use of illicit drugs. The
post World War II increase in the availability of heroin in the United
States was accompanied by a resurgence of heroin use. This was
recorded in the yearly reports of the Federal Bureau of Narcotics, the
major law enforcement agency focusing on the problem in the United
States. Their data were collected from the various states in a somewhat
haphazard fashion and included primarily those who were severely
addicted and who, as a result of their use of a legally proscribed drug,
came to the attention of law enforcement agencies. The intermittent
user, the regular heroin user who did not have to commit crimes against
property to support his habit, and those who managed to escape
detection despite illegal activities would not be included in the federal
figures. Thus, the federal figures represented only crude and admittedly
imprecise prevalence figures. Despite these problems, a profile of the
typical heroin user could be constructed. There was a disproportionately
high percentage of blacks relative to their numbers in the population;
one-half the addicts were black, but blacks constituted only one-tenth of
the US population. There was also an inordinately large number of
Spanish-speaking individuals (Puerto Ricans in the eastern United
States and Chicanos in the south-western part of the country). The ratio
of male to female in the addict population in federal and other studies
ranged from 4:1 to 9:1, and the average age was 25–30 years in the late
1920s. For the most part, the addict population was confined to the
economically deprived living in the large urban centres. Indeed, until

the mid-1960s, the collected data showed that approximately one-half of all known addicts in the United States resided in New York City.

In the mid-1960s the drug scene changed dramatically. Starting on the college campuses, a new type of drug abuse surfaced and, through the efficient technology of the communications media, spread rapidly throughout the country. Unlike the inner-city drug abusers, the young, better-educated, more affluent individuals were interested primarily in hallucinogens and euphoriants, LSD and cannabis being the most popular agents.

It was inevitable that the two initially disparate groups would, over a period of time, become less distinct, and this happened in the late 1960s and early 1970s. In the economically deprived communities, cannabis, depressants and opiates were found to be the agents of choice; among more affluent young persons, cannabis, LSD and depressants were used extensively. Additionally, in both types of drug abuse communities, oral amphetamine stimulants were quite popular and intravenous stimulants, both cocaine and methamphetamines, were used to a variable extent.

THE NEW JERSEY EPIDEMIOLOGICAL STUDIES

In the late 1960s, a substantial number of epidemiologic studies were carried out throughout the United States, in England and Canada. The results were astoundingly convergent. The studies performed at the New Jersey Medical School between 1969 and 1974 will be used to illustrate the general findings. These, like most of the other studies, were carried out by an anonymous, self-administered questionnaire technique. The results from the questionnaire studies have, in general, yielded similar data when compared with detailed personal interviews. Our questionnaire initially had 80 components, and this was subsequently increased to 120, the questions focusing primarily on demographic data, pertinent familial information, prevalence patterns and attitudes. Each major question was asked at least twice in different parts of the questionnaire, and the computer was programmed to pick up any discrepancies. Questionnaires with discrepancies, when identified by the computer, were referred to the biostatistical unit for review.

Initially, students were given the questionnaire on a specific school day and allowed to sit together as they completed it, but it soon became apparent that they were discussing questions and potential answers. Thereafter, the students were seated in a manner such that there was a vacant seat between them. Questionnaires that were insolubly discrepant, scatological, blank or facetiously answered were excluded, but in no school studied did the exclusions amount to more than a few percent.

When students were asked why they used illicit drugs, the answers were monotonously similar from school to school. The 3 major reasons listed were peer group pressure ('it's the thing to do'), pleasure and curiosity. Specific risk factors associated with drug use included the following:

Broken family
Unhappy family relationships
Not practicing any religion
Regular parental use of depressants
Parental use of one pack or more of cigarettes per day
Excessive alcohol use by parents
Poor academic achievement
Low self esteem
Lack of ambition for the future
Non-participation in extracurricular activities
Involvement in "political" or protest movements
Drug use amongst one's friends
Regular cigarette use
Sibling use of illicit drugs

These and other risk factors were examined by multivariate statistical analysis. The results indicated that pressure of the peer group outweighed all other risk factors we studied, even if all the other risk factors were considered together.

The use of licit drugs and intoxicants by the parents merits special mention. The regular use of mood-altering agents such as tranquilizers by either parent was associated with a two-to seven-fold greater likelihood that their children would use some illicit drug during the late 1960s and early 1970s when such drugs were readily available. Interestingly, it did not matter whether parental use was under rigid medical surveillance or whether it represented promiscuous and uncalled for use of such agents. The relationship between parental tobacco use and the use of illicit drugs by their children was also impressive. Whereas moderate alcohol use by the parents (moderate as perceived by their children) did not appear to influence illicit drug use patterns, heavy cigarette use by either parent was a significant risk factor for their children. Blum's elegant studies show that the more permissive a parent is in regard to use of medicaments for physical or psychological problems, the more likely it is that the child will subsequently engage in illicit drug use (Blum, 1969).

It is not unreasonable to look at illicit drug use as the end result of a series of familial or individual attitudes or behaviour patterns. Thus, if the parents are particularly ready to use drugs to handle their own physical or mental problems, then they are more likely to be permissive in regard to administration of licit drugs to their children, and this, in turn, is a risk factor in regard to subsequent involvement in the illicit drug scene. If these parents smoke regularly and heavily, the risk to their children is further augmented. The child that smokes tobacco at the age of 11–13 is far more likely to try cannabis at age 14–16 than the child who does not smoke tobacco. It is intriguing that school administrations often look on cannabis use with horror, but react insouciantly to the fact that 13–20 per cent of high school students we have studied are smoking one-half a pack of cigarettes or more each day. Yet it is clear that such tobacco-smoking behaviour constitutes a significant risk factor for subsequent illicit drug use.

Risk factor analysis permits an investigator to take a virgin population and identify a relatively small subset of individuals who account for a large proportion of the drug-using population. Using the risk factor profile outlined above, we have been able to identify about 50 per cent of the drug users in 10 per cent of a newly studied school population. Such information is enormously valuable for those involved in intervention and prevention campaigns. It is also important to stress the obverse; risk factor analysis did not identify 50 per cent of the users. What this means is that use of illicit mind-altering drugs is so prevalent in our society that many persons who are happy, functioning well, originating from effective family units, and with ample self-esteem will still use drugs such as cannabis. Although most of these persons will be transient experimenters or infrequent users, some will be regular users, particularly of milder pharmacologic agents such as marijuana.

When non-users were asked why they avoided the drug scene, there were striking differences among the populations studied. Lack of curiosity and fear of physical or mental harm were listed frequently, the latter particularly in relation to the more potent hallucinogens and opiates. Parental influence was not considered an important reason for abstinence by the students. The results in regard to fears of apprehension by the law varied profoundly from community to community. In some communities, fear of the law appeared to play no major role at all in student decisions; in other demographically similar and contiguous communities, fear of getting caught was at the top of the list of reasons cited for avoidance of the illicit drug scene. The reasons for such discrepancies are not at all clear.

Prevalence data differ from area to area, but it is clear that a considerable percentage of students in the United States (perhaps 30–50 per cent) will at least experiment with illicit drugs. In some local areas, the figure is higher, in the 60–70 per cent range. It is also clear that questionnaire surveys, although imprecise, are far more accurate than less formal community estimates of drug use patterns. For example, in the initial New Jersey Medical School studies, one of the communities was in a state of panic because of recent reports of rampant drug abuse in the high school. An accusatory newspaper story indicated that an informal survey of the school students showed that over 90 per cent were involved in the drug scene. This was confirmed by the local constabulary who insisted that over 80 per cent of the student body were heavy drug users. A local physician, who served as advisor to the community heroin rehabilitation unit, confirmed these extraordinary figures. Our anonymous questionnaire indicated that approximately one-third of the students used cannabis and 3 per cent had any heroin experience. Although these figures may have been somewhat underestimated, it was clear the the drug problem was not nearly so severe as suggested by the informal surveys. This knowledge permitted the school administration to approach the issue with far greater confidence and calm. In evaluating the emotionally-charged drug scene, the objective questionnaire approach has much to offer over the subjective informal estimate.

One of the many unanswered questions in the area of drug abuse is why some of those who experiment or become committed to drugs stop using them. No study has given satisfactory answers; for the most part, the users just appear to tire of the drug scene. In some cases, change of the peer group, alteration in life circumstances, or improvement in psychological status appear to be of major importance.

SEQUENTIAL PATTERNS OF DRUG ABUSE

There are sequential patterns of individual and of community use that merit some emphasis. In the suburban areas we have studied, the young person is likely first to smoke tobacco and next utilize marijuana. Many who use tobacco will not smoke marijuana, and most of those who smoke marijuana will not utilize more dangerous drugs to any extent except for use of other forms of cannabis and, in some cases, a very limited use of oral stimulants or depressants. The minority who subsequently become involved with more dangerous drugs ordinarily do so in a predictable sequence, first ingesting lysergic acid diethylamide, then injecting methamphetamines or other stimulants, and finally turning to heroin. Although patterns vary from area to area, this is perhaps the most frequent sequence for the multi-drug user in relatively affluent communities. Sniffing glue, or ingesting stimulants, tranquillizers or depressants fits in early in the sequence, the precise pattern varying widely from community to community. Thus, in economically advantaged communities, intravenous opiate use is the end of the line. Very few (well under 1 per cent) of those who start with tobacco and cannabis ever reach the stage of injecting heroin and likewise very few become habituated to injected stimulants. The community sequential pattern of use has real meaning for the counselor or physician. Many young persons progress from casual cannabis use to more intensive involvement and then to multi-drug use, but ordinarily they follow the documented, sequential community pattern. If they deviate, there may be a great deal of significance in the specific patterns, as demonstrated by the following case study. An 18-year-old heroin habituee disclosed that he smoked cannabis, ingested barbiturates and injected heroin. He did not, however, use LSD or stimulants. In other words, he arrived at heroin abuse without following the pattern of escalation indigenous to the community. This, in turn, suggested that there was a specific nexus among the drugs he chose to use. Further interviewing revealed that this tormented young man had no real drug problem. What he suffered from was an overwhelming identity crisis far beyond the confines of the normal adolescent identity crisis. His inability to understand who he was or where he was going resulted in severe depression; this in turn was manifested as incapacitating anxiety and whenever his anxiety exceeded his limited ability to cope with it, he would take a drug that had the capacity to alleviate those tensions. Each of the drugs he used possessed such pharmacologic potential; this also explained the fact that he eschewed hallucinogens or stimulants which would only have promoted further anxiety.

One of the judgments any person dealing with the drug scene or with an individual user must be prepared to make is whether the problem is the drug or the underlying psychological structure. In the case cited, the problem was not heroin; rather it was the identity crisis. Attention primarily to the drugs in that case would likely have produced horrendous results.

The sequence described of sequential use is different in the inner city. There cigarettes, glue, marijuana and pills are used early, often before the age of 12, and then those who will be involved with increasingly dangerous agents tend to go directly to heroin or methadone, usually avoiding hallucinogens. One particularly interesting pattern has been observed in the Haight-Ashbury district of San Francisco. This avant-garde area was inundated, indeed virtually taken over, by the so-called 'flower children' in the mid-and late-1960s. Initially, these easily-influenced young people espoused the gurus of mind expansion and the drugs of choice were cannabis and hallucinogens, particularly LSD. Other hallucinogens, including mescaline, psilocybin, dimethyl tryptamine and STP (a methoxy methyl amphetamine) were also utilized to a considerable extent. Within a 2-year period, stimulants had been introduced into the community, probably as a result of the influx of a cadre of violent, stimulant-using motor bike riders whose primary interest was in the sexual availability of the young women of the flower children movement. In a surprisingly short period of time, the cannabis-stimulant pattern became as prevalent as the use of cannabis and hallucinogens. Opinion is divided as to the reasons for the next change in pattern of use. Some believe that the young people of the Haight-Ashbury found by self-experimentation that heroin was an excellent antidote to the toxic effects of methamphetamine. Others feel that the proximity of a deprived urban heroin-using area and the availability of the young women for sexual activities resulted in heroin introduction into the Haight-Ashbury. Whatever the mechanism, by the late 1960s, a heroin epidemic ravaged the community, and this in turn was replaced by a pattern of virtually indiscriminate multi-drug use by 1972–1973.

One unexpected and disturbing pattern has recently been observed in some urban areas. This is the use of heroin by young persons as the first illicit drug with which the individual experiments. Thus far, this pattern has been observed infrequently.

EPIDEMIOLOGICAL PATTERNS

Examination of the epidemiological patterns in local communities has led Patrick Hughes and his colleagues, as well as others, to view heroin abuse as similar in many ways to a communicable infectious disease (Hughes, 1972). This concept, rejected by many, is based primarily on two observations. First, local incidence trends tend to follow an epidemic rather than an endemic pattern with clusters of new cases appearing over a brief period of time. Second, the evidence clearly shows that spread is for the most part from new user to the uninitiated rather than recruitment by older, established addicts or venal purveyors. Some of those advocates of the communicable disease model call heroin the *agent*, and non-users the susceptible *host* with addicts serving as the *reservoir*. Although there are evident problems in attempting to fit heroin abuse rigidly into a communicable infectious disease model, there can be little quarrel with the evidence of person-to-person spread (with recent converts playing a major role) or with the data showing true epidemic patterns in localized areas involving relatively few people (mini-epidemics) or in larger geographic areas involving a large number of people. In the United States, small epidemics have been particularly well described in Chicago, and major epidemics have been delineated in San Francisco and Washington, DC.

The major advantage of using the communicable disease framework is its capacity to serve as an intervention model. Hughes (1972) developed epidemiologic field teams based on the notion that identification of one heroin user would lead to identification of many others and that small epidemics could be handled effectively by finding new cases quickly and providing community-based treatment programs. In Washington, DC, the epidemic has allegedly been brought under control primarily by the availability of methadone maintenance. It may well be, however, that the rise and fall of heroin abuse in Washington, DC may relate to changes in availability of the drug, changes in fads or other factors and not to the fact that a certain treatment approach was offered. In other words, if one wishes to use the communicable disease model, then one must acknowledge that sudden rises in incidence and later decreases in incidence may well represent the natural course of the epidemic rather than the efficacy of therapy. This in no way contravenes the concept of Hughes that the most effective approach is to detect a given mini or maxi epidemic early, initiate extensive case finding, and intervene by identifying new cases and their immediate contacts, offering them a variety of treatment approaches within their own circumscribed geographic areas. It should be emphasized that in addition to epidemics, there are major foci of endemic, chronic heroin use in virtually every major city in the United States.

PATTERNS OF DRUG ABUSE AMONGST STUDENTS

Epidemiologic data from the years 1974–1975 suggest that in suburban, more affluent areas the student pattern is as follows:

(a) By the time of graduation from high school, one-third to two-thirds of the students will have at least experimented with cannabis.

(b) There has been in 1973–1975 a profound increase in use of alcoholic beverages, particularly in the regular ingestion of beer. In some grades, regular beer use has increased an astounding six-fold in an eighteen month period.

(c) Use of LSD and other hallucinogens is diminishing, and there is no evidence of a significant increase in the use of oral stimulants, but there does appear to be a somewhat greater use of ingested depressants or tranquillizers.

(d) Intravenous amphetamines and opiates are also less popular than they were two years previously.

(e) The rate of increase in marijuana experimentation has slackened, but there continues to be a yearly increase in the percentage of high school students using cannabis, at least transiently.

(f) The ratio of regular use to experimentation for cannabis remains for the most part unchanged, varying from 25 to 45 per cent. However, in some schools or school grades, the percentage of experimenters who become regular (i.e., weekly) users has diminished substantially. Whether these are stable or ephemeral trends is currently uncertain.

(g) Cigarette (nicotine) smoking continues to be a monumental and inadequately handled drug problem. In the high schools we have studied, 13 to 20 per cent of male and female students in grades 10 to 12 smoke 10 or more cigarettes per day. Clearly, the educational campaigns and warnings on packages of cigarettes have not succeeded in diminishing this problem among young people. In part, the educational programs have been counter-balanced by advertising suggesting that cigarette smoking is one way for young women to demonstrate that they are indeed liberated.

(h) The girls have caught up with, or exceeded, the boys in prevalence of use of illicit drugs and cigarettes and are rapidly closing the gap in regard to alcoholic beverages.

(i) There are pockets of excessive use in many communities that conflict with the overall pattern. For example, a community with a stable drug problem may have one class in a given school, or one among several schools, in which cocaine, heroin or hallucinogen use is surprisingly frequent.

(j) Among those using illicit drugs, the use of alcohol is greater than among non-users of such drugs or past users. There is no evidence that young persons are eschewing illicit drugs in favor of alcohol. Rather, the multi-drug user is also likely to use alcohol.

The 1974–1975 data suggests strongly that the two major drug problems facing our society are once again tobacco and alcohol. The illicit drugs have more spectacular effects, but are currently of less importance than the legal intoxicants, whose use we encourage.

MARIJUANA USE AND EXPERIMENTATION WITH MORE DANGEROUS DRUGS

One unsettled and acrimony-inducing issue in the drug scene is the relationship, if any, between use of marijuana and experimentation with more dangerous agents, such as LSD or heroin. In the 1930s and 1940s, law enforcement personnel insisted with considerable asperity that marijuana led directly to involvement with heroin. These statements appeared rather surprising because there were in the world perhaps 200 million cannabis users and only a small number of heroin habituees. Those supporting the hypothesis of a relationship between the two drugs argued that 85 to over 95 per cent of heroin users first used marijuana, but this argument is not sound epidemiologically unless it includes an analysis of the overwhelming majority of cannabis smokers who never try more dangerous agents.

In the mid-1960s, several groups began to look at the relationship between marijuana use and subsequent experimentation with LSD. We have carried out three such studies. In one of these studies it was found that if an individual smoked cannabis occasionally, the likelihood of LSD experimentation was found to be 4 per cent. Monthly marijuana use increased the chances of LSD use to 9 per cent. The weekly marijuana smoker had a 22 per cent likelihood of LSD experimentation, and the twice a week cannabis user had a 44 per cent chance of using LSD. For the daily marijuana smoker, there was a 68–85 per cent likelihood of LSD experimentation. Thus, the evidence showed that the more frequently the individual used marijuana, the greater was the likelihood that that person would use a more dangerous drug such as LSD. It is important to emphasize that these studies do not imply that marijuana forces anyone to experiment with LSD; indeed, most cannabis users will not subsequently use LSD. Furthermore, the studies do not suggest that those who experiment with LSD after use of marijuana will become committed to the more dangerous drug. But there does seem to be a connection between the frequency of marijuana smoking and the subsequent use of more dangerous drugs. There are a variety of factors that might account for this relationship including pressure from a multi-drug using peer group, curiosity, or hedonism. Additionally, those experiencing one illegal drug, marijuana, may then be more inclined to experience the thrill of using other illegal substances. Furthermore, for many, the same seller offers cannabis as well as a farrago of other agents, including LSD, stimulants and narcotics. It would also appear that those with underlying psychological problems, whether covert or overt, are more likely to become multi-drug users. It might also be that some as yet undetermined biochemical or physiological reactions to one drug such as cannabis might promote the subsequent use of another drug, such as LSD. Whatever the underlying mechanisms, it does appear that there is some escalation from the milder cannabis to more potent and more dangerous mind-altering substances. Such observations are obviously of considerable importance in making a judgement as to whether or not to add cannabis to the list of currently available legal intoxicants.

The current epidemiologic data suggest that the relationship between marijuana and LSD may not be stable and may diminish with time. These data also suggest that a careful analysis will have to be made of the relationship of cannabis to depressant pill use.

REHABILITATION PROGRAMS

Finally, it is important to stress that far too little is known about the epidemiological aspects of rehabilitation of those dependent on legal or illegal intoxicants. The initial efforts at extra-mural evaluation of rehabilitation programs was undertaken by Dr. Frances Gearing of the Columbia University School of Public Health and Administrative Medicine in New York City. She and her colleagues took data provided them by New York City methadone programs and assessed efficacy of the drug as a rehabilitative tool (Gearing, 1974). At the New Jersey Medical School, we have modified the approach to evaluation and have attempted to conduct totally impartial extra-mural assessment of a variety of in-patient and out-patient treatment programs. Each heroin-dependent individual entering the system is processed by personnel of the Drug Abuse Division and then each patient is followed through therapy utilizing specially-trained personnel and a computerized track-ing system. Initial efforts were directed to relating retention in a given treatment modality to nine demographic characteristics: age, sex, occupation, ethnicity, education, residence, duration of drug use, age of onset of illegal drug use and previous treatment. It was assumed, on the basis of several previous studies, that addicts leaving treatment within a 1-year period would almost certainly return to drugs within a brief period of time. The retention rates in six different modalities are shown in Figure 1. Retention rates in the six programs studied ranged from over 60 to less than 5 per cent. In general, the most effective approach (by the criterion of 1-year retention) was methadone maintenance. Re-sidential therapeutic communities varied markedly in retention rates whereas the two out-patient programs showed minimal patient re-tention at the 1-year interval. Interestingly, the only one of the nine demographic variables used that correlated with retention in the six programs was the level of education. In one of the three in-patient therapeutic communities, those who were high school drop-outs had a

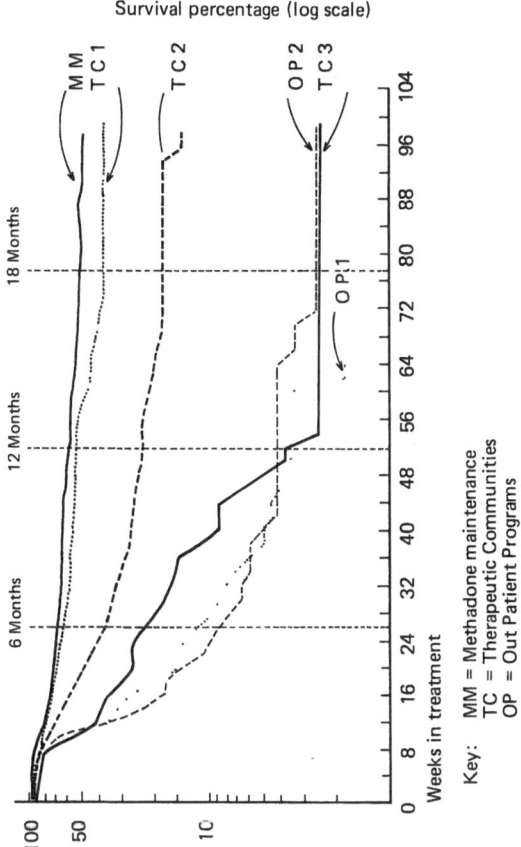

Survival percentage (log scale)

Figure 1 Retention rates in 6 different heroin rehabilitation programs Those leaving each program within 4 weeks are excluded.

significantly lower retention rate when compared to those who had completed high school. Currently, demographic analysis had been augmented by a detailed psycho-social questionnaire and by intensive investigations of the inter-relationship between a given addict and a specific treatment program that might contribute to either success or failure. The idea, of course, is to begin to dissect the variables that make for successful rehabilitation in the many individual treatment programs available to the addict population. At present, there are many more

addicts than there are places in well-run treatment programs; furthermore, many of the addicts fail in treatment and are recycled in the same
or different therapeutic programs. By looking carefully at epidemiologic aspects of rehabilitation, it may be possible to define the variables
that contribute to treatment success or failure. Once such variables are
better defined, they can be used prospectively for predictive purposes,
thereby matching any given drug-dependent individual to that treatment approach (or specific program) that speaks best to the needs of that
particular patient. In the field of drug abuse, epidemiologic principles
and analysis must be applied to an understanding of the genesis and
nature of the problem and equally to efforts at rehabilitating those who
suffer as a consequence of their commitment to the drug scene.

REFERENCES

Blum, R. *et al.* (1969). *Students and Drugs II: College and High School
    Observations.* (Jossey-Bass: San Francisco)
Einstein, S. and Allen, S. Eds. (1972). *Proceedings of the First International
    Conference on Student Drug Surveys.* (Baywood Publishing Company, Inc:
    New York)
Gay, A. C. and Gay, G. R. (1971). Haight-Ashbury: evolution of a drug culture
    in a decade of mendacity. *J. Psychedel. Drugs,* **4**, 81
Gearing, F. R. (1974). An Epidemiologic Evaluation of Long-Term Metha-
    done Maintenance Treatment for Heroin Addiction. *Amer. J. Epidemiol.,*
    100, 101
Hughes, P. H., Senoy, E. C. and Parker, R. (1972). The medical management
    of a heroin epidemic. *Arch. Gen. Psychiat.,* **27**, 585
Lavenhar, M. A. and Sheffet, A. (1973). Recent trends in non-medical use of
    drugs reported by students in two suburban New Jersey communities.
    Prevent. Med., **2**, 490
Newmeyer, J. A. (1973). Five years after: drug use and exposure to heroin
    amongst the Haight-Ashbury free medical clinic clientele. *J. Psychedel.
    Drugs: Drug Abuse*
Sheffet, A., Hickey, R. F., Lavenhar, M. A., Wolfson, E. A., Duval, H.,
    Millman, D. and Louria, D. B. (1973). A model for drug abuse treatment
    program evaluation. *Prevent. Med.,* **2**, 510

CHAPTER 5

The interaction between alcohol and other forms of drug taking

E. B. RITSON AND M. A. PLANT

INTRODUCTION

This chapter sets out to describe the problems of illegal drug taking in a culture where alcohol and tobacco have been long established as the domesticated drugs of use and abuse. Our experience derives mainly from Scotland, but most of the trends we describe are evident in other industrialized countries. We review evidence about recent patterns of drug abuse amongst young adults, examine the overlap that exists between the use of alcohol and other drugs and consider the social policy implications posed by the arrival of a profusion of new drugs in a society where alcohol continues to be the major problem drug.

HISTORICAL BACKGROUND

'Many in this Kingdom have had such a continual use of taking this unsavoury smoke, they are not now able to resist the same, no more than an old drunkard can abide to be long sober.' (James VI, King of Scotland, 1604).

It is rare for Royalty to enter into the debate about the dangers of drug abuse, but this counterblast from a Seventeenth Century King of Scots contains three recurrent influences on Scottish attitudes. The first is the message itself which is characteristic of any culture's response to invasion by a foreign drug but perhaps expressed with characteristic Scottish vehemence. Secondly, the deleterious effects of alcohol are taken as the yardstick by which to judge other forms of drug abuse and the pre-eminence of alcohol as the domesticated drug is a recurrent theme in Scottish history. The third influence is embodied by the author who, as James Sixth of Scots, became James I of the joint Kingdom of Scotland and England, inextricably linking the two countries to the present day and making it at times near impossible to separate the habits of the two cultures statistically while they remain emotionally quite distinct.

In the Sixteenth Century wine and ale were widely used and abused in Scotland; by the Eighteenth Century Scotch whisky was growing in popularity but with the exception of tobacco often taken as snuff, no other drugs were commonly used. Sir Archibald Geikie (1904) in his *Scottish Reminiscences* observed during his travels in the Nineteenth Century that:

'The question is often asked why so much whisky should be consumed in Scotland. One explanation assigns as the reason the moist, chilly climate of the country and this cause may perhaps be allowed to have some considerable share in producing the national habit. No small proportion of the spirit, especially in the Highlands, is drunk by men who are certainly not at all drunkards, and who can toss off their glass without being any the worse of it, if, indeed, they are not, as they themselves maintain, a good deal the better. But it must be confessed that, especially among the working classes in the Lowlands, tipsiness is a state of pleasure to be looked forward to with avidity, to be gained as rapidly and maintained as long as possible. To many wretched beings it offers a transient escape from the miseries of life, and brings the only moments of comparative happiness which they ever enjoy. They live a double life—one part in the gloom and hardship of the workaday world, and the other in the dreamland into which whisky introduces them. The blacksmith expressed this view of life who, when remonstrated with by his clergyman for drunkenness, asked if his reverence monitor had himself ever been overcome with drink, and, on receiving a negative reply, remarked: "Ah, sir, if ye was ance richt drunk, ye wadna want ever to be sober again." '

The desire of getting quickly intoxicated is perhaps best illustrated among the miners in the great coal-fields. Thus an Ayrshire collier was heard discoursing to his comrades about a novel way he had found out of getting more rapidly drunk: 'Jist he putt in thretty draps o' lowdamer (laudanum) into your glass and he're fine an' fou' (drunk) in ten

minutes.' In the county a publican advertised the potent quality of the
liquor he sold by placing in his window a paper with this announcement:
'Drunk for three bawbees, and mortal for threepence.'

This is the less elegant face of opiate abuse which had become quite
widespread amongst the literati throughout Britain in the Eighteenth
Century. At least one Scottish physician was an enthusiastic protagonist
of the beneficial effect of opium on the imagination and there appears to
have been a cult of opiate use not dissimilar to the recent vogue for LSD
as a mind expander. The influence of opiates on the literature of this time
has been discussed by Althea Hayter (1968) in her study entitled 'Opium
and the romantic imagination'. Britain in 1830 had imported 22 000 lbs
of opium and by 1860 had quadrupled that consumption (Edwards,
1971).

The pleasure and despair of opiate abuse was vividly described by de
Quincy in his confessions of an English opium eater. De Quincy himself
was buried in an Edinburgh churchyard but a more eloquent epilogue
on the effects of opium in Nineteenth Century Scotland may be found in
the effects of opium given as a quietening syrup to babies in Edinburgh
and reported in the local medical journal.

'Feb. 10, 1816—A boy aged six months. This infant had the breast
during the first month after its birth, at which period, being deprived of
it, its mother began the pernicious practice of giving in an anodyne
every night; a practice which has been continued to the present day, and
which had induced the following effects:

The countenance has a shocking disfigured appearance; the colour is
sallow . . . . There is an entire want of that appearance of intelligence
observed in infants in general even of this age . . . . The infant is thin,
emaciated, sickly and puny and is said to be less in bulk than on the day of
its birth . . . .

May 18, 1816—. . . numerous instances . . . . The appearance has,
indeed, become quite familiar. One female infant, of five months old,
died of the effects of this baneful practice.' (Edwards, 1971)

Opium, usually in the form of Laudanum, was readily available in
Scotland throughout the Nineteenth Century; in this respect it was
probably no different from the rest of Britain.

'Few people are aware to what a frightful excess the vice of opium
eating has extended lately in this country, and how rapidly it is

increasing, both in England and Scotland; I could name one apothecary's shop, where innumerable small packets, costing only a penny, of this pernicious drug, are prepared every night, and where a crowd of the wretched purchasers, many of them women, glide silently up to the counter, deposit the price, and without uttering a word, steal away like criminals, to plunge themselves into a temporary delirium, followed by those agonies of mind and body by which both are at last distorted and ruined. We have all read the English Opium-Eater's Confession, who took laudanum toddy after dinner for his refreshment! The fascinations of this drug are like those of the snake, whose victims see their impending destruction, and yet cannot resist the fatal impulse to go on—an affecting instance of which is the well-known anecdote of Coleridge entreating that his friends would place him in a madhouse as his only hope of being cured; and few are capable of a high moral and religious effort, such as that eminent man successfully made, to rescue himself from the destructive propensity, afterwards using those affecting expressions, "I feel with an intensity unfathomable by words, my utter nothingness, impotence and worthlessness, in and for myself. I have learned what a sin is against an infinite, imperishable being, such as is the soul of man. I have had more than a glimpse of what is meant by death, and outer darkness, and the worm that dieth not; and that all the hell of the reprobate is no more inconsistent with the love of God than the blindness of one who has occasioned disease to eat out his is inconsistent with the light of the sun"' (Sinclair, 1875).

During the Industrial Revolution there was a drift of population from rural to urban areas. In the harsh working conditions of British manufacturing towns, alcohol sometimes laced with laudanum, became the 'opium of the masses.' The pub offered a convivial escape from an otherwise bleak existence. It was the drunkenness of the time with its attendant social and economic consequences which inspired the growth of the temperance movement and the development of increasingly restrictive licensing and growing taxation on alcohol. This period has been described in detail (Harrison, 1971, Glatt, 1958).

These fiscal and legislative influences on the availability of alcohol were associated with a decline in the prevalence of British drunkenness between the close of the Nineteenth Century and the end of the First World War. It would be wrong to attribute these changes directly to restrictive policy alone since other major social upheavals were occurring simultaneously. Nonetheless it seemed that the country had entered a period of reduced alcohol abuse as evidenced by a reduction in arrests for drunkenness and deaths from hepatic cirrhosis (Kessel and Walton, 1974).

No serious attempt to regulate other forms of drug abuse was made until this Century when international pressures and a growing awareness of the hazards of abuse and addiction led to the control of opiate availability and deemed that opiate addiction should be regarded as a medical problem. The subsequent emergence of controls on the use, production or sale, of a wide range of drugs such as cannabis, hallucinogens and opiates has been in marked contrast to social policy regarding alcohol. In spite of the fact that alcohol abuse causes far more harm than any other form of drug abuse, alcohol use is penalized only when it is connected with some specific form of problem, such as drunken driving, or violent behaviour. The use of many other drugs is proscribed even if no such problems are evident (Schofield, 1971).

In 1926 a departmental committee reported to Neville Chamberlain (then Minister of Health) on morphine and heroin addiction in Britain. By that time Dangerous Drugs Acts were in force which placed restrictions on the import, export, manufacture, sale, distribution, supply and possession of opiate drugs which contained more than trace amounts of morphine (0.2 per cent) or heroin (0.1 per cent). Pharmacies were subject to inspection by the Police or Home Office Inspectors. This Committee, chaired by Sir Humphrey Rolleston, could find little evidence of opiate abuse or other addictions at that time:

'This evidence has all tended in the same direction and the collective effect is remarkably strong in support of the conclusion that, in this country, addiction to morphine or heroin is rare. Some experienced general practitioners have stated that they had never been called upon to treat such cases; others that they have only seen two or three such cases in the course of 20–30 years' practice. As might perhaps be anticipated, the cases appear to be proportionately more frequent in the great urban centres than elsewhere and persons engaged in occupations which entail much nervous and mental strain are specially liable to be affected. It appears also that a relatively high proportion of cases occurs among those who, by reason of their occupation or otherwise, have special facilities for access to the drugs.

'There is also a general concurrence of testimony to the effect that addiction has diminished in recent years, most witnesses attributing the decline in the number of cases to the operation of the Dangerous Drugs Acts which have made it difficult to obtain the drugs otherwise than from, or through, doctors.'

Three experienced Scottish physicians gave evidence to that committee and it seems that opiate abuse was little known at that time. It appears that the Dangerous Drugs Acts had forced many people to abandon the laudanum habit which was so prevalent in the previous Century.

'The effects of the restrictions are even more important in respect of the class of nervously unstable persons by whom addiction is most easily acquired, and who may be designated "potential addicts". When morphine was readily obtainable such persons were prone, on even small provocation of pain or mental stress, to seek relief in the drug, purchased on their own responsibility and addiction was thereby quickly developed. Thus the diminution in the number of addicts may be regarded as mainly due to the fact that new addicts are not being created as they were under former conditions.'

The Rolleston Committee made it clear that opiate addiction was an illness and established the foundations of what has been called the British approach to heroin addiction which has determined all subsequent attitudes towards the addict in this country. They set down the circumstances in which morphine or heroin might legitimately be prescribed to addicts as follows:

'There are two groups of persons suffering from addiction to whom administration of morphine or heroin may be regarded as legitimate medical treatment, namely:

(a) those who are undergoing treatment for cure of the addiction by the withdrawal method;
(b) persons for whom, after every effort has been made for the cure of the addiction, the drug cannot be completely withdrawn, either because:

   (i) complete withdrawal produces serious symptoms which cannot be satisfactorily treated under the ordinary conditions of private practice; or
   (ii) the patient, while capable of leading a useful and fairly

normal life so long as he takes a certain non-progressive quantity, usually small, of the drug of addiction, ceases to be able to do so when the regular allowance is withdrawn.'

These regulations sufficed to restrict opiate abuse and dependence in Scotland to a handful of well known addicts, many of whom were doctors and nurses. Throughout the first half of the Twentieth Century, police records did not reveal much trafficking of drugs in Scotland. Bromide abuse seems to have been quite common and the clinical features of 'bromism' were detailed in most psychiatric texts.

Self-poisoning, which has reached near epidemic proportions in Scotland in recent years, was uncommon. Records for the first half of the present Century indicated that coal gas and lysol poisoning were in vogue, contrasting with the near ubiquitous choice of barbiturates or aspirins in recent years. Alcohol use has long been associated with self-poisoning (Stengel, 1969).

The way in which the British drug scene suddenly surfaced and became a cause for public concern during the 1960's is well known and has been described elsewhere (Spear, 1969; Judson, 1974). Britain changed the regulations governing the prescription of heroin: in 1968 clinics were established for the treatment of known opiate dependents and maintenance supplies of heroin and allied drugs could only be obtained from licensed doctors, most of whom were consultant psychiatrists.

The drug treatment clinics were situated in metropolitan areas, notably in London and Birmingham. In addition, licensed prescribers were designated throughout Britain, including Scotland.

STUDIES OF DRUGTAKERS IN SCOTLAND

Any discussion of the abuse of alcohol and other drugs is limited by the partial information that is available.

Most British studies have been carried out in England. Information about drugtaking is related largely to drugtakers known to 'official agencies' such as the police or medical treatment institutions. In addition, a number of surveys have been carried out, but these have been mainly small scale exercises restricted to accessible, relatively homogeneous groups such as University students (Kosviner, Hawks and Webb, 1973) or school children (Weiner, 1970).

CLINICAL STUDIES

A number of studies have described the biographical characteristics and patterns of drug use of people treated for drug dependence or for other reasons connected with drug misuse.

In 1966, 12 morphine dependent patients were admitted to a Glasgow hospital. This followed the theft of morphine from a local hospital. These patients were mainly intelligent young males who had not fulfilled early educational promise and who had preexistant behavioural problems. During the period 1966–1970 approximately 60 cases of heroin or morphine dependence were treated in Glasgow (Mullen, 1975).

Bennie and Sclare (1966) reported that the type of heroin addiction amongst young people found in London during the 1960's was also apparent in Glasgow. They described three patients at the Eastern District Hospital and suggested that these three might be: 'only a fragment of the local problem'. All three were males and had used a wide range of drugs and all had obtained heroin from non-medical sources, such as other addicts.

Whittet (1967) reviewing psychiatric problems in the highlands and islands where alcoholism is particularly common, found that during 1963–64 only seven admissions at Craig Dunain Hospital, Inverness, were classified as drug addicts.

Evans (1971) commenting upon the incidence of drug abuse amongst patients at a Young People's Unit, in Edinburgh between 1967–68, stated:

'During that period some 15 per cent of adolescents referred to our unit were drug abusers ... . Thereafter, the incidence dropped to 10 per cent although within the past 10 months the picture has changed dramatically so that at least 20 out of our recent 100 referrals have been involved in drug abuse, while 10 per cent have indulged in severe drug abuse with social deterioration ... . In my experience, the drug which is used most often by young people is alcohol. Next is cannabis.'

Woodside (1973) reviewed the first 100 referrals to the drug addiction treatment centre at the Royal Edinburgh Hospital. She found that virtually all drug patients were young: 82.0 per cent being aged 15–24. Eighty per cent were born in Scotland. Almost half the group had a disturbed family background:

'As children they grew up in poverty in loveless homes, characterised by parental "arguments", drunken quarrels and scenes of violence.'

Many were clearly multi-problem individuals. Eighty had drug convictions and 41 had committed non-drug offences. Many were described as sexually promiscuous and amoral. Self-reported drug data indicated that the patients were poly-drugtakers, using whatever drugs they get. Nevertheless, few appeared to conform to the stereotype of the 'real' heroin dependent. Withdrawal symptoms were rare and none seemed very ill. It was concluded that patients attended the treatment centre for the following reasons:

1. To obtain drugs.
2. Because they were on a court charge, or were in trouble with the police.
3. Because of a social crisis, such as their parents putting them out of the home.
4. Because of a fright such as a bad LSD trip or amphetamine psychosis.

Forrest and Tarala (1973a) reviewed 252 consecutive cases of drug abuse admitted to the Regional Poisoning Treatment Centre (RPTC) in Edinburgh during 1971 and 1972. Sixty per cent of these cases were manual workers and it was concluded that few required social and psychiatric support. A wide range of drugs had been used, 35 per cent reporting that alcohol had been taken in conjunction with another drug. Overall, drug abusers constituted 7.0 per cent of total admissions to the RPTC. Three quarters of the abusers were males. Forrest and Tarala commented:

'This study shows that drug abusers place a significant work load on the police and hospital services.'

Forrest and Tarala (1973b) also reviewed 60 cases of young people who had been admitted to Edinburgh Royal Infirmary due to bad LSD trips. Their evidence made it clear that hallucinogenic drugtaking, as noted elsewhere in Britain (Ritson *et al.*, 1973, Plant, 1975a) was a cause of medical problems, though not of true drug dependence. Most of these studies reported drug abuse against a background of continuing alcohol use which was often excessive. There was no evidence that young abusers characteristically eschewed alcohol.

Clinical studies deal with only the casualties of drugtaking, not with a representative group of all those using illegal drugs. The evidence suggests that a high proportion of young adults who require medical treatment in connection with their drug abuse are disturbed multi-problem individuals who are indiscriminate in their abuse of legal and illegal drugs. True addiction—physical dependence to a specific drug—is the exception rather than the rule amongst those in clinical populations. Ritson *et al.*, (1973) found in Nottingham:

'Drugs were usually started in a spirit of imitation or experiment rather than in an attempt to cope with intra-psychic stress. From the start dependence seemed to rest more on the subculture—"The Drug Scene"—than on any particular drug.'

Most of those who require medical treatment for drug abuse are deeply involved with the lifestyle of the drug scene and many appear to find great social support within the networks of their fellow drugtakers. There is a continuum of involvement with drugtaking. Many of these drugtakers known to medical agencies have used a wide range of drugs and appear to take whatever substances are available, including alcohol. It appears that those with least conventional social status such as unskilled workers are especially likely to adopt the drug scene as their main reference point. In addition, individuals with disturbed biographies such as familial, marital or educational difficulties appear to find the free and easy lifestyle of the drug scene attractive.

SURVEYS

Most surveys of drugtaking have collected information through single contact interviews. This is an excellent method of collecting data from large populations, but is seldom possible to validate.

In 1968 a sub-committee of the Chief Medical Officers Consultative Committee of Medical Officers of Health in Scotland was set up to assess the prevalence of Scottish drug misuse. Letters were sent to medical officers of health, directors of social work and the medical officers of universities and colleges of education. Most reported that they were aware of drugtaking in their areas.

'Among the thirty-one directors of education who replied to our request for information eighteen indicated that small numbers of school pupils or young persons in further education colleges had been found misusing drugs. The misuse was generally cannabis, but LSD, methalqualone and barbiturates were also mentioned. Another form of drug misuse which was reported . . . was solvent sniffing, either of quick-setting glues or of cleaning fluids or hairsprays.'

The same enquiry indicated that few school children used drugs, but that a minority of university students did, using largely cannabis, LSD and mescaline.

Dean (1971) reported the findings of a questionnaire survey of general practitioners in Edinburgh. Completed questionnaires were returned by 274 general practitioners giving details of their knowledge of drug abuse amongst their 608 073 patients. Ten known or suspect heroin dependents were reported. Eighty-two of the 274 doctors stated that they knew of drug abuse amongst their patients and this abuse involved 204 'known' and more than 90 'suspect' cases. Most of the cases involving a specific drug involved amphetamines.

In the Times Educational Supplement (29th January 1971) it was reported that the Dundee University Student Association had found that 10.0 per cent of students in the University smoked cannabis once or twice a week. This contrasted with a similar enquiry made by the medical officer of the Dundee Student Health Service in 1968 which concluded that only 1.0 per cent of students were regular users (Ward, 1971).

McKay, Hawthorne and McCartney (1973) carried out a survey of medical students at Glasgow University. Questionnaires were completed by 1236 students, of whom 179 (14.5 per cent) admitted having used drugs such as cannabis and LSD.

'Marijuana and hashish were by far the most commonly used drugs, the use of 'harder' drugs being limited. Almost half of the students acknowledged the regular use of alcohol, and approximately a fifth were regular tobacco smokers. Those who took drugs were predominantly males who tended to smoke and drink more than other students. They also came from homes where the parents no longer lived together and tended to live away from home more than other students. Exposure to drugs increased between 1971 and 1972, but the number accepting drugs did not.'

Fish *et al.* (1974) carried out a survey using a self-administered questionnaire to determine the prevalence of non-medical drug taking within the age group 16–24 in the following groups: school pupils, university/college students, trainee nurses, patients attending VD clinics, casualty patients and young offenders. Data were collected from 2809 young people of whom 886 (31.5 per cent) reported that they had at some time used drugs non-medically. Cannabis was the most frequently misused drug and heroin the least used. As in other studies, the pattern was of experimentation with several types of drug including LSD, sleeping pills, amphetamines and tranquillisers.

Watson (1974) carried out a comprehensive investigation of solvent or hydrocarbon sniffing in Lanarkshire 1973–74. Following press reports of individual cases of solvent sniffing, she sent questionnaires to social workers, police, medical and educational officials and parents of schoolchildren. This study found that solvent sniffing amongst school-children, including young children, was a problem in Lanarkshire. During 1973, the Western Infirmary, Glasgow, examined 15 self-confessed glue sniffers and one Glasgow youth died due to solvent inhalation. Dr. Watson concluded that instances of solvent abuse were generally concealed by families and friends, reducing the significance of official records. She found that solvent sniffers were generally younger than other drug abusers and suggested that there may be a progression from the abuse of solvents to the abuse of alcohol.

POLICE STATISTICS

An important source of information about drug misuse is provided by the Home Office annual statistics of convictions for drug offences. These show that the offence of possessing cannabis has become rapidly more prevalent and that other drug offences (such as those relating to LSD) have also increased. Police figures may reflect the growth of police zeal in enforcing the drug control laws, rather than the actual increase in drugtaking in the community. Edinburgh and Glasgow are the centres of drug misuse convictions, but these occur in virtually all other areas of Scotland. In Scotland as a whole, the number of drug prosecutions (mainly related to cannabis) rose from 112 to 766 between 1968 and 1973.

This increase was roughly in keeping with the trend throughout Britain, though the Scottish rate of drug convictions per 10 000 population is rather lower than that in England and Wales. Conviction rates vary locally. They are especially high in Edinburgh (in 1971 the Edinburgh: Glasgow rates were in a ratio of 2.5: 1). In Edinburgh during 1972, 242 charges were made relating to cannabis and 25 persons were arrested or reported on charges of illegal possession of morphine, heroin, opium and other synthetic drugs. Information provided by the Edinburgh Police suggests that many of those convicted of drug offences are male low status unemployed or manual workers amongst whom experimentation with several types of drug is commonplace. These arrest figures may be contrasted with more than two thousand arrests for drunkenness each year in Edinburgh (Flint, 1974).

The majority of drugtakers remain undetected by the police. It is likely that the minority who are charged with or convicted of drug offences are more conspicious and deeply involved with drugtaking than the majority who are not. The same is even more likely with alcohol abuse.

THE DRIFT TO LONDON

Opiate addiction in the United Kingdom is largely an urban phenomenon and 80.0 per cent of known addicts live in the London area or in other towns with easy access to London. There is a black market in Chinese heroin which is important in other cities, such as Southampton (Reeves, 1973) and official figures certainly show only part of the picture. There is considerable mobility amongst young adults in Britain and drug fashions are rapidly taken from one area to another. It has been suggested that young Scots tend to move South when they get involved with the drug scene, or that they may become drug dependent after they move South, especially into London. A leading article in the Scottish Medical Journal (1971) stated:

'Most of the Scottish opiate addicts have acquired their habit in the London drug culture.'

Woodside (1973) found evidence to support this in her review of Edinburgh patients:
'Among the confirmed opiate-takers, there was evidence that contact with London was of noxious significance. Of the 45 so assigned, 37 were

native born Scots who had stayed in London for varying periods: the remaining 8 had been born in London or the South. An association was also observed between these hard-core addicts, life in London and a known criminal record. This constellation of factors was found in 22 out of the 45 cases and would probably have been higher had full criminal histories been available.... . Treatment in London hospitals was reported by 25 patients.'

THE OFFICIAL RESPONSE TO DRUG ABUSE

Following the Annual Representative Meeting of the British Medical Association in 1970, local medical committees began resolutions urging a voluntary ban on amphetamine prescribing. A significant reduction in the prescribing of amphetamines was achieved. Also during 1970, the Scottish Health Education Unit and the Pharmaceutical Society organised a campaign to collect and destroy unwanted drugs. Over 4 000 000 tablets were collected, mainly in Edinburgh and Aberdeen. A number of local drug liaison committees were established and by 1971, there were 10 of these in Scotland. Apart from these measures, national legislation introduced special drug treatment centres which opened in April 1968 and the Misuse of Drugs Act (1971) provided for the investigation of excessive prescribing of controlled drugs and controlled the security of drug storage at pharmacies.

The tightening up of legal supplies of drugs has been followed by an increased black market in illegal drugs. In spite of the increased security of pharmacies, break-ins continue. In Edinburgh two-thirds of all chemists were raided by drug thieves between 1964 and 1974. The Solicitor General of Scotland stated in 1974 that Edinburgh had an especially serious drug problem and that in Scotland generally, the misuse of drugs had become widespread.

The main official response to drug misuse is through augmented police activity as reflected by steadily rising conviction figures. Drug experimentation in its many forms is now widespread amongst young adults in widely varying social positions in all areas of Scotland. Most do not attract the notice of either police or medical authorities. Drugtaking is fostered by strong peer pressures, as are alcohol and tobacco use. Evidence indicates that young people who use drugs are recruited largely from the same groups who use alcohol and tobacco. Most drugtaking is prompted by curiosity and social pressure. Most use is casual and does not appear to be problematic. Nevertheless, many of those most deeply involved with the abuse of legal and illegal drugs are clearly very disturbed both socially and psychologically.

Apart from measures designed to limit availability the main area through which social policy might fruitfully be implemented is education. At present there is no clear educational policy and little is done to ensure that young people receive accurate information (not scare propaganda) and few confidential counselling services are available to young people who are not students at universities and colleges of higher and further education. In addition, the policy of restricting the prescribing of amphetamines could usefully be extended to limit the supply of barbiturates. Barbiturate abuse is widespread and dependence is an all too frequent complication of regular use.

THE CLINICAL RESPONSE TO DRUG ABUSE

Scotland is a small country of approximately 5 million people, most of whom live in the central belt between Glasgow and Edinburgh. Much of the country, particularly the North, is sparsely populated. The Scottish Office, which retains some independence from Westminster administration, is responsible for the organisation and provision of health care through the National Health Service which employs most doctors. The size of Scotland facilitates communication between professionals about drug abuse. Few Scottish doctors outside the main cities have been involved in the treatment of opiate dependents.

A small number of heroin addicts, mainly in Glasgow, have been enrolled into methadone maintenance programs. Treatment focuses on using regular supplies of methadone as a means of forming a relationship with the patient and encouraging a return to work and to other social activities. Patients attending the out-patient clinic in Glasgow have been encouraged to come into hospital for reduction of, or withdrawal from, their opiate use. The Glasgow in-patient service functions as a means of reducing drug usage to a possible maintenance level.

The principal form of treatment offered at the Royal Edinburgh

Hospital was in-patient withdrawal and social support and rehabilitation. If abstinence is used as the principal measure of success the effort of clinicians appear to be conspicuously unsuccessful (Woodside, 1973).

Maintenance treatment has remained uncommon in Scotland. The reasons for this vary from one clinic to another. Part of the explanation lies in the small numbers of physically dependent addicts who attend for treatment. Also some doctors are reluctant to offer an additional drug to individuals with long histories of drug abuse. An important factor is the fear of inducing real physical drug dependence in someone who is dependent upon the lifestyle of the drug scene, but not yet dependent upon any one drug. It has been suggested earlier that the Scots' relative reluctance to prescribe has forced addicts to move South to London if they wish to find a legitimate source of heroin; and that the parsimony of the clinics forces the remaining addicts into the black market. There is no conclusive evidence to support either of these views. The drift to London seems to be a feature of disaffected young Scots who are present amongst London's homeless, as well as its alcoholic and drug dependent population. It is likely that this drift may be curtailed better by improving Scottish social and economic conditions than by providing more opiates.

There is growing recognition that the abuse of drugs or more often alcohol by adolescents in Scotland is often one aspect, a presenting symptom, of more widespread disturbance.

Illicit drugtaking is now a common feature in the life histories of disturbed adolescents. Often it is of incidental significance while in others it appears to be the chosen mode of escape and handling life crises. In either case, the clinicians have tended to focus on the underlying interpersonal and social difficulties rather than the drugs themselves. There are very few voluntary services specifically geared to the drug abuser although some youth work agencies show a particular concern for the drug sub-culture and a small number of self help communities devoted to attaining a drug free life have opened in rural areas.

THE ROLE OF ALCOHOL

The non-medical use of drugs such as cannabis, LSD and opiates has received great publicity during the past fifteen years. Many of the illegal drugs are exotic and some were largely unknown before their adoption by young adults. We have reviewed the recent Scottish literature on this topic in some detail but in spite of enormous attention focussed on the use by young people of illegal drugs, the main drug problem in Scotland continues to be, as it has long been, alcohol abuse and alcohol addiction.

The evidence indicates that Scotland has an alcoholism rate four or five times as great as that in England and Wales (Plant, 1975b; Scottish Health Education Unit, 1976). Many possible reasons have been put forward to explain this disparity; the ambivalence of Scots towards the use of alcohol, the distillery trade, highland unemployment, Calvinism, or the climate. There is no doubt at all that alcohol is very important in Scotland's culture, especially in the highlands and islands, where the alcoholism rate is particularly high.

Only 9.0 per cent of Scottish adults report that they do not sometimes use alcohol (Dight, 1976). Research in Glasgow (Davies and Stacey, 1972) examined a sample of 1321 teenagers aged 14 to 17. The findings showed that 92.0 per cent of the boys and 85.0 per cent of the girls had at least some experience of alcohol by the age of 14 years. Also, by the age of 17 years 91.0 per cent of the boys and 61.0 per cent of the girls admitted illegal under age drinking in public houses or other public places. The extent of such illegal alcohol use far exeeeds any estimate of other illegal drug use, apart from that of tobacco.

Flint (1974) reviewing the evidence about the problems of teenage drinking, traces the steady rise in drunkenness convictions amongst Scottish teenagers. Between 1966 and 1971 the numbers of those aged 14 to 18 who were convicted of such offences grew from 273 to 445. Flint cites considerable evidence that alcohol abuse is a far more serious problem than the abuse of cannabis and other proscribed drugs. Considerable press coverage has been given to alcohol abuse by young people during recent years. The Times (January, 28th, 1974) published an article entitled 'Drunkenness in Under 18's Doubled in Seven Years'.

Flint points out that the dramatic increase in drunkenness amongst the young is parallelled by a general increase in alcohol consumption. Consumer spending on alcohol in Britain increased by 43.0 per cent between 1961 and 1971, in spite of a 7.0 per cent decline on expenditure on tobacco. Even so, the evidence indicates that teenage alcohol abuse is increasing more rapidly than amongst the general population. Alcohol abuse has long been a serious problem in Scotland—more so than elsewhere in Britain. The arrival of new drugs of abuse has rather distracted attention from the main drug problem. Current evidence suggests that many young drug abusers are indiscriminate in their choice of psychotropic substances and that many use alcohol and other drugs in conjunction. Many young people tire of illegal drug use and revert to more traditional drugs of abuse. The identity of particular drugs may not be important, but it is manifestly evidence that more problems are caused by alcohol than by all the other drugs combined.

ALCOHOL AND OTHER DRUGS

As noted above there is considerable evidence that Scotland has a much higher rate of alcoholism and drink-related problems than the rest of Britain. Alcohol is Scotland's traditional recreational drug, and continues to cause far more problems than any of the more recently adopted substances such as cannabis, hallucinogens or opiates.

Most young adults in Scotland begin to drink at a relatively early age, and regard drinking as a mark of maturity and toughness (Davies and Stacey, 1972). While the population as a whole are consuming more alcohol, and experiencing growing difficulties related to drinking, this increase is especially great amongst young adults. Teenage drunkenness and other forms of alcohol abuse are causing increased concern (Flint, 1974).

A number of studies have shown that some of the heaviest users of illegal drugs are also heavy alcohol users (Blum, 1969; Simon and Gagnon, 1970; Goode, 1970; Weschler and Thum, 1973). Berg (1976) in a review of 69 American surveys found that in most, though not all, studies, the heaviest drugtakers were the heaviest drinkers, though this relationship was not reciprocal. Similar conclusions were also reached by Tec (1973), Rockwell (1973) and Plant (1975a).

As Hindmarch *et al.* (1975) noted, there is similar evidence linking the use of tobacco and other drugs;

'... Blum (1969), Bogg *et al.* (1968) and Goode (1969; 1972) have shown that tobacco usage and the use of all illicit drugs are closely related Smart (1970), Lavenhar (1972) and Smart and Fejer (1972) have shown that both parents and peers of cannabis and other drug users are more likely to be smokers of tobacco. Individual interviews with 153 admitted drug users (Hindmarch *et al.*, 1970) showed that cannabis users were heavy cigarette smokers, while Weitman *et al.* (1972) claimed that the use of alcohol and tobacco correlated with the use of other illicit drugs especially cannabis. McKay *et al.* (1973) concluded that "drug users" were males who smoked and drank alcohol more frequently than the norm. Einstein *et al.* (1974) also found that chronic users of cannabis tended to be heavy tobacco and alcohol users, and they showed that the tendency to "try" cannabis was also associated with heavy use of alcohol and tobacco.'

A similar concomitance was noted by Plant (1975a) in his participant observation study of drugtakers in Cheltenham, Gloucestershire;

'Many individuals, especially those who were unemployed, spent a great deal of their time in public houses, which were amongst their favourite haunts. The low status unemployed and manual workers spent most evenings at a number of public houses, where many regularly drank to intoxication. Heavy drinking was an approved form of social behaviour amongst this sub-group and I often observed those from working-class backgrounds to be drunk. Several respondents had fathers who were also heavy drinkers . . . . The low-status sub-group often used other drugs in conjunction with alcohol. Barbiturates, Mandrax, amphetamine sulphate, cough linctuses and inhalers were regularly taken with alcohol, and cannabis was smoked with conspicuous regularity in some public houses . . . . My general conclusion is that young people who use illegal drugs such as cannabis are broadly the same as those who abuse alcohol and tobacco.' (Plant, 1975a, pp. 138–139)

Fieldwork during the same study indicated that many unemployed or manual workers were extremely catholic in their use of legal and illegal substances. One construction worker described his alcohol–drug use in these terms;

'Yes, I get drunk quite often, mainly at weekends. I usually swallow a . . . (type of inhaler), or maybe two. They give a bit of a speedy buzz. I get drunk easily, but last weekend I had ten to twelve pints a night. My chick (girl-friend) drinks like a fish too. She can drink me under the table. Sometimes we take a couple of Mandrax, or some kind of barbiturates. We sometimes get newted on barbs, if we can't afford alcohol.' (Plant, 1975a, p. 139) This is very reminiscent of the Ayrshire miners quoted earlier in the chapter.

Following on from these observations of drug–alcohol use amongst young working-class drugtakers in Gloucestershire, Plant (1976) reviewed the case notes of 100 young drug and alcohol abusers attending the Royal Edinburgh Hospital between 1st January 1972 and 31st January 1974. Each of these individuals had attended the Hospital, either as an out-patient or as an in-patient and had been classified as either drug or alcohol dependent. All those examined were younger than 30.

Only two individuals had been recorded by the Hospital on the International Diseases Codes as dependent upon both drugs and alcohol. Case notes revealed that a further 32 individuals had used illegal drugs and were also noted to be excessive drinkers or alcohol abusers. This examination showed that while these drugs and alcohol abusers were not necessarily physically dependent upon both alcohol and other drugs, there was a considerable overlap of the abuse of these substances. Eighty of the 100 individuals whose case notes were reviewed were either unemployed or were manual workers, in marked contrast to most other patients at the Royal Edinburgh Hospital, 70.5 per cent of whom were non-manual workers during 1973. While this study does not in itself form a basis for generalisation, it is consistent with existing evidence that alcohol is frequently included in the poly-drug usage of some young adults. In addition, in both the Cheltenham and Edinburgh studies those who had injected drugs were significantly more likely than other drugtakers to be classified as heavy drinkers, alcohol abusers or as alcoholics. These studies indicate that excessive alcohol use is frequently in conjunction with great involvement with other forms of drug abuse.

A familial connection between alcohol and illegal drugs has been noted by Goode (1972) in his American field research:

'One regularity that has been empirically supported in a number of different studies in various locates is the *general continuity* in drug use. Parents who use legal drugs—cigarettes, alcohol and prescription drugs such as barbiturates and amphetamines—are most likely to have children who use illegal drugs, marijuana included. This does not mean every drinking family will raise children who inevitably become junkies; it means simply that on the whole there will be important statistical differences between drinking families and abstemious families.' (Goode, 1972, p. 34)

Goode elaborates this point by commenting that alcohol and other drugs are only 'partial competitors';

'Young adults who drink liquor and smoke cigarettes are much more likely to try marijuana and other drugs. That is, people who use illegal drugs, marijuana especially, are *fundamentally the same people* who use alcohol and cigarettes—they are just a little further along the same continuum. People who abstain from liquor and cigarettes are far less likely to use marijuana than people who smoke and/or drink.' (Goode, 1972, p. 35)

Jessor and Jessor (1972) in a survey of 388 United States' school pupils found that problem drinkers '... had more tolerant attitudes toward transgression, indicated greater social support for drinking, and engaged more in various other behaviours such as marijuana use and sexual intercourse.'

From the evidence cited above it seems clear that alcohol and the illegal drugs are not necessarily mutually exclusive. It has been suggested that alcohol is the 'traditional' drug in western countries and that cannabis and other illegal substances are adopted as alcohol substitutes. In fact it appears that many young adults have added the newer, illegal drugs to the traditional legal ones, alcohol and tobacco, frequently taking these in conjunction. There is also some evidence to suggest that a person's intensity of involvement with illegal drugs is paralleled by intense involvement with alcohol and, perhaps, with tobacco. This is also reflected in a willingness to abuse drugs and engage in other delinquent activities. As Erich Goode has commented, the illegal drugs have many similarities to the legal ones; they are simply a little further along the same continuum. Socially acceptable alcohol use does not constitute a legal, or indeed any kind of problem, whereas even sporadic illicit drug taking is by definition illegal and in that narrow sense deviant. Both legal and illegal drugtaking generally begin the same way, due to peer pressure and as symbols of maturity and independence from parental norms and authority. Most drug use, whether legal or illegal, is social rather than solitary, and many groups of teenagers approve of and encourage the use of a wide range of psychotropic substances. The illegal drugs have been fitted into youthful leisure time alongside their predecessors, and coexist within a subculture which approves of both, together with a mixture of other old and new beliefs and activities. For most young people, any drug use is casual and not a central pre-occupation. For a minority alcohol and/or drug are used excessively and abuse is correlated with a range of other problems. A growing pre-occupation with drugs and alcohol in the young is often a symptom of far reaching social and psychological malaise (Hassall and Ritson, 1971). Few young people in Britain become physically dependent upon a single substance, but may become deeply preoccupied with the drug–alcohol way of life as an escape, support or source of prestige. In view of the obviously catholic tastes of many young people in regard to how they achieve their chosen highs, it is no longer appropriate to make a rigid distinction between their abuse of alcohol and other drugs.

PREVENTION

Preventive strategies are naturally closely allied to national campaigns and policies. Scotland has retained an understandable concern with preventing or minimising the growing problem of alcohol abuse amongst young people. Research has been directed at examining the ways in which young people learn to drink (Jahoda, 1972) and the Scottish Health Education Unit and Scottish Council on Alcoholism have jointly initiated training programmes in the recognition and management of problem drinking.

There is no national policy of education concerning drug abuse. Far less is spent upon education than upon advertising alcohol and tobacco. Health Education efforts have been piecemeal, unco-ordinated and lack financial resources.

Preventive campaigns have been mostly directed at schoolchildren. This is logical enough, since it is easier to mould attitudes before habits are formed. Nonetheless there is no convincing evidence that such strategies are effective in changing attitudes. A varied selection of films and talks have been used, which have adopted tactics varying from the presentation of medical evidence to 'horror films'. Health education about drugs has frequently been given by people who themselves know little of the subject. Some films are outmoded or present inaccurate information. Drug abuse has often been regarded as the province of clergymen or policemen. These may or may not be well informed. Alcohol and tobacco use have often escaped this treatment and are presented in health issues—it seems only consistent that the use of all psychoactive substances traditional or novel should be presented as part of the same curriculum.

Young people are influenced by the drug use of their parents and other important people in their lives. Most young people begin use and abuse of drugs because of peer pressure or curiosity. Research (Plant, 1975a, Davies and Stacey, 1972) has shown that both legal and illegal drugs abuse is especially commonplace amongst people from families where legal drugs are used heavily. Neither teetotal nor heavily drinking parents are able to set an example of controlled drug use. Alcoholism tends to be most prevalent where there are many abstainers as well as many heavy drinkers. Scotland is traditionally ambivalent about alcohol use.

Deviant patterns of drugtaking perpetuate themselves. Young people are likely to be more influenced by their peers than by 'official' drug educators. The key to controlling abuse is likely to be the example of the judicious use of legal drugs.

Drug education should be related to the characteristics and needs of the specific groups to whom programmes are directed. If schoolchildren in the Orkney Islands have never heard of LSD, there may be little use in warning them about its misuse. Limited, relevant, and above all, *accurate* information should be presented in an attractive way. Discussion should be fostered. In the past, drug educators have too often directed a one-way flow of views and information at schoolchildren. As a corollary to any drug education, there should be some mechanism for confidential counselling not necessarily by teachers.

Realistic education must take into account how attitudes and behaviour are formed and influenced. At present, what education exists is often dispersed in a vacuum from the realities of drug use at home, in medicine and amongst friends. Health education stands a better chance of success if the social determinants of legal or illegal drug use are frankly considered.

Looking back at the history of alcohol and drug misuse in Scotland it seems that those measures which have sought to influence availability have proved more effective than attempts to exort change in attitudes and behaviour of the population. The introduction of stricter licencing laws and ever increasing taxation of alcohol, have both had a profound effect on the drinking habits of the population. When the availability of intravenous methyl amphetamine was severely restricted the incidence of abuse dropped away. A similar trend has been observed since family doctors in Scotland have mostly agreed on a voluntary restriction on amphetamine prescription. This has meant that the chemist shops no longer stock such drugs and even if a burglary occurs the cupboard (at least as far as amphetamine is concerned) is usually bare.

It is perhaps surprising that against this background of attempts to limit availability, a recent committee reviewing Scottish Licencing Law recommended changes that would appear to enhance availability. The thinking behind this revision is to diminish the 'pressure to drink' by, for instance, encouraging public houses to become places where one may drink in the company of one's family in a more relaxed and less intense manner no longer with an eye to the clock. This should lead to fewer people drinking heavily within the relatively short period of evening opening and then staggering to their cars in a state which can only precipitate more road accidents and domestic disharmony when the husband arrives home drunk at 10.30 in the evening.

It is interesting that the same moderate opinion which supports increased availability of alcohol with extended licencing hours looks askance at any measure which enhances the availability of illegal drugs. This is a clear example of the paradox which enables society to treat drugs which may be very similar in their psychological effects in totally different ways because of the customs of their country, and the social meaning ascribed to their consumption. A culture's response to a particular drug tells us more of that culture's history and political make-up than it does of the pharmacology of the drug or the psychopathology of the drug taker.

The legitimate use of psychoactive drugs notably tranquillisers and antidepressants, is, of course, a prominent feature of Scottish society. Distress, anxiety and depression, which have long been regarded as legitimate responses to human suffering and crises, are now seen as material for pharmaco-therapy. It would be interesting to speculate how far the intervention of a doctor in legitimating drug taking significantly alters the relationship between the drug and the user. It seems that society allows the use of drugs if the user will admit to being sick but prohibits them if the user takes the medicine into his own hands and becomes his own physician or, worse still, takes them merely for pleasure. There is growing anxiety about the boundaries of legitimate drug prescribing, and many recent campaigns have endeavoured to dissuade doctors from prescribing commonly abused drugs such as barbiturates but there has been no serious attempt to question the criteria on which prescriptions are based. Opportunity and the chance meeting with a particular practitioner or a particular group of friends is a major determinant of behaviour and yet should that chance lead to the choice of an illicit drug the consequences for the individual may profoundly influence his subsequent life. The evidence which we have presented above suggests that the young drug and alcohol abusers are not fundamentally different and yet society's reaction may be worlds apart.

REFERENCES

Bennie, E. H. and Sclare, A. B. (1966). Heroin Addiction in Glasgow. *Scot. med. J.*, **11**, 319
Berg, D. (1970). The Non-Medical Use of Drugs in the United States: A Comprehensive Review. *Intern. J. Addict.*, **5**, 799
Blum, R. H. (1969). Drugs and Students (Jossey Bass: San Francisco)
Bogg, R. A., Smith, R. G. and Russel, S. (1968). Drugs and Michegan High School Students (Mimeograph)
Davies, J. and Stacey, B. (1972). Teenagers and Alcohol: A developmental study in Glasgow. Vol. **II** (HMSO: London)
Dean, N. M. B. (1968). Amphetamine and Other Drug Dependence in Edinburgh. *Health Bull.*, **XXVI**, 7
Department of Health. (1926). Report of the Committee on Morphine and Heroin Addiction (HMSO: London)
Dight, S. E. (1976). Scottish Drinking Habits. *Social Survey Division, Office of Population Censuses and Surveys*
Edwards, G. (1971). Unreason in an Age of Reason (Royal Society of Medicine: London)
Edwards, G., Hawker, A. and Williamson, V. (1966). London's Skid Row. *Lancet*, **1**, 249
Einstein, R., Hughes, I. and Hindmarch, I. (unpublished) Patterns of use of alcohol, cannabis, and tobacco in a student population
Evans, J. (1971). Drug taking in adolescents. *Scot. med. J.*, **16**, 369
Fish, F., Wells, B. W. P., Bindeman, S., Bunney, J. E. and Jordon, M. M. (1974). Prevalence of Drug Misuse Among Young People in Glasgow 1970–72. *Brit. J. Addict.*, **69**, 343
Flint, R. (1974). Teenage Drinking: a cause for concern? (Edinburgh Corporation)
Forrest, J. A. H. and Tarala, R. A. (1973). Abuse of Drugs for Kicks: A Review of 252 Admissions. *Brit. med. J.*, **4**, 136

Forrest, J. A. H. and Tarala, R. A. (1973). 60 Hospital Admissions Due to Reactions to Lysergide L.S.D.) *Lancet*, **ii**, 1310

Geike, Sir A. (1904). Scottish Reminiscences (Maclehose: Glasgow)

Glatt, M. M. (1958). The English Drink Problem: its rise and decline through the ages. *Brit. J. Addict.*, **55**, 51

Goode, E. (1969). Multiple Drug Use Among Marijuana Smokers. *Social Problems* **17**, 48

Goode, E. (1970). The Marijuana Smokers (Basic Books: New York)

Goode, E. (1972). Cigarette Smoking and Drug Use on a College Campus. *Intern. J. Addict.*, **7**, 133

Goode, E. (1972). Drugs in American Society (Alfred A. Knopf: New York)

Harrison, B. (1971). Drink and the Victorians. (Faber and Faber: London)

Hayter, A. (1968). Opium and the Romantic Imagination (Faber and Faber: London)

Hindmarch, I., Hughes, I. and Einstein, R. (1975). Attitudes to drug users and to the use of alcohol, tobacco and cannabis on the campus of a provincial university. *Bull. Narcot.*, **XXVII**, 27

Jahoda, G. (1972). Children and Alcohol: a developmental study in Glasgow (HMSO: London)

James VI (Scotland) and I (England). (1604). Counterblaste to Tobacco (London)

Jessor, R. and Jessor, S. L. (19). Problem Drinking in Youth: Personality, Social and Behavioural Antecedents and Correlates. Institute of Behavioural Science, University of Colorado, Publications 144, p 3

Judson, H. F. (1974). Heroin Addiction in Britain (Harcourt Brace Jovanovich: London)

Kessel, N. and Walton, H. J. (1974). Alcoholism, p. 54 (Pelican: Harmondsworth)

Kosviner, A., Hawks, D. and Webb, M. G. T. (1973). Cannabis Use Amongst British University Students. *Brit. J. Addict.*, **69**, 35

Lancet Editorial (1949). *Lancet*, **1**, 310

Lavenhar, M. A., Wolfson, E. A., Sheffet, A., Einstein, S. and Louria, D. B. (1972). Survey of Drug Abuse in Six New Jersey High Schools: II Characteristics of Drug Users and Non Users. *In* Student Drug Surveys (ed. Einstein, S. and Allen, M.) (Baywood: New York)

McKay, A. J., Hawthorne, V. M. and McCartney, H. N. (1973). Drug Taking Among Medical Students at Glasgow University. *Brit. med. J.*, **1**, 540

Mitcheson, M. (1973). Reported in *Health Bulletin*, **XXXI**, 86

Mullen, P. (1975). Personal communication

Plant, M. A. (1975a). Drugtakers in an English Town (Tavistock: London)

Plant, M. A. (1975b). Alcoholism in Scotland. *New Psychiatry*, **2**, 12

Plant, M. A. (1976). Young Drug and Alcohol Casualties Compared: Review of 100 Patients at a Scottish Psychiatric Hospital. *Brit. J. Addict.*, **71**, 31

Reeves, C. E. (1973). Sociological Aspects of Drugtaking in Southern Hampshire. Paper presented to 2nd International Conference on Alcoholism and Drug Dependence, Liverpool

Ritson, E. B. (1971). Drug Use in the Provinces. *Drugs and Society*, **2**, 19
Ritson, E. B. and Hassall, C. (1971). The Management of Alcoholism (Edinburgh: Livingston)
Ritson, E. B., Toller, P. and Harding, F. (1973). Drug Abuse in the East Midlands: A Study of 139 Patients Referred to an Addiction Unit. *Brit. J. Addict.*, **68**, 65
Rockwell, D. A. (1973). Alcohol and Marijuana—Social Problems Perspective. *Brit. J. Addict.*, **68**, 209
Schofield, M. (1971). The Strange Case of Pot (Pelican: Harmondsworth)
Leading Article (1966). The Problem of Drug Addiction. *Scot. med. J.*, **11**, 340
Leading Article. (1971). Drug Takers in Scotland. *Scot. med. J.*, **16**, 342
Scottish Health Education Unit (1976). Understanding Alcohol and Alcoholism in Scotland (Edinburgh)
Scottish Home and Health Department (1972). Drug Misuse in Scotland (Edinburgh)
Simon, W. and Gagnon, J. H. (1970). The End of Adolescence: The College Experience (Harper and Row: New York)
Sinclair, C. (1875). Sketches and Stories of Scotland and the Scotch (Simpkin Marshall: London)
Smart, R. G. (1970). Relationships between parental and adolescent drug use (Mimeograph)
Smart, R. G. and Fejer, D. (1972). Drug Use Among Adolescents and Their Parents. *J. Abnorm. Psychol.*, **79**, 153
Spear, H. B. (1969). The Growth of Heroin Addiction in the United Kingdom. *Brit. J. Addict.*, **64**, 245
Stengel, E. (1969). Suicide and Attempted Suicide, p. 63 (Pelican: Harmondsworth)
Stimson, G. V. (1973). Heroin and Behaviour (Irish University Press: London)
Tec, N. (1973). A Clarification of the Relationship Between Alcohol and Marihuana. *Brit. J. Addict.*, **68**, 191
Ward, J. A. (1971). The drug scene in Scotland. *Scot. med. J.*, **16**, 376
Watson, J. M. (1974). A Study of Solvent Sniffing in Lanarkshire 1973/4 Diploma in Public Health Dissertation, Glasgow University
Weitman, M., Scheble, R., Johnson, K. G. and Abbey, H. (1972). Survey of Adolescent Drug Use. Correlations Among Use of Drugs. *Amer. J. Pub. Health*, **62**, 166
Weschler, H. and Thum, D. (1973). Teenage Drinking, Drug Use and Social Correlates. *Quart. J. Stud. Alcohol*. December, 1220
Weiner, R. S. P. (1970). Drugs and Schoolchildren (Longman: London)
Whittet, M. M. (1967). Highland and Island psychiatric reflections. *Brit. J. med. Psychol.*, **40**, 1
Woodside, M. (1973). The First 100 Referrals to a Scottish Drug Treatment Centre. *Brit. J. Addict.*, **68**, 231

PART II

Medical Complications

CHAPTER 6

The medical complications
of drug abuse

D. LOURIA

As the prevalence of drug abuse around the world increases, so does the
incidence of medical complications. It is clear that no drug used illicitly
for mind altering purposes is free of medical complications. It is equally
clear that the following list for each of the major categories of drugs used
currently will be expanded in future years as more persons become
involved in the drug scene and more of the consequences are recognized
and recorded in the medical literature.

HEROIN AND OTHER ILLICITLY USED OPIATES

OVERDOSE

The most feared consequence of heroin injection is so-called 'overdose'.
This may be experienced by the veteran heroin user as well as the
neophyte. There continues to be an angry debate about the nature of
overdose, but it would appear that the overdose syndrome can be
divided clinically into three groups.

Respiratory depression

First there are those who experience profound respiratory depression
and in some of these cases, apnoea ensues. There are no adequate data
indicating the incidence of respiratory depression after heroin; presumably it occurs relatively infrequently but the overwhelming majority of long term heroin abusers experience 'overdose' at least once.
There are many who feel that the use of the term overdose is
unacceptable for this syndrome on the grounds that among those dying
from so-called overdose, tissue opiate levels may be surprisingly small.

Additionally they point out that 'overdose' may supervene in a chronic heroin user who presumably ought to be tolerant and therefore able to withstand enormous amounts of the drug given intravenously. But their arguments cannot contravene the fact that in this form of overdose, something is depressing the respiratory center, presumably the opiate, since opiates are known to so affect the brain. Furthermore the treatment of choice in cases of profound heroin-induced respiratory depression is an opiate antagonist, including nalorphine, levallorphan or naloxone. When these medicaments are administered, the respiratory rate increases promptly; this in itself strongly supports the notion that the respiratory depression was due to an opiate.

Acute pulmonary edema

The second form of overdose is acute pulmonary edema of non-cardiac origin. This may kill so rapidly that at autopsy the needle is found still in the vein. In most cases the pulmonary edema occurs within two hours after heroin injection but occasionally its onset may be delayed for four to six hours. If the drug is taken by the nasal route, pulmonary edema may on rare occasions appear up to 48 hours after heroin use.

In these patients, the respiratory rate ranges from less than 5 to more than 60 per minute. Physical examination usually shows a stuporous individual with severely constricted pupils. Examination of the lungs reveals no dullness to percussion and no evidence of consolidation, but on auscultation bilateral rales and rhonchi are evident. Chest roentgen-ogram usually shows bilateral infiltrates radiating from the hilum, mimicking cardiogenic pulmonary edema, but there is in most instances no increase in central venous pressure, no cardiomegaly and no pathological evidence in those who die of significant cardiac dysfunction.

In some cases an important clue to the correct diagnosis is a normal or slowed respiratory rate in the presence of extensive bilateral infiltrates on chest x-ray. In such circumstances, the respiratory rate ought to be profoundly increased; if it is not this suggests depression of the respiratory center. If the respiratory rate is increased, the diagnosis can be suspected by a history of heroin use and by the presence of needle marks and constricted pupils. It is well to remember that pupillary constriction can also follow brain trauma and that profound hypoxia can cause pupils that otherwise might be constricted to dilate.

In almost all cases, there is laboratory evidence of marked hypoxia, the partial pressure of oxygen falling to as low as 40 mm Hg. Consequently the administration of oxygen is of paramount importance in treating the overdose pulmonary edema syndrome. Some investigators feel that the pulmonary edema is totally consequent to the hypoxia but there is little firm evidence to support this hypothesis, and the hypoxia may, for the most part, follow the onset of pulmonary edema. There are many other possible mechanisms to account for the edema including histamine or kinin release, acute allergic response, or direct drug-induced vascular spasm. Whatever the mechanism, it is clear that profound physiological changes occur and measures of ventilatory function show that these abnormalities may persist for many weeks after the clinical manifestations of the overdose have resolved.

Treatment consists of recognition of the cause of the pulmonary edema, administration of oxygen, conventional supportive measures, and use of narcotic antagonists including naloxone (adult dosage 0.01 mg/kg), nalorphine (3–10 mg) or levallorphan (1 mg) intravenously or subcutaneously, repeating the dose 2–3 times every 15–30 minutes if the response is not deemed adequate. Ordinarily after administration of antagonists, the pupils dilate and the respiratory rate increases promptly. Especially if long acting opiates, such as methadone, have been taken, the shorter acting antagonists may have to be administered repeatedly during the initial 24 hours of observation. Particularly in cases of methadone intoxication treated with naloxone, the patient may improve strikingly, leave the hospital after a few hours and then experience recurrent respiratory depression hours later. Consequently, if possible, cases of overdose should be held under observation for a minimum period of 24 hours.

Patients suffering from heroin overdose with pulmonary edema may have substantial fever and a peripheral blood leukocytosis of up to 30 000/mm^3. Ordinarily patients become afebrile within 48 hours and concomitantly the white blood cell count returns to normal levels. Should the fever and leukocytosis continue for over 48 hours, the assumption must be made that the patient either has aspiration pneumonia or secondary bacterial infection. In these cases a second x-ray taken 48 hours after hospitalization should show a localized infiltrate and disappearance of the generalized lung edema. It is well to stress that in the overwhelming majority of cases, no antimicrobials are needed.

In most cases the central venous pressure is normal, so that there is no need for administration of digitalis or diuretics. Of course, if there is evidence of congestive failure, such medicaments should be given.

It is well to remember that any opiate has the capacity to induce pulmonary edema. Indeed, the first description of this abnormality was by Sir William Osler in 1880, some 15 years before the synthesis of diacetylmorphine (heroin). In Osler's case, unilateral lung edema supervened after morphine was administered, but usually the edema is bilateral. Although heroin causes most of the cases of pulmonary edema, an increasing number of cases have recently been ascribed to methadone, taken either by mouth or vein by non-tolerant individuals. In some cases young children have mistakenly ingested their parent's therapeutic methadone with catastrophic results.

Acute cardiac arrhythmia

The third form of overdose is acute and potentially lethal cardiac arrhythmia due, not to the heroin, but rather to the quinine frequently employed as an adulterant. The abnormality in cardiac rhythm should resolve after conventional treatment, the particular regimen depending on the specific arrhythmia induced.

ENDOCARDITIS

Those who inject drugs in egregiously unhygienic fashion are at great risk from a variety of infections. An increasing number of cases of endocarditis have been reported in the past decade. In the earlier reports enterococci and staphylococci were the microbes given most attention in the literature.

In the mid-1960s, the syndrome of recurrent septic emboli from the tricuspid valve was emphasized, the hallmark of this entity being sequential involvement of different parts of the lung. In these cases, the staphylococcus was thought always to be the causative micro-organism. Several studies have stressed that there are two distinct clinical patterns. In some cases, there is little to point to the heart valves and the major manifestations are related to the lung emboli; in these patients there is no murmur suggesting tricuspid disease or only an insubstantial systolic bruit that does not suggest organic disease. In other cases, lung findings are minimal and there are both cardiac and peripheral evidences suggesting endocarditis including a murmur increasing during the inspiratory phase of respiration, petechiae, clubbing and peripheral embolization.

In the late 1960s, the emphasis changed back from the right side to the left side. Several investigators found that left-sided valvular disease was more frequently observed than right-sided disease in autopsy series. But as of the mid 1970s, most reports suggest a clear predominance of right-sided disease among intravenous drug users. It is also clear that the staphylococcus is not the only organism responsible for right sided infection; strains of pseudomonas are increasingly the etiologic agent and occasionally alpha streptococci, enterococci, *Candida sp.* enterobacters and serratias have been isolated. A small number of cases of pulmonic valve involvement have been described in which the responsible micro-organisms were either staphylococci or strains of pseudomonas. The more recent data also suggest that the ostensibly divergent data on prevalence of right sided as contrasted to left sided disease were not in actuality contradictory; it would appear that studies of living patient populations will show a preponderance of right-sided valvular involvement whereas autopsy studies will tend to show left-sided predominance because the mortality from left-sided valvular infection appears to be substantially higher. This would in turn appear to be related to two factors: first, those with aortic valve insufficiency are more likely to suffer from congestive heart failure; second, many of those acquiring left sided infection have previously damaged valves whereas in the overwhelming majority of drug users with tricuspid or pulmonic valve infection, there is no evidence of prior valve damage.

Staphylococci are responsible for at least half the heart valve infections in intravenous drug abusers; other organisms isolated frequently include strains of pseudomonas and enterobacter. Enterococci are currently responsible for only a small number of endocarditis cases. Recent evidence indicates that approximately 10 per cent of cases are due to species of Candida and an additional 10 per cent of cases are caused by alpha streptococci. Interestingly, in about 1/3 of those with infections due to either Candida or alpha streptococci, there is no evidence of underlying valvular abnormality, a surprising observation since these organisms ordinarily possess little capacity to invade an undamaged valve. It is well to recognize that any species of Candida can cause endocarditis; consequently the term 'non-pathogenic' species of Candida must be viewed in the context of the clinical situation. It is true that *Candida guilliermondii* or *C. parapsilosis* will not cause progressive disease after injection into experimental animals, but in man any species can cause not only endocarditis but even disseminated candidosis of the renal-myocardial type if host defenses are markedly impaired. Patients have been left untreated for substantial periods of time because the laboratory reported only a candida 'contaminant' in blood cultures. This is of course a clinical, not a laboratory, judgement especially if the patient uses illicit drugs intravenously. In approximately 5 per cent of cases dual heart valve infections are present, either involving a single or multiple valves. Thus, for example, a patient may have both pseudomonas and Candida organisms in aortic valve vegetations. In other instances a staphylococcus has caused right-sided infection and simultaneously an enterobacter has invaded the aortic valve. In any addict who fails to respond to appropriate therapy, this possibility must be given careful consideration and repeated blood cultures obtained.

Those with tricuspid disease should be treated on admission (before culture results are known) with a regimen such as a semi-synthetic penicillin and gentamicin because the two organisms most likely to be the etiologic agents are *Staphylococcus aureus* and strains of pseudomonas. Frequently the clinical course is stormy for a period of days or even weeks despite appropriate therapy, but most eventually recover.

INFECTIOUS HEPATITIS

It remains uncertain how frequently those who inject heroin by vein develop infection due to hepatitis B virus (serum hepatitis). Among those dying of other causes at a young age, at least half show histologic abnormalities in the liver. However, studies of Australia antigen in an unselected heroin-using population showed that only about 2 per cent were positive. This discrepancy may be related to the techniques then in use for determination of Australia antigen or antibody. It is clear that the radio immuno assay is currently by far the most sensitive method for detecting hepatitis B infection. More sensitive techniques, such as immune adherence hemagglutination, are in the developmental stages. It would appear likely that when antigen and antibody are measured by the most sensitive techniques, the data will converge and will support the older pathologic data, indicating that in the range of half the heroin using population suffer liver dysfunction, most of which is due to hepatitis B infection. A second question relates to the frequency with which progressive liver disease occurs among those who use heroin for a prolonged period. The accumulating data strongly suggest that if the transaminase levels remain elevated or if Australia antigen persists in serum, biopsies will show active or aggressive hepatitis. If on the other hand, antibody to Australia antigen is found but there is no antigen present, then the prognosis is good. A small amount of preliminary and tenuous evidence suggests that those with persisting hepatitis may progress to fibrosis and cirrhosis.

In addition to subtle and/or chronic hepatitis, the heroin user may suffer from severe, occasionally lethal acute hepatitis. Interestingly, overt hepatitis is primarily a disease of the young drug user and is far less frequently seen among those who have been addicted for more than five years.

Recently there has been increasing interest in the role of alcohol in the liver dysfunction found in heroin addicts. In the United States there is no longer a monolithic focus by the user on a single category of intoxicating drugs. In the mid-1960s one could conveniently separate opiate abusers from those who indulged in cannabis or LSD, and both these were separate from a much larger third group that employed alcohol as its intoxicant. Currently multiple drug use is the norm, the majority of the users taking two or more drugs in large amounts. Studies by Stimmel, Vernace and Tobias suggest that the liver damage seen on biopsy in heroin abusers may be either due to the effects of alcohol or hepatitis B virus or a combination of the two.

TETANUS

Among those injecting heroin subcutaneously (skin poppers), a small number of cases of tetanus are seen each year. This is hardly surprising since the multiple inflammatory subcutaneous lesions that characterize the chronic skin popper provide an ideal mileau for the growth of *Cl. tetani*. Treatment consists of debridement, antibiotics and the administration of human anti-toxin but even with prompt and appropriate therapy the mortality in the addict population is fearsome, ranging from 50 to over 75 per cent in different series.

MALARIA

In the 1930s a few hundred cases of falciparum malaria were observed in heroin addicts. In many, the cerebral form supervened and this was associated with a considerable mortality. Perhaps because of the widespread use of quinine as an adulterant, malaria virtually disappeared as a complication of heroin use but recently there has been a re-crudescence of this infection. Epidemiologic studies show that these mini-epidemics have been initiated by heroin users who have returned from Vietnam bringing both their heroin habit and their malaria with them. Thus far only a small number of cases have occurred, all have been due to *Plasmodium vivax*, and all have responded to chloroquine therapy (in these cases because there is no exo-erthyrocytic phase, chloroquine alone is perfectly satisfactory therapy).

NEUROLOGICAL COMPLICATIONS

Immediately following overdose associated with pulmonary edema, the addict may have transient paresis that ordinarily resolves in a 48–72 hour period. In a small number of cases repetitive use of heroin may be followed by thoracic cord degeneration. In some, this is accompanied by limb paralysis that gradually improves. Others are left with significant residual neurological defects and in some cases the transverse myelitis is fatal. The precise mechanism underlying the cord destruction has not been satisfactorily elucidated.

RENAL DYSFUNCTION

A small number of cases have been reported of nephrotic syndrome with deposition of immunoglobulin M (and smaller amounts of immunoglo-bulin G) in the kidneys. This would appear most likely to be due to an adulterant in the heroin or to an allergic response to a microbial infection but thus far the latter has not been demonstrated and no unusual adulterants have been found in the heroin. Since this association with addiction has only recently been described, the long range consequences of this renal abnormality are not yet fully understood.

Following the administration of heroin, the user may become stuporous with resultant soft tissue compression; this in turn can result in myoglobinemia, myoglobinuria and in some cases in acute renal failure.

Treatment consists of conventional supportive measures and this should result in complete recovery in most cases.

MISCELLANEOUS

Recently a considerable number of cases have been reported of septic arthritis due to staphylococci, strains of pseudomonas or species of Candida. The same organisms have also caused osteomyelitis in the addict population. The injection of heroin in unhygienic fashion may result not only in bone and joint sepsis, but also in severe purulent myositis; in these cases the responsible microorganisms are staphylococci, gram negative bacilli or a combination of these organisms.

Those injecting contaminated heroin may also suffer from embolic lung infections, manifested as focal pneumonitis, single or multiple lung abscesses, empyema or pyopneumothorax. In most instances, streptococci or staphylococci are isolated but increasingly gram negative organisms are being isolated from blood or empyema fluid.

The intravenous heroin user is also said to be susceptible to upper respiratory tract-acquired bacterial pneumonia. In these cases, the lower lobes are usually affected, the responsible organism is usually the pneumococcus and conventional antimicrobial therapy is ordinarily successful. The epidemiological data are presently so limited that it is uncertain whether the incidence of bacterial pneumonia is actually increased or whether the incidence is unchanged but the severity of the pneumonia is greater and therefore more likely to result in hospitalization.

CENTRAL STIMULANTS OF THE METHAMPHETAMINE, PHENMETRAZINE OR METHYLPHENIDATE TYPES

CARDIOVASCULAR

It has long been known that those inadvertently or intentionally ingesting or injecting large amounts of central stimulants may die shortly thereafter. Presumably the mechanism of death is marked cardiac arrhythmia. Large amounts of central stimulants can also induce profound hypertension and this in turn may result in incapacitating or lethal cerebrovascular accidents. Although such alarming elevations in blood pressure have been observed more frequently after intravenous injection of methamphetamine in extraordinary dosage (100 mg to 1000 mg per injection), this has also been reported occasionally after the ingestion of large amounts of the drug.

A small number of cases of diffuse vasculitis have been attributed to injection of methamphetamine. Most, but not all, such cases have been found in a localized area in the western part of the United States. Because this has not been observed over a wide geographic area and because it has not been reported in certain communities noted for their large coterie of intravenous stimulant habituees, the assumption has been made that the angiitis is due not to the methamphetamine but rather to an adulterant popular in that particular geographic area. Thus far no specific adulterant has been incriminated and the significance of the findings remain uncertain.

INFECTIONS

The heavy intravenous stimulant user often suffers extraordinary weight loss and emaciation due primarily to a reduced inclination to eat while taking the stimulant. Perhaps as a result, such individuals appear particularly susceptible to skin and subcutaneous infection due to the usual farrago of microorganisms. The intravenous central stimulant habituee also appears to be susceptible to the same endocardial and hepatic infections reported in the heroin abuser.

It is difficult to separate the roles of different drugs in these infectious complications because most intravenous stimulant users also inject a variety of other drugs. Thus in one extensive epidemiologic survey in an affluent suburban area of the United States, approximately 75 per cent of the intravenous methamphetamine users also injected heroin. However, presently there is no reason to believe that infections arising in methamphetamine users are due to drug induced defects in host defense mechanisms; rather it seems likely that the cardiac and hepatic infections result primarily from needle contamination with bacteria, yeasts and viruses.

BRAIN DAMAGE

The question of stimulant induced chronic brain damage remains unsettled. Some Japanese and Swedish observers reported what they believed to be an organic mental syndrome in some habituees who took gargantuan doses of central stimulants by vein for a considerable period of time. These clinical observations have been buttressed by findings of persistent electroencephalographic changes in some patients and by biochemical changes in brain tissue slices of animals given substantial doses of stimulants. Many authorities remain sceptical about the existence of a chronic brain syndrome. In the United States, the prevailing opinion, based on studies in communities that have suffered major stimulant epidemics, is that most habituees never show evidence of organic brain damage. Some do indeed manifest such a syndrome but recover completely over a period of months; in an occasional individual recovery may require one to two years and in a small number of cases abnormalities suggesting an organic brain syndrome persist. Thus, although there are no corroborative anatomical data, the clinical observations suggest that large amounts of central stimulants taken for a prolonged period can cause brain damage in a very small percentage of the habituees.

HALLUCINOGENS

Lysergic acid diethylamide is the prototype of the potent hallucination causing drugs. The major controversy revolves around the capacity of the drug to cause teratogenic or chromosomal aberrations. Although the data are convincing in neither area, what information is available should at least cause the potential user to approach the drug with caution. A small number of cases have been reported in which the use of LSD, prior to conception or early in pregnancy, has been associated with severe deformity in the fetus, usually involving the extremities. Additionally, in one study of women undergoing therapeutic abortions, those who had used LSD showed a striking increase in fetal defects, many involving the nervous system. However in another series of similar size, focusing on birth defects in live-born offspring, there was no evidence of LSD-induced fetal abnormalities. In both studies, use of LSD was associated with an increased prevalence of spontaneous abortions.

The data on chromosomal defects are equally confusing. It would appear that pure LSD causes very limited, and usually reversible, abnormalities in the chromosomes, consisting of breaks and occasionally the potentially more-serious rearrangements. On the other hand, street LSD, which is frequently adulterated and use of which is usually combined with self administration of other mind altering agents, is associated with an increased frequency of breaks and rearrangements; the incidence of such abnormalities is increased about 50 per cent compared to a control population. The significance of these chromosomal abnormalities for the LSD users or their progeny is not clear. It has been shown that in some persons the aberrations may persist for years and that the offspring of LSD taking mothers may also show the defects; here again the abnormalities may persist for at least two years. Of some concern is the observation that a small number of cases of leukemia or lymphoma have followed LSD use; this may be mere coincidence but possibly the observations might have more serious import.

LSD use has also been associated with subsequent trauma; under the influence of the drug people have jumped out of windows, run in front of cars and even jumped into fires. In part, these self-destructive actions appear to result from a gross misinterpretation of the environment and in certain cases, this self-destructive behavior is abetted by LSD's known analgesic actions.

A few cases of homicide have also occurred under the influence of LSD as have a small number of suicides consequent to despair over the unpleasant effects felt during recurrent LSD 'flashbacks'.

Additionally, LSD has been associated with peripheral gangrene and with an apparent reduced ability to handle a superficial infection, both presumably secondary to the drugs effects on blood vessels. LSD may also be implicated in small artery occlusive disease in the brain.

CANNABIS

There is increasing evidence that cannabis smoking causes aberrations in time and space perception and as a result users are at risk when driving an automobile. The initial studies suggesting that cannabis was innocuous as far as automobile driving was concerned have now been controverted by several investigations of simulated and actual driving that show braking and judgemental defects as well as erratic and often dangerous driving.

In recent years, five physical effects of cannabis have been described that remain the focus of frequently acrimonious debate:

Liver damage

One study showed hepatic dysfunction but this has not been confirmed and the investigators did not have at their disposal tests for Australia antigen or antibody. Consequently, hepatitis B was not ruled out and the current consensus is that cannabis does not by itself cause liver damage.

Chromosomal abnormalities

Despite the repeated contention that cannabis can hurt human chromosomes, there is at present not a single bit of evidence that this is so.

Teratogenic effects

In experimental animals, crude extracts of cannabis caused resorptions and a variety of fetal abnormalities. But in at least some of these experiments, the subsequent use of pure tetrahydrocannabinol produced no such fetal abnormalities. In mice that inhaled cannabis during pregnancy, the offspring showed cleft palate. But there is no evidence that cannabis exerts teratogenic effects in man.

Cerebral atrophy

Studies in the United Kingdom using pneumoencephalography showed evidence of cerebral atrophy in 10 cannabis users. These interesting data are, as noted by the authors, open to two criticisms. First, most of the subjects were multiple drug users even though cannabis seemed to predominate. Second, it is difficult to obtain adequate controls for this kind of study. Consequently, the preliminary data on cerebral atrophy should be interpreted with great caution until ample confirmatory studies are available.

Organic brain syndrome

Two American psychiatrists on the basis of a limited experience have insisted that the similarity of patterns of personality disturbance they observed in cannabis users indicates organic brain damage. To most observers this conclusion appears to be stretching the data too far. There is simply no convincing evidence that cannabis results in organic brain damage. Earlier studies from Greece drew the same conclusion, but impartial observers reviewing the data felt that there was evidence of substantial personality deterioration but not of specific brain damage.

Cannabis has been associated with an acute anaphylactic reaction and there is at least one case in which smoking of a great amount was followed by death; no other drug was isolated from tissues at autopsy. Among chronic heavy smokers, bronchitis or evidence of airway obstruction may supervene. Other than these, there is no convincing evidence of physical abnormalities incurred as a consequence of smoking cannabis.

Injection of cannabis can result in transient hypotension and thrombocytopenia.

MISCELLANEOUS MIND ALTERING DRUGS

MDA

MDA is an amphetamine derivative that can produce muscle rigidity, fever and according to some observers, severe, even lethal, cardiac arrhythmias.

PHENCYCLIDINE HYDROCHLORIDE

Phencyclidine hydrochloride is a veterinary anesthetic. It is perhaps the· drug most frequently used in the United States to adulterate or substitute for potent hallucinogens. Thus, for example, what is sold on the street as tetrahydrocannabinol or mescaline in America is very likely to be phencyclidine. This agent causes stupor, coma, hypertension and also may exacerbate any underlying mentation or personality disturbance.

STP

STP, (standing for serenity, tranquility and peace,) is a methoxy methyl amphetamine with atropine-like toxicity including difficulty with vision, difficulty with swallowing and impairment of respiratory mechanisms, allegedly with lethal respiratory paralysis in a few cases. One of the problems with atropine-like mind altering agents is that the mentation abnormalities can be accentuated by administration of chlorpromazine, the drug of choice in cases of LSD or methamphetamine intoxication.

Indeed, in a few cases of STP intoxication, chlorpromazine treatment supposedly resulted in cardiovascular collapse. Thus if there is any significant chance that the patient ingested an atropine-like agent, chlorpromazine should not be given; in these cases diazepam, chlordiazepoxide or short acting barbiturates are probably the agents of choice.

SOLVENT SNIFFING

A variety of substances have been mis-used including gasoline, glue, deodorants, foot sprays and cleaning fluids. On rare occasions severe cerebral edema may occur as may bone marrow depression if the substance contains a benzine base. Some of the substances can cause hepatic and renal dysfunction that ranges from mild to severe. Solvent sniffers also may die, presumably from cardiac arrhythmias, especially if the victim has indulged in moderate to strenuous physical exertion after solvent use.

Although most chronic solvent inhalers suffer no serious effects if they avoid dangerous judgemental errors, some cases have been described with what appears to be an organic mental syndrome.

BARBITURATES

Administration of large amounts of barbiturates can of course cause coma and death. Injection of barbiturates may also be followed by local abscesses at or adjacent to the site of injection if the barbiturate has infiltrated the perivascular soft tissues.

Withdrawal from barbiturates must be carried out with great caution, for abrupt withdrawal can be followed by fever, stupor, convulsions, coma and even death.

PULMONARY AND EYE GRANULOMAS

The injection of drugs meant to be taken by mouth may cause pulmonary granulomatosis, fibrosis, and in some cases, obliterative endarteritis. This is caused by a reaction to the talc used as a filler in many pills and capsules including methadone and methylphenidate.

The pulmonary ventilatory and physiologic aberrations range from mild to severe and may on occasion result in death. Those injecting talc or cornstarch may also develop eye granulomas, and this may result in significant visual impairment in the more severe cases.

NEONATAL DEPENDENCE ON OPIATES AND BARBITURATES

It has long been known that heroin addicts are far more likely than controls to have underweight babies, and that their infants will in about 50 per cent of cases show clinical evidence of opiate dependency. In these cases, withdrawal usually starts within 48 hours and is characterized by failure to thrive, restlessness, fever, a high pitched cry, hyperreflexia, vomiting, sneezing and yawning. If not treated, seizures, coma and even death may supervene. Treatment of 14 days is usually sufficient but in some cases, up to 8 weeks of therapy is required.

Recent data show that maternal use of barbiturates even in dosages as low as 60 mg daily can result in neonatal dependence. The manifestations are similar to those described for opiates, but the time of onset is usually later ranging from less than one hour to 14 days after birth. Abnormal behavior may persist for as long as two to six months, the manifestations including irritability, hyperacusis sweating and hyperphagia. Unlike the babies of heroin-addicted mothers, the birth weight of barbiturate-dependent infants is usually in the normal range. Treatment consists of administration of chlorpromazine or phenobarbital.

REFERENCES

Bass, M. (1970). Sudden sniffing death. *J. Amer. med. Ass.* **212**, 2075
Cherubin, C. E., Kane, S., Weinberger, D. R., Wolfe, E. and McGinn, T. G. (1972). Persistence of transaminase abnormalities in former drug addicts. *Ann. intern. Med.* **76**, 385
Cherubin, C. E., Rosenthal, W. S., Stenger, R. E., Prince, A. M., Baden, M., Strauss, R. and McGinn, T. G. Chronic liver disease in asymptomatic narcotic addicts. *Ann. intern. Med.* **76**, 391

Citron, B. P., Halpern, M., McCarron, M., Lundberg, G. D., McCormick, R., Pincus, I. J., Tatter, D. and Haverback, G. J. Necrotizing angiitis in drug addicts. *New Eng. J. Med.*, **283**, 1003

Jacobson, C. B. and Berlin, C. M. (1972). Possible Reproductive Detriment in LSD Users. *J. Amer. med. Assoc.* **222**, 1367

Louria, D. B., Hensle, T. and Rose, J. (1967). The major medical complications of heroin addiction. *Ann. intern. Med.* **67**, 1

McGlothlin, W. H., Sparkes, R. S. and Arnold, D. O. (1970). Effect of LSD in human pregnancy. *J. Amer. med. Assoc.* **212**, 1483

Perlmutter, J. F. (1967). Drug addiction in pregnant women. *J. Obstet. Gyn.* **99**, 569

Ramsey, R. G., Gunnar, R. M. and Tobin, J. R. Jr. (1970). Endocarditis in the drug addict. *Amer. J. Cardiol.* **25**, 608

Richter, R. W. and Rosenberg, R. N. (1966). Transverse myelitis associated with heroin addiction. *J. Amer. med. Assoc.* **206**, 1255

PART III
Treatment

CHAPTER 7

Psychotherapy of drug dependents and alcoholics

R. BATTEGAY

GENERAL CONSIDERATIONS

The increasing use and abuse of drugs since the Second World War has led to a growing interest amongst psychiatrists and society as a whole in the associated problems. This interest has arisen not only because of the increasing number of drug dependents but also because of the psychological and sociological causes and consequences of drug abuse. It has become increasingly clear that drug dependencies—such as alcoholism—originate not only in the pharmacological effects of the drugs but also (and possibly mainly) in constitutional, psychological and sociological factors. With the progress of time the spread of drug dependencies has changed. Furthermore, the scientific view of, and theories about, drug-and alcohol-dependencies have developed further. In former times the addictions, and especially alcoholism, were seen as vices provoked by the individual himself. Today, they are considered as illnesses which we have to treat by medical means (Kielholz, 1949, 1962, 1964, 1965, 1971; Zurukzoglu, 1963). We know, for instance, that childhood plays an important role in the psychological development of man and especially in laying the ground for alcoholism and drug dependence.

In an inquiry in 31 Swiss military schools, in which 4 082 20-year-old healthy men were examined during the years 1972–1973, the marital status of the parents until the age of 15 of the examined subjects was found to play an important role in determining alcohol consumption, drug intake and the smoking habits of the subjects (Battegay *et al.*, 1975a,b).

Table 1 shows that sons of unmarried mothers, parents married after the child's birth, or parents living separated or divorced run a relatively

Table 1 Parental status, subject's age at beginning of disturbed situations and % representation of upper consumption classes

Parental status and subject's age at beginning of situations	subjects (sum of line)	% of n = 3988	% representation of upper consumption classes								
			> 350 g alcohol (100%) week	relative risk		> 24 g tobacco/day	relative risk		totally > 6 drug intakes	relative risk	
			%	esti-mate	95% interval of reliability	%	esti-mate	95% interval of reliability	%	esti-mate	95% interval of reliability
Parents married	3311	83.0	8.0	1.0	–	16.3	1.0	–	9.8	1.0	–
Parents married after birth of subject	63	1.6	17.5	2.2	1.23–3.61	23.8	1.5	0.91–2.20	13.3	1.4	0.70–2.44
Father absent	282	7.1	9.6	1.2	0.81–1.72	17.7	1.1	0.82–1.40	12.4	1.3	0.90–1.73
—Mother single	(41)	(1.0)	7.3	0.9	–	17.1	1.0	–	24.4	2.5	–
—Father deceased											
subj. 5–15 years	(135)	(3.4)	9.6	1.2	–	20.7	1.3	–	15.4	1.6	–
subj. 15 years	(106)	(2.7)	10.4	1.3	–	14.0	0.9	–	3.8	0.4	–

	112	2.8	4.5	0.6	0.23–1.27	25.9	1.6	1.13–2.15	11.6	1.2	0.69–1.94
Mother absent 1)											
—Mother deceased											
subj. 0–4 years	(18)	(0.4)	5.6	0.7	—	50.0	3.1	—	16.7	1.7	—
subj. 5–15 years	(52)	(1.3)	1.9	0.2	—	21.2	1.3	—	13.7	1.4	—
subj. > 15 years	(42)	(1.1)	7.2	0.9	—	21.4	1.3	—	7.3	0.7	—
Parents separated or divorced	220	5.5	14.1	1.8	1.23–2.45	26.8	1.6	1.29–2.05	15.5	1.6	1.13–2.16
subj. 0–4 years	(54)	(1.3)	16.7	2.1	—	27.3	1.7	—	20.8	2.1	—
subj. 5–15 years	(119)	(3.0)	12.6	1.6	—	29.4	1.8	—	16.1	1.5	—
subj. > 15 years	(47)	(1.2)	14.9	1.6	—	19.1	1.2	—	10.7	1.1	—
sum of column	$n = 3988$	100.0									
Other and incomplete answers	94	$Total\ N = 4082$									

1) in 13 cases both parents deceased

great risk of falling into a high consumption class for alcohol (more than
350 g 100 per cent alcohol a week, an amount corresponding to 9 litres of
beer, 4½ litres of wine, 1 litre of liqueur), for tobacco (more than 40 g
tobacco per day, an amount corresponding to 24 cigarettes) and for
other drugs (more than 6–220 drug intakes during the whole life).

It is interesting that sons of mothers who died before the subjects' age
of 5 show a greater percentage in the high consumption class of tobacco:
with this exception, such subjects are not overrepresented in the higher
consumption classes. It seems, therefore, that anxiety-provoking conditions in childhood are much more harmful than the death of one
parent. When the sons of mothers who died early in the childhood of the
subjects show a higher percentage of strong cigarette consumers we may
assume that the early loss of the mother still produces considerable
trauma in our society, and that cigarette consumption represents a legal
way of trying to overcome the oral frustration linked to it.

The socio-psychological findings have indicated that alcoholism and
other drug dependencies are also correlated with sociological circumstances (Wieser 1972, 1973). In a pilot-study on 2558 patients (Battegay
et al., 1975 a, b, c) who came in the year 1968 to the Basle Psychiatric
University Out-Patient Clinic we found that the alcoholics among them
came significantly more frequently from a densely populated area
($p < 0.01$). Drug dependents showed an inverse spread, these patients
coming significantly more frequently from a region of low population
($p < 0.01$). This corresponded to findings previously reported by
Kielholz and Battegay (1967), showing that among alcoholics representatives of lower, and among drug-dependents of higher, socioeconomic classes were overrepresented.

We can see, therefore, that alcoholism and drug dependencies are not
only symptoms of the individual, but also symptoms of the social
surroundings. We may view in this context the drinking habits which
occur in our culture and which are so resistant to change, and the
prejudices which exist towards non-drinking people and towards new
drinking habits. These are not only accidental manifestations but
certainly also the result of general flight- and false autotherapy tendencies. The members of our society very often suffer from problems of
communication following fear of contact, fear of judgement and of
prejudices by other people, introversion, and the reduction of verbal
capacities as a result of permanent passive perception of mass media.

Alcohol helps them to loosen their tongues. Such individuals, by drinking, lose inhibitions and are able to enter into contact with other people.

When we consider that in the 31 Swiss military schools in which 4082 20-year-old recruits were examined, 89.6 per cent had experience with alcohol, 45.6 per cent with cigarettes and 23.0 per cent with drugs, and that 72.5 per cent reported up to 50 or more drunken bouts in their lives, we can say that the motive of solving reality problems by drinking alcohol, taking drugs, or smoking is not only an isolated problem of some individuals, but spreads throughout a considerable portion of the population.

As Glatt and Hills (1968) report, in a study of drinking habits of teenagers aged 15–20, carried out in 1960 and 1961 by postgraduate students of the Public Health Department of the London School of Hygiene and Tropical Medicine, 6 per cent of the total (630 boys, 480 girls) had taken alcohol by the age of 10, and 90 per cent of both sexes had done so by the age of 15. This number corresponds closely with that found by us in military schools. These numbers also suggest that the use of alcohol is a phenomenon which characterises almost all members of our society. Furthermore we found that the earlier the examined individuals began to drink, to smoke or to take drugs the higher was the risk that they would have a high alcohol-, tobacco- or drug consumption (Battegay and Mühlemann 1973; Battegay *et al.*, 1975a, b).

In a study by Weidmann *et al.* (1973) with Basle school boys of 16–20 years ($n = 1\,733$) 26 per cent reported experiences with different drugs (cannabis, hallucinogens, amphetamines, opiates, glue-sniffing). These numbers also indicate that drug use and abuse is a problem not only of the individual but of the whole society.

We have also to bear in mind that at the present time juveniles are always confronted with different norms within the various groups in which they have to live—the family, the school class, the sports team, leisure group etc. No longer are all groups of society submitted to one traditional norm: each group has its own norm, and juveniles are always in middle of a conflict of such norms.

It has to be taken into account that at the present time many young people will, as children, have received from their parents all the material pleasures which they wanted. They were "orally spoiled" and consequently expect that during their whole life they will always receive more oral pleasure. When they enter society, already in the higher school classes, and they have to fulfil more and more of the demands of society, they may try to escape from this urging outside reality by taking drugs.

Both those who take alcohol and those who take drugs—and many juvenile drug-users also take alcohol—build up a world of illusions in which they believe that they enter into closer contact with other human beings. They are not conscious of the fact that in their intoxicated state they cannot overcome their communication difficulties and cannot build a bridge over the space which separates them from other human beings through the use of alcohol or other drugs.

Since, therefore, the causes of the development of drug and alcohol dependencies are to be sought not only in the individual himself but also in the immediate and distant surroundings, it is clear that we cannot only treat these patients as isolated human beings. We also have to consider their social context. We should not therefore use only an individual approach; we have also to reach the patients within a social framework.

In spite of the fact that it is principally indicated that the patient should be left as long as possible in his natural surroundings it is not often possible to withdraw alcohol and drugs with the patients remaining in their family or in a substitute milieu. This is not only because physical dependency hinders the elimination of drug-taking when the patient is not treated in a hospital with well-trained staff, but also because the environment at home may reinforce drinking and drug taking habits. It may, therefore, be necessary to take the patients out of their usual surroundings, at least for a certain time. Especially for alcoholics it is almost impossible for them to stay in their old environment and to terminate their alcohol drinking because their acquaintances attempt to keep them in their role as alcoholics. It is necessary to lead the patient to a full alcohol abstinence (Battegay, 1966; Kielholz and Battegay, 1967; Wieser, 1972, 1973) and this cannot be attained if the patient remains in his usual environment at the beginning of the treatment. The alcoholic can generally not remain a moderate drinker. The first glass is in general the first step on the way to loss of control which leads shortly to inebriation and ultimately to a relapse to alcoholism. Also when psychotherapy is combined with medical treatment, e.g., with a treatment by disulfiram (Antabus), calcium–carbamide–citrate (Dipsan) or metronidazole (Flagyl) the treatment should be commenced in a hospital setting, because of possible initial somatic complications (side effects).

It is, in principle, possible to arrange for part-time hospitalization, with patients being taken to night or day clinics, to clubs where they can gather together, and to voluntary associations such as Alcoholics Anonymous. When we want to take young drug dependents out of their milieu we have to try to admit them into special departments of general hospitals or psychiatric in-patient institutions. Very often, however, it is not easy to hold them, with their manifold adaptation difficulties, within an ordered environment. They frequently disturb the hospital atmosphere and tend to smuggle drugs into the institution. Because of this it is useful to have special facilities such as 'Drop-ins' and communities in which a treatment program is fulfilled with the young drug dependents in a specially tolerant atmosphere. On the one hand, with this approach they can continue to live in their own subculture and, on the other hand, they can be trained to live without their drugs.

The growing number of juveniles being commited for trial for drug offences (see Table 2) not only shows an increase of juvenile drug abuse in Switzerland but also the more pointed reaction of society. It indicates too that prohibitive measures are not able, by themselves, to prevent the spread of drug use.

Table 2 Number of persons being prosecuted because of an offence against the narcotic law in Switzerland

Year	No. of prosecutions
1966	16
1967	11
1968	123
1969	367
1970	900
1971	2518
1972	3113
1973	3458
1974	5094

Therefore we should ask ourselves whether possibilities of experimenting with drugs should be created at special legalised institutions, authorised by the government where juveniles could take determined quantities of clean drugs under medical control. In this way they could be protected from criminal drug traffickers. They would not get addicted to drugs through the reinforcement effect of prohibitions and prejudices and they could enter in contact with the doctors.

Let us now come to the different special forms of psychotherapy of alcoholics and drug dependents. There are several forms of therapeutic technique between which we must differentiate.

THERAPEUTIC TECHNIQUES

INDIVIDUAL PSYCHOTHERAPY

Supportive psychotherapy

When we treat alcoholics and drug dependents we cannot approach them from the standpoint of a social norm and expect them to adapt unconditionally to the demands of society. Especially, we cannot take away their only source of support—the alcohol or the drugs (which are, of course, very doubtful supports)—without giving them by our therapy something that is able to lead them out of their distorted view of life. In psychotherapy, therefore, we have to consider that the drug dependents have not only to be lead away from their dependency but should also experience a participating human relationship.

It is important that the patients themselves are motivated for psychotherapy. It is scarcely possible to build up confidence in the doctor-patient relationship when the alcohol- or drug-dependent patient is not ready to cooperate. The treatment of alcoholics and drug dependents should be principally on a voluntary basis. Without the patient having at least a partial insight that his way of escaping reality is inappropriate, psychotherapy will be very difficult. Even then it is not easy to withdraw the patients from the alcohol or the drugs. Often only when they have suffered many recurrences or when they have been seriously ill (e.g. after recovering from a severe virus-hepatitis) will patients recognise that they reached a critical point in their life and that they have to make up their mind to leave the illusionary world of chronic alcohol or drug effects. It is not, however, always possible to base therapy on this voluntary participation by the patients. The self-destructive tendencies, the tendency to repeat their evasive patterns, their psychological and very often physical dependency hinders them from becoming sufficiently detached to gain the necessary insight into the deleterious aspects of their dependency. With patients being sent involuntarily to special treatment units, a prepsychotherapy phase will be necessary in which the staff have to prepare the patient for real psychotherapy, to create the confidence which opens up the patient to the doctor. In this initial prepsychotherapy phase it is inopportune to ask the patients about all details of their alcohol- or drug-abuse. The patients might feel such a procedure to be more like police procedure than a method that should create a solid relationship between the doctor and the patient.

Only when this atmosphere of confidence is created is a real psychotherapeutic approach possible. We have therefore to differentiate from the psychotherapeutic work a preparative state in which we try very delicately with these highly sensitive patients to give them a new appreciation of a meaningful human relationship.

Psychotherapy does not necessarily mean psychoanalysis. In fact, Fenichel (1945) observed that psychoanalytical work with addicts is difficult or even impossible before or shortly after withdrawal of the addictive substances. Their defence-mechanisms, their narcissistic personality disorders in the sense of a weak self assertion (Kohut, 1971), their distrust, their tendency towards correction of reality, their resignation and loss of tenacity, their insufficient staying power and their intolerance for frustrations make it very difficult, or even impossible, to maintain the necessary psychoanalytical distance. Therefore the psychotherapeutic approach cannot generally be an analytical one, especially not in a primary phase of psychotherapy, even when there is a neurotic basis for alcohol- or drug dependence. In examinations at the Basle Psychiatric University Hospital we saw that only 11.1 per cent of 207 drug dependents of the barbiturate type and only 4.1 per cent of 122 alcoholics were real neurotics (Kielholz and Battegay 1967). But independently of the question of whether the basis of the drug- or alcohol-abuse is a healthy personality, a psychopathic personality in the European sense (character disorder in the American sense), a conscious abnormal psychic development in the sense of Binder (1960) as it may occur after a chronic or intermittent stress situation, or a real neurosis, it is generally not possible for the patient to undergo analytical psychotherapy, especially not before or shortly after withdrawal. We have to accompany the patient through this difficult phase which comes after the withdrawal of alcohol and drugs, and we have to give support to the weak, or weakened, ego in encouraging him to make his mind up for a life without alcohol or drugs. In the beginning these patients will satisfy all their dependency needs in the contact with the therapist. It is important not to frustrate these individuals in this state. Only when the patients are allowed to experience these regressive needs in the relation with the therapist will they feel sure enough to make the first steps towards a new future. In this phase of psychotherapy we have to see the patient often. When he is still in hospital we have to let him come each day, for at least 15 minutes. When treated as an outpatient he should have the opportunity of seeing the doctor at least three times a week for 30 minutes. The patient must have the justified impression that he can always reach his doctor when he is confronted with problems. During the initial hospital stay only the beginning of psychotherapy can be done. Following the hospital treatment comes the more important psychotherapeutic aftercare which has to be done in addition and which must be coordinated with the after-care by a social worker. It is important that the psychotherapeutic methods do not end when the patient leaves the protected atmosphere of the hospital. It is especially necessary to have established a strong doctor–patient relationship when the previous alcohol-or drug-dependent encounters new difficulties and is in danger of flying to his old means of evasion of reality. With the possibility of finding understanding by the psychotherapist it is possible that he will remain away from alcohol and drugs. In this respect the therapist really becomes a valid substitute for alcohol and drugs. These patients must have a psychotherapeutic support over a long time-span.

Therefore alcoholics and drug dependents need in general a supportive-directive psychotherapeutic approach and not a psychoanalytical one. Directive does not mean that the doctor himself always behaves actively. It means only that he tries to avoid the frustrations which would be linked with analytical psychotherapy and that he tends to lead the psychotherapy not only by means of interpretation but also by means of pedagogic influence on the patients.

Psychotherapy of alcoholics and drug dependents always includes pedagogic measures. The psychotherapist has to help his patient to find his way in the social reality. As we have already stressed, the therapist will have to strengthen the often very weak ego of these patients so that they are better able to get over the stress situations and the frustrations of every-day life. The doctor has to give these individuals a supportive psychotherapy which includes practical pedagogic aspects concerning social learning processes.

In the literature the question appears repeatedly whether we can lead alcoholics to moderate, 'normal' drinking. We have to say that our experiences (which correspond to the majority of other authors) show that we have to insist upon total alcohol-abstinence by these individuals (Bleuler 1969). It is difficult, if not impossible, to teach the alcoholic to get acquainted with moderate drinking patterns. Similarly, as drug effects change personality—at least temporarily—in very disturbing ways, we cannot try to get the patient onto a moderate drug-taking regime. They have in general to stop totally with their drug intake. The Methadone maintenance treatment programs should be the exception when we have tried, in vain, other ways of treatment, because Methadone also implies a physical and psychological dependence which limits, in a dangerous way, human freedom.

Analytical psychotherapy

In some individual patients who really suffer from neuroses and who are motivated for psychotherapy we can try to approach them psychoanalytically. But it is absolutely necessary that the patients abstain from alcohol or drugs during a period of several months before they are taken in for psychoanalysis. Psychoanalytical treatment does not succeed when the patient has been under the effect of alcohol or drugs during this time.

We had the opportunity to observe a patient—a doctor—taking alcohol and drugs during a period of several years undergoing psychoanalysis. He had never ceased to take alcohol and hypnotics in an excessive manner. The analytical treatment did not succeed and he became deeper and deeper enmeshed in his drug-and alcohol-dependency. It progressed so far that he had to spend most of the time in a psychiatric hospital and there was a danger that he would never again be able to earn his living. But the doctors of the hospital did not give up their colleague and tried to help him, giving him the opportunity of remaining in contact with the outside world. A director of an out-patient clinic even gave him the chance of working there as a doctor. The patient suffered many relapses, but after several months, held by the supportive treatment of a psychiatrist and the moral support of the director of the out-patient clinic, he succeeded in overcoming his alcoholism and his drug use and could continue in his medical work and in the world.

The analytical work with alcohol- and drug-dependents is very difficult. Their oral fixation, their narcissistic deficiency in self-esteem and their secondary conditioning on avoiding frustrations and on seeking oral pleasures as well as self assertion from outside makes it difficult to treat these patients analytically. The technique must be in the beginning almost the same as we use with other alcohol- or drug dependents or with psychotics. Therefore initially we cannot be as frustrative with these patients as with other neurotics. We have to give them first the opportunity for reliving their regressive tendencies within the analytical situation, as is the case with all pregenital neuroses and with the narcissistic neuroses in the sense of Kohut (1971). Only when we have given them the opportunity to experience an acceptance on their regressive level will we have to go a step further to real analytical work. In the treatment of such a patient there is always the danger of an infinite analysis, as Freud has shown. Even when we enter into an analytical working through we have to help the alcoholic- or the drug-dependent to strengthen his ego and by this his will and his self-assertion. Considering these necessities in the analytical treatment of alcoholics and drug dependents we would say with Solms (1960), Bräutigam (1958) and other authors, that classical psychoanalysis has very often been disappointing in the field of alcohol- and drug-dependency. As we have stressed, many alcoholics and drug dependents are not able to bear frustrations and gain insight. Alcoholics are not seldom not differentiated enough, are not sufficiently able to use their brains and have also very often an insufficient capacity for verbalising their conflicts. As we and others have shown alcoholics come mostly from the lower socioeconomic classes and possess therefore only the verbal abilities of their social levels. We say also that psychoanalysis, which demands a high level of verbalisation, is in general not the most suitable method of treating these patients. It is only for a few alcoholics with neurotic conflicts and with good intelligence and the possession of a differentiated verbalisation, that psychoanalysis is indicated. Drug dependents are often too sensitive for psychoanalysis and not tolerant enough of the frustrations which are linked with this treatment even when we modify our method and give them much more affective support than in the classical procedure as it is recommended by Kohut (1971) with patients suffering from narcissistic disturbances, in spite of the fact that their intelligence and verbalisation-capacity would in general be high enough.

Hypnosis

J. H. Schultz (1952), Wallerstein (1957) and other authors have tried to treat certain alcoholics by hypnosis. We can say that hypnosis seems to be successful only in the case of passive dependent individuals who are motivated for treatment. Hypnosis was also tried in groups. By this group-hypnotherapy (Wallerstein, 1957) the effects of hypnosis could be reinforced by the group.

Behaviour therapy

For many authors alcoholism and drug dependence represent forms of conditioned behaviour. Therefore methods have been used of conditioning e.g. an aversion towards alcohol mainly with apomorphine. The patients always received, together with alcohol, an injection of apomorphine. This method was dropped by most of the treating centres because it was found to be very distressing not only for the patients, but also for the staff. Newer methods use other ways of conditioning or deconditioning. For example the patient is allowed to come to a bar where he can receive drinks and when he wants to take the glass he receives an electric shock. But all these methods which are related to behaviour theory do not profoundly change the personality of the drinker. They are based on the theory that, by a deconditioning of the pathological behaviour and by inhibition of the drinking pattern, the individual is able to develop himself into new dimensions.

PSYCHOTHERAPIES IN WHICH THE INDIVIDUAL IS SEEN
IN HIS SOCIAL CONTEXT

Group psychotherapy

At the Basle Psychiatric University Clinic we have taken alcoholics and drug-dependents in diagnostically mixed groups since 1955, and since

1957 in diagnostic homogeneous groups (Battegay, 1958). We have observed that these patients are much more amenable to treatment in a psychotherapeutic group than in a dual psychotherapy situation. The group gives these patients a bit of the security which they missed in their childhood or which they received in an overwhelming manner from their mothers. The group gives them a community in which they feel emotionally reborn. They feel also something of the security which often they could not experience in their childhood.

We observe in the group treatment of alcoholics and drug dependents that they often experience the group as a Great Mother (Neumann, 1956) who should support them, feed them and always understand them. But it is not only characteristic of alcoholics and drug dependents that they go through a regressive phase during group treatment. Other patients also behave, in the initial period of group treatment, in a regressive manner. The group activates infantile patterns on the transference level. However, the drug users and the alcoholics tend to be fixed in a regressive relationship towards the group. They become really dependent on the group. We think, however, that this group de-pendence should not be hindered by the therapist, since it may replace drug and alcohol dependence. We see that patients can be approached by group psychotherapy who were not to be reached by individual psychotherapy. The group gives them, because of the reinforcement effect of the group on the emotions of the participants, the possibility of going through a much deeper regression than in individual psychotherapy. The feelings of the different members influence each other in such a way that all are touched and activated emotionally by them. Flight away from these group emotions is almost impossible, since the colleagues in the group tend to break resistance. Rationalizations do not help, whereas in individual psychotherapy of drug dependents and alcoholics we are often confronted with a whole system of defence mechanisms which cannot be questioned because emotions do not get the same intensity as in the group. But it is true that, for these patients, the group as a whole becomes a mother, of whom they expect an unconditional approval and support.

At the Basle Psychiatric University Hospital, we ran a group of middle-aged women who had partly drunk too much, partly abused analgesics of hypnotics together with alcohol. After long initial difficulties they cooperated generally very well, some for more than 10 years (1957–1967), but after we had to stop the group treatment because of outside reasons, most of the participants relapsed into alcohol- or drug-abuse. Thus, we recognized that we would have to accompany these patients throughout a long period of their life if we wanted to help them decisively. We cannot foresee when we could end group treatment with them. Indeed, we have to be aware of the fact, that group therapy of all kind of dependents tends to last indefinitely, as Freud (1961) has described it as a danger for individual analysis. But I think that in respect to these patients we have indeed to accompany them and to give them a constant support over a long length of time in such a way that they can bear the frustrations of the outside world.

Not only in the named hospital group, but also in a treatment group of alcoholics which we had in our Psychiatric Out-Patient Clinic, we observed that we can lead some patients, after we have fulfilled their regressive expectations for a certain time, slowly to take over some responsibilities for themselves and other patients. They become spontaneously, from time to time, into the position of a co-therapist, giving the other patients advice, asking them about their conflicts and showing them that they themselves have problems. The behaviour as a co-therapist helps them in the sense of "noblesse oblige". They slowly acquire more ego-strength.

Other patients remain over a longer time deep in their regression. In the group, they often speak in a most disapproving way of their wives, of the surroundings, of society etc. Often, they repeat these accusations almost in a stereotyped manner. Other patients also adopt this tone and bring their own resentments against the frustrative family or other groups of the environment. We can have, session after session, cathartic abreactions of hostile feelings towards the surroundings. In general, we ask them after some sessions if they think that all their failure is caused by their relatives and the surroundings. In general, the alcoholics and the drug dependents recognize, at this moment at least a little of their projection-tendencies and begin to think over their own attitudes and expectations: but also, at this point they wish to have their problems solved by the therapist. On the one hand, we have to give them, in their regressive needs and their resentments against a frustrating world, a comprehension almost without borders, on the other hand we have to train them to be able to bear frustrations.

We can also reach, with alcoholics and drug dependents, a stage at which they become ready for insight. Even in this phase, however, they will never renounce their regressive needs. It is still more difficult to come to the next phase of development, that of change of attitudes and behaviour patterns. We even observed that alcoholics praised drinking in a group session which activated their emotions shortly after they had expressed before the session that they would never touch a glass of alcohol again. They drunk the non-alcoholic apple-juice offered to them as if it were wine. In this group of hospitalised men, which was formed only by alcoholics and which we led for more than 10 years, we always offered non-alcoholic beverages—and small cigars—in order to show them that we did not only want to take something away from them, but wanted to replace the alcohol by less dangerous beverages (Battegay, 1958; 1966).

Drug dependents also need (as our experience with a group of juvenile drug-users in our Psychiatric Out-Patient Department since 1971 shows) an affective support by the group before they can renounce on the drugs. In the beginning, the participants still took their drugs before they came to the sessions, or even during the sessions. Only when they experienced contact with the two leaders, a young doctor and a social worker, as well as with the co-patients, did they slowly start to avoid taking drugs, apparently because they recognized that the drugs disturbed their possibilities of contact with other human beings.

We further observed that the young drug users could learn within the framework of the group to gain social experience and to go through a social learning process. They recognized in this group, that not all adults behave in the repressive manner they expected, and that the two representatives of society, the doctor and the social worker, are also human beings, with whom it is possible to enter in contact.

It appeared that the young drug dependents, mainly cannabis-, amphetamine-, LSD-, mescaline- and opiate-abusers, were mostly disturbed in the field of communications. Often they could not enter spontaneously into contact with others. They had high passive expectations towards the leaders but could not contribute actively to the group process. Often they waited until the moderators began to speak and to activate them. In the early days of our experience, we were astonished to recognize how much most of these participants respected the authority of the therapist and of other representatives of society. In the group discussions we got the impression that the young drug-users are not at all asocial or even antisocial. They seemed to us to be hindered bourgeois who were not able to bear the frustrations usually linked with social life. They did not have enough criticism towards authority, towards the therapist, and because of this fact, they had to suffer many frustrations, which they could not bear. As a sign of their intolerance towards frustrations it may be mentioned that two members who had had a quarrel with one another did not appear for the next session. Some of the participants avoided injections of amphetamine and of opiates after some sessions of the therapeutic group. Some of them were totally abstinent, others still smoked cannabis.

All the participants were very eager to make coffee together with the moderators, and even to pay the expenses. The oral pleasure linked with the coffee seemed to be a common denominator which facilitated the identification of the group members with each other. This identification process was, as we have described it, in the beginning not easy. They lived initially in a mass-existence, without link to the others. Only step by step, partly also by the common preparing and drinking of coffee, they became a group with cohesive-centripetal forces.

The therapeutic group gives them at least some of the emotions which they did not have in their past and which they need so much. As we have mentioned, it gives them a Great Mother (Neumann, 1956) and even a surrogate of a real mother. In this maternal milieu, they can on the one hand recognize their early frustrations, and on the other hand receive emotional support. In the first stages of group psychotherapy with drug- and alcohol-abusers, we have indeed to feed them, to give them emotional support. This state may last more than one year. Most impressive is the fact that in the beginning the participation in the group is very irregular. We always see other participants. This symptom we would like to call the 'revolving stage phenomenon' of the initial phase of group psychotherapy of alcoholics and drug dependents. In general, it lasted several months of weekly sessions of $1\frac{1}{2}$ hours, until the participation became more constant.

From these descriptions of group psychotherapy it is clear that it is impossible to work in a purely analytical way with drug dependents and alcoholics. These patients are not able to bear the frustrations linked with analytical therapy and they are also therefore initially not able to work the conflicts through and to gain insight. Signs of regression can be seen much more often than in groups with common neurotics. In these

groups we can learn how much these patients demand to be supported
by the outside world and how much they are dependent on other human
beings. Indeed, they tend almost to swallow persons who are devoted to
them.

After this long initial phase we may reach a state in which the patients
themselves take responsibilities, helping, as described, to make coffee for
the others, and finding solutions for their problems and the conflicts of
the others. Often, however, they want very soon to get praise for the
responsibilities they have taken over. They want a narcissistic support.
Since they are not tolerant of frustrations, the working through in this
state is also very difficult. Thus, the therapeutic group composed of drug
dependents or alcoholics cannot work in the same way as with common
neurotics, for again and again some members of the group or the group
as a whole come into a state in which they need emotional support. In
these moments, they are not able to work their conflicts seriously
through. Group psychotherapy with drug dependents and alcoholics
means therefore not purely analytical work though using analytical
knowledge. It must be a more supportive, directive treatment, in the
sense that the therapists always have to intervene when they recognize
that the participants come to the borderline of their tolerance for
frustrations.

Practicing group psychotherapy with drug- and alcohol-dependents,
we also come to the problem of counter-transference of the therapist. In
the treatment of these patients who tend to demonstrate such a degree of
regression, there is always the danger—especially for young
therapists—that they become too leader-centered and, because of their
own compensatory unconscious needs, consider the group-members
more as children needing parental leadership than as patients. It may
happen that the leader feels too well in the group. From our control of
young group therapists and from our own training period, we know
that the therapist may experience unconsciously a group of young drug
dependents as undeveloped sides of himself or of his own children,
brothers or sisters, etc. This means that the therapist may identify too
much with the group and lose the distance necessary for treating this
kind of patient. With alcoholics, this identification of the therapist with
the patients cannot in general be so strong. They generally come to
treatment in a much later state and, as an effect of chronic alcohol abuse,
they are much more hollow in their emotions than the young drug

dependents. The doctors who treat these patients must know that they exercise a very strong appeal on the paternalistic or maternalistic needs of the therapists as well as on own desires which could not be lived enough in the therapist's life. Group psychotherapy, especially with drug dependents and alcoholics, demands of the therapist that he is able to control his own unconscious needs, his counter-transference. In spite of the fact that these groups cannot be led on an entirely analytical basis, the therapists need analytical formation and knowledge to get aware of the strong dependency needs of the patients and of his own unconscious tendencies which are activated in the contact with these groups.

Family therapy

Especially in the case of alcoholics we observe that the treatment often cannot be effective unless the whole family is included in the therapy. The individual who drinks is often only a symptom of an unbalanced family (Balint, 1963). Family therapy gives us the possibility of incorporating more than one member of the relationship at the same time, but often we cannot cooperate with the relatives for external reasons. They are often not all prepared to come to a therapy session. However, we have observed that we can bring about some change in a family living quietly at the cost of the alcoholic. In this case, we have to recognize the pseudo-equilibrium of the family and help the patient to come out of the role of the black sheep. In other family situations, we shall have to seek for a sedation of the family and by this to take care that the patient loses the guilt feelings which reinforce drinking. Our personal experience with family therapy of alcoholics is very modest. It is perhaps easy to send for the wife of a drinking man, but it is more difficult to reach the husband of a drinking woman. It is still more difficult to have the cooperation of other relatives.

In one family, the very dominating woman drank quietly at home. Her daughter had had some schizophrenic attacks. The son suffers from a very severe neurosis. The father has nothing to say at home. He only brings the money home. Since this mother was also keeping the whole family group orally captive, we sought in family therapy—which we led together with another doctor and a social worker—to motivate her for a half-time job as a waitress in the alcohol free canteen of a factory. We thought, that she would then be able to live her oral tendencies partly in the contact with the persons she served. At the same time, the other members of the family would be more free. Indeed, she could spread her maternal desires over the new occupational milieu, and the family members had the opportunity to develop more freedom. Especially the schizophrenic daughter learned to be more active, even to work half days in her profession. But after some weeks our patient abandoned her occupation and remained again at home. It was now again more difficult for the rest of the family to feel free and to take its responsibilities.

Often, however, it is not possible to bring the family together. We therefore have to seek for other methods in order to come into contact with family members. Our experiences with a group of spouses of alcoholics have shown us that they are more than ready to come together in a group. It became openly apparent how these women fight for their husbands. They are like mothers who know about all the possible difficulties of their husbands and want to protect them. It became also evident that perhaps this tendency to over-protection may provoke the husbands to turn into opposition and to drink still more. We therefore have to work through with these spouses of alcoholics their overwhelming tendencies to care in a maternal way for their husbands.

It was, as already mentioned, much more difficult to gather the husbands of alcoholic women. They had enough with one session in which they explained, mostly in a very distant manner, how their wives drank. The husbands of alcoholic women patients were almost never so cooperative or motivated that they could be of great help to us and by this for their spouses.

Therapeutic community—Community therapy

If the drug dependents and the alcoholics are sent to an institution, it is important that they are in a department which is organized as a therapeutic community (Jones, 1962; Basaglia, 1971). Between 1955 and 1957, we observed that drug dependents and alcoholics who were hospitalised in a ward of 20 to 25 patients, slowly learnt to take over responsibilities when they became motivated by the other patients. Therefore, it is important to organize the whole department in such a way that all members contribute to the administration of the ward.

Also if the patients remain in their surroundings, it is indicated to integrate them in a therapeutic community or at least in a therapeutic social club (Bierer, 1955). It is important for the alcoholics to have a support within the social frame of a group or a community, which facilitates them to overcome the frustrations of outside social life. In a therapeutic group of alcoholics at our psychiatric out-patient clinic, we can see that this circle allows them for the time they spend in the group to withdraw from the interactions in the outside and by this of the temptations and frustrations of society. Here, they get listeners and understanding, without coming in danger by alcoholic beverages. In this group, they also get, in a therapeutic-experimental form, social experience. If we may use an image, we would say that the therapeutic community or another group, for example a therapeutic social club, or as we have seen, a therapeutic group of out-patients may be a milieu of active immunisation against the danger of drinking. By this, we do not mean that these groups should always talk about alcohol. On the contrary. But we can observe that the patients learn with the help of the others to overcome more easily their own problems and the frustrations linked with the demands of a social environment. In the group treatment of young juvenile drug dependents, we have seen that we can mobilise social valencies which may lead on one hand to dependencies of the group but on the other hand let them even really overcome their drug abuse.

In 1971 we had the opportunity of observing a therapeutic community of juvenile drug dependents in Norway, in an institution linked to a State Hospital for Drug Dependents (Statens Klinikk for Narkomane, Hov i land, Director: Dr. Arnfinn Teigen). A number of 7 to 9 young boys and girls lived on a farm not too far from the hospital and had to carry out all the work concerning cattle and agriculture. Already the fact that the cows for example demanded regular milking seemed to have the effect to turn the community members away from the pleasure principle towards outside reality. Moreover, the experience of belonging to a community of which all have the same responsibility, enabled them to communicate with one another. There was no full-time doctor there, only a man who instead of entering the Army absolved a civil service, and acted as a part of the community. He did not behave as a leader but as one of the members. This really democratic community did not only help the participants to feel like human beings, but stimulated them also to see the responsibilities which are linked to community-life. When a problem was very acute and regularly every week, the chief of the hospital came and sat together with the community in a very informal way. They developed towards him and the other members of the community a real feeling of belonging.

Many similar trials have been done and most have shown good results. In the United States, too (Fischmann, 1968; Costello *et al.*, 1973, and others) the method of therapeutic community for rehabilitation of drug dependents seems to have at least more success in handling the different problems of drug addiction than the former way of "classical incarceration".

There should not, however, be only therapeutic communities created. The whole community of a certain region should recognize that the drug problem is not only the symptom of the persons involved in it, but also a symptom of the community and of society as a whole. Therefore, more stress is needed, to convince every community to develop programs to deal with the field of drug abusers (Costello *et al.*, 1973). These programs should seek new ways of approaching the drug abusers and new ways of prophylaxis. Methods of mental hygiene should be the responsibility of the whole community. Initially in the kindergarten, and later on in the schools and high-schools, the whole youth should be helped by offering them weekly regular sessions for working through their conflicts. When the community is really ready to encounter its juveniles with their problems in an open way, then one of the conditions of an effective prophylaxis of drug dependence is provided. Our effort has to begin very early and to include everyone who has to grow into society. The whole community must realise that we cannot only treat the symptom "drug dependence", but that we also have to recognize that real prophylaxis must begin with the readiness for confrontation with the problems of youth.

REFERENCES

Baden, M. M. (1970). Methadone related deaths in New York City, *Intern. J. Addict.*, **5**, 489

Balint, M. v. E. (1963). Psychotherapeutische Techniken in der Medizin. Huber/Klett: Bern (1963)

Basaglia, F. (ed.) (1971). Die negierte Institution oder die Gemeinschaft der Ausgeschlossenen. Ein Experiment der psychiatrischen Klinik in Görz. Aus dem Italienischen von Ascheri-Osterlow, Anneheide, Suhrkamp, Frankfurt a. Main

Battegay, R. (1958). Group therapy with alcoholics and analgesic addicts. *Int. J. Grouppsychother.* **8**, 428

Battegay, R. (1966) Neuere Aspekte der Genese und Behandlung des Alkoholismus. *Praxis* **55**, 185

Battegay, R., Rauchfleisch, V., Grafton von Schieffen, H. (1972). Soziooko mische Determinantes der Inanspruchnehme der Psychiatrischen Universitats Poliklinik Basel, Scloez. *Arch. Neurol. Neurochir. Psychiat.*, **111**, 67

Battegay, R. and Mühlemann, R. (1973). Pilot-Studie in einer Rekrutenschule betreffend Alkoholkonsum, Drogenerfahrungen und Rauchergewohnheiten. *Schweizer Archiv. für Neurol., Neurochirurg. und Psychiat.*, **113**, 109

Battegay, R., Mühlemann, R., and Zehnder, R. (1975a). Comparative investigations of the abuse of alcohol, drugs, and nicotine for a representative group of 4082 men of age 20. *Compreh. Psychiat.* **16**, 247

Battegay, R., Mühlemann, R., Zehnder, R., and Dillinger, A. (1975b). Erheburg (1975). 31 Rekrutenschulen über den Alkohol-, Tabak- und Drogenkonsum. *Bull. Eidg. gesundheitsamt Beilage*, **21**, 6

Bierer, T. (1955) Die therapeutischen Social Clubs. *Z. Psychotherapy* **5**, 58

Binder, H. (1960) Die psychopathischen Dauerzustande und die abnormen seelischen Reaktionen und Entwicklungen, In *Psychiatric der gegenwart* **2**, 180 (Springer: Berlin/Gottingen/Heidelberg)

Bleuler, E. (1969) Lehrbuch der Psychiatric, II Aufl., umgear beitet von Bleuber, M. (Springer: Berlin/Heidelberg/New York)

Bloom, W. A. and Sudderth, E. W. (1970). Methadone in New Orleans; patients problems and police. *Intern. J. of the Addict.*, **5**, 465

Bräutigam, W. (1958). Psychotherapie bei Süchtigen. *Nervenarzt*, **10**, 445

Costello, R. M., Bechtel, T. E. and Giffen, M. B. (1973) A Community's Efforts to Attack the Problem of Alcoholism II Base Rate Data for Future Program Evaluation. *Intern. J. Addict*, **8**, 875

Davis, E. P. (1970). The Man Alive Programme: *Int. J. Addict.*, **5**, 421

Dole, V. P. (1970). Research on Methadone maintenance treatment. *Intern. J. Addict.*, **5**, 359

Fenichel, O. (1945). The Psychoanalytic Theory of Neuroses. Norton: New York

Fischmann, V. S. (1968). Drug addicts in a therapeutic community: Outline of the California rehabilitation center program, Corona. *Intern. J. Addict.* **3**, 351

Freedman, A. M., Zaks, A., Resnick, R. and Fink, M. (1970). Blockade with Methadone, Clyclazocine and Naloxone: *Intern. J. Addict.* **5**, 507

Freud, S. (1961). Die endliche und die unendliche Analyse. *In* "Gesammelte Werke" Vol. 16. Fischer: Frankfurt a. Main

Gearing, F. (1970). Evaluation of Methadone maintenance treatment program. *Intern. J. Addict.* **5**, 517

Glatt, M. M. and Hills, D. R. (1968). Alcohol abuse and alcoholism in the young. *Brit. J. Addict.* **63**, 183

Hoogerbeets, J. (1970). Methadone in Miami. *Intern. J. Addict.*, **5**, 499

Jaffe, J. H. (1970). Further experience with Methadone in the treatment of narcotics users. *Intern. J. Addict.*, **5**, 375

Jones, M. (1962). Social psychiatry, in the community, in hospitals and in prisons. Charles C. Thomas: Springfield

Kielholz, P. (1949). Behandlung des chronischen Alkoholismus mit Curéthyl. *Der Fürsorger* **17**, 46

Kielholz, P. (1962). Merkblatt für die Behandlung des chronischen Alkoholismus. *Bulletin des Eidg. Gesundheitsamtes* No. 6.

Kielholz, P. (1964). Erfahrungen in der Schweiz. *In*: "Sucht und Missbrauch" (Laubenthal, F. ed.) Georg Thieme: Stuttgart

Kielholz, P. (1965). Chronischer Alkoholismus und Alkoholpsychosen. *In*: "Psychiatrische Pharmakotherapie in Klinik und Praxis" (Kielholz, P. ed.) Hans Huber: Bern

Kielholz, P. (1971). Diagnostik und Therapie der Depressionen für den Praktiker. Lehmanns 3. vollständig überarbeitete Aufl., München

Kielholz, P. and Battegay, R. (1967). Vergleichende Untersuchungen über die Genese und den Verlauf der Drogenabhängigkeit und des Alkoholismus. *Schweiz. med. Wschr.*, **97**, 89 und 944

Kielholz, P., Battegay, R. and Mühlemann, R. (1973). Alkohol und Verkehr. *Schweiz. med. Wschr.*, **103**, 21

Kleber, H. (1970). The New Haven Methadone maintenance program. *Intern. J. Addict.* **5**, 449

Knowles, R., Lahiri, S. and Anderson, G. (1970) Methadone maintenance in St. Louis. *Intern. J. Addict.*, **5**, 407

Kohut, H. (1971). The Analysis of the Self. Int. University Press: New York

Kolton, M. S., Dosher, A. and Dwarshuis, L. (1972). Community drug-abuse programs for youth: A conceptual model. *Internat. J. Addict.*, **7**, 333

Langrod, J. (1970). A bibliography of the methadone maintenance treatment of heroin addiction. *Intern. J. Addict.* **5**, 581.

Martin, W. R. (1970). Commentary on the Second National Conference on Methadone Treatment. *Intern. J. Addict.*, **5**, 545

Maslansky, R. (1970). Methadone maintenance programs in Minneapolis. *Intern. J. Addict.*, **5**, 391

Mühlemann, R. und Battegay, R. (1975) Inkonsistenz in der Beautwortung eines Fragebogens über Alkohol-, Nikotin- und Drogenkonsum. Ausmass der dadurch bedington Vertzenung der gesamtresultate. *Z. Prao. Med.*, **20**, 19–20

Neumann, E. (1956). Die Grosse Mutter. Rhein-Verlag: Zürich

Schultz, J. H. (1952). Hypnosetechnik. Piscator: Stuttgart

Solms, H. (1960). Die Behandlung der akuten Alkoholvergiftung und der akuten und chronischen Formen des Alkoholismus. *In*: "Psychiatrie der Gegenwart", Vol. 2. Springer: Berlin

Trussel, R. E. (1970). Treatment of narcotic addicts in New York City. *Intern. J. Addict.*, **5**, 347

Wallerstein, R. S., Chotlos, J. W., Friend, M. B., Hammersley, B. W.,

Perlswig, E. A. and Winship, G. M. (1957). Hospital treatment of alcoholism. Basic Books: New York

Weidmann, M., Ladewig, D., Faust, V., Gastpar, M., Heise, H., Hobi, V., Mayer-Boss, Sybille and Wyss, P. (1973). Drogengebrauch von Basler Schülern—ein Beitrag zur Epidemiologie. *Schweiz. med. Wschr.* **103**, 121

Wieland, W. F., and Chambers, C. D. (1970). Two methods of utilizing Methadone in the outpatient treatment of narcotic addicts. *Intern. J. Addict.*, **5**, 431

Wieser, S. (1972). Psychotherapie und Sozialtherapie des Alkoholismus. *In*: "Psychiatrie der Gegenwart", Vol. 2. Springer: Berlin

Wieser, S. (1973). Das Trinkverhalten der Deutschen. Nicolai: Herford

Williams, H. R. (1970). Low and high Methadone maintenance in the outpatient treatment of the hard core heroin addict. *Intern. J. Addict.*, **5**, 439

Zurukzoglu, S. (1963). Ist Trunksucht eine Krankheit? Beih. z. Alkoholfrage in der Schweiz. Benno Schwabe: Basel

CHAPTER 8

New and innovative techniques in the treatment of drug abuse

P. G. BOURNE

INTRODUCTION

Treatment of drug abuse has in the last several years grown to involve a wide variety of new concepts and approaches. Until relatively recently, there were in the United States four major treatment modalities: longterm hospitalization, methadone maintenance, therapeutic communities, and detoxification with methadone or other pharmacological agents followed by outpatient counseling. There was heavy emphasis on the use of professionally trained personnel to provide the treatment, and also a strong orientation towards a basically medical model.

Part of the motivation for the continuing search for new techniques is tied to a belief by some people that drug abuse in the final analysis can be found to be attributable to a single cause, and that somewhere there is a single treatment technique, which, if discovered, would be the answer to all the problems of drug abuse.

Few experienced workers in the field would admit to sharing this belief. However, this thinking has been pervasive through most of the drug abuse literature. The second motivation for the research for any new treatment techniques came from a frustration felt by many people with the present approaches. Methadone maintenance, in particular, failed to fulfill its earlier promises, and to a certain extent, the same was true with therapeutic communities. There has also been increasing recognition that the problems of drug abuse are not homogenous, but are symptoms associated with a wide variety of causes and human problems. Therefore, treatment for individuals involved with drugs needed to offer not only two or three approaches, but also a wide variety of modalities geared to highly specific needs that go beyond merely dealing with a person's propensity to consume drugs. In the search to find modalities that would be new and innovative, a number of key requirements for any new treatment approach have been defined:

(a) that it be more acceptable to patients and community groups;
(b) that it have a higher success rate than previous modalities;
(c) that it be cheaper to carry out than existing modalities;
(d) that it meet the special needs of certain addict subgroups;
(e) that it is more adaptable to the changing patterns of drug abuse in the country than present approaches.

For a new modality to have any validity, it should meet at least one of these criteria. Some new approaches to treatment relate specifically to the issue of drug abuse, and are methodologies which result in a resolution of the drug using behavior itself, or its medical side-effects such as new approaches to detoxification. Other modalities which are considered new or innovative deal with broader social rehabilitative issues, which are less specific for the drug abuser but which are of particular consequence to the drug using individual because he must overcome them if he is to become a recovered and functioning member of society again. With these latter techniques, which are not of exclusive value only to drug addicts, it is to be hoped in the long run that they may be of value to a variety of individuals, particularly the mentally ill, for whom the same rehabilitative needs exist. Because of the heavy emphasis and concern with drug abuse in recent years, and the availability of federal support, a unique opportunity exists in the drug abuse area to develop and refine these general rehabilitative techniques which then can be subsequently applied much more broadly to the entire social service field.

Although we talk about 'new treatment techniques' much of what is put in this category does not strictly fit into this definition. In fact, it is probably more accurate to consider three distinct categories:

1. Completely new techniques used exclusively for treatment of drug abuse such as the development of new antagonist drugs;
2. Treatment techniques that have been available for some time and applied to other medical or psychological conditions, but which are now for the first time being applied to the field of drug abuse. This includes acupuncture, hypnosis, biofeedback, transcendental

meditation and Darvon-N, as well as a number of other methods
that are currently being used with addicts;

3 New techniques which represent no new technology but instead
   are a new approach to the delivery of treatment services. This
   category includes Health Maintenance Organizations, and many
   of the programs geared to meeting the needs of certain special
   populations.

Although these distinctions may not seem consequential, they do help
to underscore the fact that there are very few, if any, completely new
and revolutionary approaches to drug abuse treatment that have been
developed in recent years. Instead, the primary issue is how best to apply
and make accessible the knowledge and techniques we already have
available so as to maximize the impact and efficacy of our treatment
efforts.

EVALUATION OF NEW TECHNIQUES

Many of the newer techniques and approaches to treatment were
generated by the intense enthusiasms of people in various programs
around the world to meet the perceived needs of their clients. Many of
those who developed these projects did not have any training in research
or evaluative techniques. Acceptance of the new approach by the
community they serve, and the apparent success of a certain percentage
of the patients they treated is in many instances enough to convince these
individuals that what they are doing was worthwhile. Often they have
little interest in collecting data for formal scientific analysis. For their
needs, there is little reason to expend large amounts of their limited and
precious time and resources on evaluation as long as general local
acceptance of the technique continues.

   Lack of data and limited concern with evaluation proves to be a major
problem in assessing the efficacy of many of these approaches. In some
instances, it is impossible to determine adequately whether a specific
technique is efficacious or not, merely because there is insufficient data on
which to make any definitive determination. Too often therefore, one is
forced to make judgments based on one's own experience, and what
limited data is available as to whether a technique validly accomplishes

what is claimed for it. Every attempt has to be made to allow for the overwhelming enthusiasm of some program operators for their technique which is no substitute for hard data.

The problems in obtaining data are attributable to a number of factors. New treatment techniques are by definition inherently 'new' and, as a result, many programs have been in operation for very short periods of time and have no follow-up or outcome data. This is particularly true in the case of acupuncture and some of the newer pharmacological techniques. In some instances, adequate preparations have been made to perform the follow-up studies and time alone is all that is needed for an adequate evaluation to be performed. A second problem is that those operating some of the innovative programs lack the professional background or knowledge to understand either the need for evaluation or the appropriate methodology. In some instances, there is the sense that the ability to sell a program by generating local enthusiasm is an adequate substitute for outcome research. Also in a few instances one has the sense that those running programs fear evaluation and outcome studies and are determined to thwart any attempt to critically examine the efficacy of what they are doing. An additional difficulty is that many of the techniques, particularly in the social rehabilitative area, are not amenable to traditional evaluation methodology. The procedures in such techniques as nutritional therapy or certain special job training programs are hard to define and outcomes are difficult to quantify. It is unlikely that it will ever be possible to perform an adequate scientific evaluation in some of these areas and we remain dependent on our own best subjective assessment.

Certain areas have been approached with a greater emphasis on scientific method than others. Biofeedback, for instance, had physiological measurement built in as one assessment parameter and investigators using this modality are generally well versed in research methodology. Similarly, this is the case for the more medically based treatment modalities including the pharmacological approaches to treatment. As one gets into areas such as acupuncture and transcendental meditation this is less true, and the social rehabilitative areas are frequently devoid of any emphasis on research methodology.

One of the most glaring needs in the entire area of new treatment techniques is for more and better evaluative studies and the development of assessment tools which can be uniformly applied across a spectrum of treatment modalities. Too often the consensus appears to be that an approach appears to have tremendous potential but there is no way of scientifically documenting a subjective impression. There is some concern that lack of adequate studies will be interpreted as meaning that a given technique is not effective when, in fact, this is not the case. Additional carefully designed studies to produce definitive data should therefore be a top priority for this entire field.

CONCEPTUALIZATION OF NEW TREATMENT TECHNIQUES

The more recent developments in the drug abuse treatment field can be conceptualized in a number of ways. One approach is to look at those treatments that relate specifically to the physiological aspects of addiction, and those that relate to social rehabilitation. Particularly in the physiological area there are certain natural clusterings which can help provide understanding of the interrelationship between different approaches.

Probably the most interesting and significant new developments are in the physiological area. Some individuals would argue that these techniques have specific neurological effects on a 'craving' center in the hypothalamus. Viewed schematically, these approaches can be considered to be on a continuum according to their specificity of action in the brain as shown in the following diagram.

Heroin maintenance → Methadone maintenance → Darvon-N → Apormorphine →

Propanalol → Acupuncture → Electrosleep →

Biofeedback → Hypnosis → Meditation

Heroin, or other drug maintenance, can be considered the most specific approach for drug seeking behavior for that particular substance. Other pharmacological approaches as one proceeds along the continuum are of gradually decreasing specificity. Acupuncture is no longer a pharmacological agent, but is an external agent with apparently specific neurophysiological effects. Biofeedback and electrosleep represent a further decrease in specificity with basically self-induced physiological changes with the aid of external influences. Hypnosis and meditation represent further progressions to the point where the individual by himself is inducing body changes that may alter his drug seeking behavior.

The last four approaches, acupuncture, biofeedback, hypnosis and meditation and to some extent electrosleep, may be considered together as a cluster, because of the apparent relative similarity of their mechanisms of action. All presumably have a relaxing or other anxiety relieving effect which may to varying degrees induce biochemical changes in the brain and more specifically in the hypothalamus.

ACUPUNCTURE

The use of acupuncture in the treatment of addiction is a relatively new event and represents the application of a very old treatment technique to a new condition. The recent use of acupuncture in the treatment of addiction dates from the work of Dr. H. L. Wen in Hong Kong in 1972 (Wen and Cheung, 1973). Dr. Wen successfully alleviated withdrawal symptoms in a series of forty heroin and opium addicts, treated on an inpatient basis over periods ranging from one to three weeks. Wen's technique involves applying acupuncture needles to the 'lung' points of the ears, and then attaching to the needles an electro-stimulator which provides stimulation for periods of approximately thirty minutes. This procedure rapidly alleviates withdrawal symptoms and, although it has to be repeated with steadily decreasing frequency over a period of several days, it appears to be very effective in maintaining the patients in a state of relative comfort.

The patients described a general sense of well being while undergoing the treatment. They rapidly became less lethargic, ceased to crave narcotics, and generally felt relaxed but alert. After 10 to 15 minutes of stimulation, lacrimation had ceased, their noses stopped running, and there was relief from other symptoms such as aching limbs, wheezing, cramps in the stomach, cold sensation, and irritability. Interestingly, there was increased thirst and urination during treatment suggesting that the stimulation has a diuretic effect.

Between treatments they were less drowsy, more alert, and increasingly involved with their surroundings. Although the withdrawal symptoms returned periodically, it was with steadily diminishing frequency, with in general, a greater overall freedom from discomfort than with the more traditional pharmacological withdrawal procedures. While it is difficult to determine for certain the exact level of addiction or tolerance that these patients had, it is estimated that in general their daily use of heroin substantially exceeded that of the average heroin addict in the United States. Although the overwhelming majority of Dr. Wen's patients were Chinese men, two patients were occidental, one of them a woman.

Although the evidence is convincing that the patients treated by Wen experienced a substantial alleviation in their withdrawal symptoms, there is by Wen's own account no solid data yet to determine what the long-term recidivism rate is with these addicts. At present, Wen and his team are planning to conduct a careful follow-up and outcome study with those patients who have been through his program in the last two years.

ACUPUNCTURE IN THE UNITED STATES

Awareness of Dr. Wen's work with heroin addicts occurred in the United States at about the same time that the general awakening of interest in acupuncture as a medical procedure took place. A number of individuals, particularly in San Francisco and Los Angeles, became interested in using the procedure; however, there was considerably more intellectual enthusiasm than actual practice with a number of individuals using acupuncture on a few patients largely to satisfy their own curiosity and then not pursuing it. The key programs that have been identified as involving a substantial ongoing effort are the following:

At Lincoln Hospital in New York a program has been operating since February 1974 under the direction of Dr. Michael Smith. Since that time they have treated over 200 patients using Wen's technique. Although they report 80–90 per cent success in alleviating withdrawal symptoms, they have no hard data on follow-up with their patients (Smith, 1973).

Others in the United States who have used acupuncture with at least a few patients, include Dr. J. Bradshaw at the Palister Lodge Clinic in Detroit, Dr. Charles Becker at San Francisco General Hospital, Dr.

Joyce Lowinson at Beth Israel Hospital, Dr. Timothy Smith at the Center for Special Studies in San Francisco and Dr. Joseph Okimoto in Seattle.

Of particular significance is the work of Dr. Lester Sacks in Torrance, California, who has developed a substantial program using a variation of the standard acupuncture technique (Sacks, 1974). In an attempt to overcome the problem of the need for repeated treatment during the acute phase of withdrawal, Sacks developed the 'Staple-Puncture' technique, which while not technically acupuncture in the traditional sense, appears to use the same physiological mechanism for its effect. A surgical staple is placed in the ear and the patient is instructed to stimulate it by manipulation with his finger. The staple can safely be left in for up to three months, and periodic added effect can be obtained by using electrostimulation through staples in a manner similar to that used by Wen. Although follow-up data is lacking, Sacks has treated in excess of 100 patients with apparently at least short-term success in alleviating withdrawal symptoms.

Dr. Lorenz K. Ng who is responsible for coordinating acupuncture research at the National Institute on Drug Abuse, is one of the few people to have conducted basic research on acupuncture and electrostimulation as a treatment for addiction. He has been able to demonstrate significant attenuation of withdrawal symptoms in addicted rats by means of these techniques (Ng, 1974). He also is establishing a clinical research program for acupuncture and addiction at the Veteran's Administration Hospital in Washington, D.C.

OTHER ACUPUNCTURE PROGRAMS OUTSIDE THE UNITED STATES

Acupuncture has had considerable appeal as a treatment for addiction in a number of places outside the United States since Dr. Wen first received widespread publicity. Its appeal is based, firstly, on the fact that it is inexpensive. Although there is the assumption among workers in the United States that methadone or other pharmacological approaches are inexpensive, this is only true by American standards. Elsewhere in the world, the cost of methadone maintenance is regarded as prohibitive and even the cost of more traditional methods of detoxification are regarded as high. The second major attraction of acupuncture is that its use is culturally and philosophically compatible with many cultures, particularly those in the orient.

The largest such program is being operated at Phra Mougkut Khlao Hospital in Bangkok, Thailand by Dr. Aroon Showanasai. In the last year he has treated more than 800 patients. Other programs have been started in Mauritius (Rajah, 1974), in England (Dr. Margaret Patterson) and in Vientianne, Laos (Dr. Soudalay).

Acupuncture has been regarded by the general public in the last few years both with unbridled enthusiasm and considerable scepticism. In the drug field many felt it was highly improbable that acupuncture was really effective or could have anything to offer the field.

Part of the problem encountered by those advocating the use of acupuncture is that to those educated in the Western medical tradition there seems to be no immediately apparent physiological explanation of why it works, if it does. Many workers in the drug field are willing to accept that empirically acupuncture may have some effect, but they are unwilling to accept or get involved in the traditional oriental explanations of how acupuncture works and particularly the philosophical concepts that have surrounded it in the past.

The evidence from the several programs around the world now using acupuncture suggests overwhelmingly that the procedure does have some impact in alleviating the withdrawal symptoms from narcotics. Although the mechanism of action is unclear or at least unconfirmed, Wen has suggested that stimulation of the vagus nerve through its distribution in the ear is crucial. Stimulation of central nervous centers through the vagus, he argues, results in the discharge of neurochemical substances that have a β-adrenergic blocking effect suppressing parasympathetic nervous system function and specifically the symptoms of withdrawal which appear to be largely the result of parasympathetic activity. It has also been hypothesized that the stimulation by acupuncture might have a direct effect on a 'craving' center in the hypothalamus which results in a reduction in the individuals desire for drugs over a prolonged period of time. There is very little data to support or refute these hypotheses and it is clear substantial additional research is needed to elucidate the mechanism by which acupuncture acts (Bourne, 1974).

Although the data is convincing that acute withdrawal symptoms are significantly relieved in most instances by acupuncture, there is to date no evidence that acupuncture reduces recidivism or that people detoxified by this method are any less likely to return to drugs than those detoxified by any other method. There have been repeated claims by those using acupuncture that it did reduce subsequent drug use.

However, so far there appears to have been no scientifically valid follow-up study that would answer this question. The development of outcome studies looking at drug using behavior over a six-month to one-year period of time or even longer should be a high priority for those working with acupuncture.

BIOFEEDBACK

Biofeedback appears to be part of the same constellation of techniques which include acupuncture, hypnosis, meditation, and electrosleep, all of which are aimed at inducing a degree of relaxation and which may also result in certain biochemical correlates affecting the physiological elements of the addictive process in the brain.

Biofeedback training is a method of improving individuals' capacity for discernment and control of their physiological processes. The physiological processes to be brought under control, such as heart rate, blood pressure, muscle tension, electroencephalic activity, palmar sweating, hand temperature and gastric acidity, are continuously monitored with instruments that are sufficiently sensitive to detect the smallest momentary fluctuations of the function. The individual is then asked to try to achieve voluntary control of these functions, using the feedback signal as an indicator of his progress.

Biofeedback is being used increasingly in the United States in the treatment of addiction. The primary arguments in its favor, according to Kamiya (1971) are:

1. That, in the process of achieving self-control of physiological activity, the individual comes to discover, by direct self-observation, many of the psychological variables of mood, atten-
   · tion level, and a variety of physiological and emotional sensations. The ability to induce various emotional and physiological states is, he suggests, highly consistent with what the drug abuser is attempting to do in his ingestion of drugs.
2. He notes that biofeedback training effectively reduces anxiety levels, a prime motivating factor in drug taking behavior of many addicts.
3. The technique is, he feels, easily adapted to drug abuse re-habilitation programs, with the equipment being conventionally

available at a reasonable cost. It is relatively innocuous and virtually free of side effects. Also, he feels that with reasonably motivated patients, the procedure can be easily learned in most instances.

According to Kamiya there are some aspects of biofeedback that should temper the enthusiasm for its use as a technique in the drug abuse field. First, it has no direct effect on drug taking behavior itself, although some might question this. Second, the issue of motivation and the willingness of addicts to become actively involved in the training process over a long period of time is one that has yet to be determined. The evidence, however, as with some other approaches described in this paper, such as hypnosis and transcendental meditation, is that there is sometimes some problem in getting addicts to elect to use this particular modality. Kamiya points out that the research in this area relating biofeedback training to addiction is only in the early stages, and it is therefore too early to draw any major conclusions about its effectiveness. There are a number of studies underway including those by Wesson in San Francisco, Fotopoulos and Graham in Missouri, Bigelow at Baltimore City Hospital, Kurty in St. Cloud, Minnesota, and Rose at the Richmond Methadone program in Virginia.

This modality is of particular significance as the research in this area is generally being carried out by trained scientists with sophisticated equipment, and the data they produce is likely to have considerable scientific validity.

For those patients who are motivated to take the time to learn this technique it appears that there is considerable efficacy in its ability to reduce drug using behavior. The key question remains however, as to how significant a number of patients can be persuaded as to the desirability of this treatment method (Kamiya, 1975).

HYPNOSIS

Hypnosis is hardly a new technique although it is only recently that it has been used to treat drug abuse. At a theoretical level it is felt that hypnosis provides an opportunity for a relearning process, for the patient to go back to the pre-drug using years, and relearn certain aspects of his acquired behavioral patterns.

Hypnosis is used in a number of specific ways (Kuska, 1975).

1. It is used to link some aspects of drug using behavior and the drug itself with nausea, anxiety, and other negative reinforcers of behavior. This in many ways parallels the use of apomorphine as a negative conditioning approach.
2. Hypnosis is used to produce a reliving of the drug experience without the injection of drugs. This, in a way, is a substitute gratification, perhaps paralleling in some respects the nutritional therapy used at Prana House, as described in the article on Drugs and Youth by Smith.
3. Hypnosis is used to remove unpleasant symptoms or phobias which the person is currently coping with instead of with drugs. This in effect is an attempt to remove some of the underlying causes of drug use, and perhaps is comparable to the use of biofeedback and other relaxing techniques to reduce anxiety, and hence, the urge to use drugs.
4. Hypnosis is used as an ancillary method of teaching muscle relaxation or for systematic desensitization. In this respect in particular, hypnosis very closely parallels the other relaxation techniques.

The data to date on hypnosis is entirely empirical. It has been used and reported on in relatively few programs, and where it has, generally very few patients have been involved, and without adequate control. In effect, there is no really significant research study at the present time to demonstrate the efficacy of this approach, particularly on a long-term basis. Future work in this area needs to focus not merely on whether hypnosis has any validity as a treatment method, but with how it compares as a relaxing modality with biofeedback, transcendental meditation and other similar approaches. It may well be that hypnosis can have special appeal to certain segments of the addict population which other approaches would not. However, further clinical evaluation in this area is required.

There is every reason to believe that hypnosis is effective with a certain percentage of highly motivated patients. However, no matter how effective it might be, it will remain almost impossible to implement on a large scale and the extent of its use will always be limited by the relatively small number of competent practitioners of hypnosis.

MEDITATION

The use of meditation and other self induced hypometabolic states in a variety of forms has been the source of considerable attention as a way of reducing drug-using behavior. The use of this modality has been dominated by Benson at Harvard whose work in this field has been meticulous (Benson, 1975).

Transcendental meditation, which originated in the ancient Vedic tradition of India involves four basic elements:

1. *A mental device*—there is a constant stimulus of a silently repeated secret sound or word called a mantra. The purpose of this repetition is to free one's self from logical, externally oriented thought. The eyes remain closed throughout the practice.
2. *A passive attitude*—if distracting thoughts do occur during repetition they should be disregarded and one's attention should be redirected to the mantra.
3. *Decreased muscle tone*—the subject should sit in a comfortable position so that minimal muscular work is required.
4. *Regular practice*—the subject is instructed to practice the technique for two daily 20-minute periods, usually before breakfast and before dinner.

The result is a relaxed, wakeful hypometabolic state. Although the method varies slightly in association with different religions or cultic groups the net effect is the same.

Herbert Benson first suggested the use of transcendental meditation in the treatment of drug abuse in 1969 (Benson, 1969). With an initial group of 20 male volunteers, 19 of whom used a variety of drugs including heroin, all reported a disinclination to use drugs after their involvement with transcendental meditation. In a study by Winquist questionnaires were given to 525 meditators concerning their drug use. He reported that more than 80 per cent stopped using drugs completely. In a larger follow-up study by Benson and Wallace (1972) with 1950 individuals decreases in drug use of similar magnitude were recorded when they underwent meditation training. Shafii et al., (1974) conducted a study with similar findings and Shapiro (1900) using meditation on patients in a methadone program felt they could lower their doses of the drug. He also suggested that meditation combined

with supportive services could form the basis for an effective rehabilitative program.

On the basis of these several retrospective studies, which admittedly
are subject to biases and various reporting errors, Benson has concluded
that 'the regular practice of transcendental meditation acts to reduce
drug taking behavior in those who are motivated to learn the technique
and those who continue to regularly practice' (Benson, 1975).

Schwartz (1974) has conducted a prospective study in which an
experimental group of 50 novice meditators were compared with 34
controls. Over six months marijuana used dropped by over 50 per cent
in the experimental group and by a minimal amount in the controls. A
study in Malmo, Sweden in 1971 showed a similar drop in drug use
between an experimental group of meditators and controls (Brautigan,
1974).

The most recent, largest and most ambitious study was conducted by
Benson et al., (1974). They investigated the usefulness of transcendental
meditation in a population of 4000 high school juniors in Massachusetts
and Michigan. Unlike previous studies there appeared to be little decline
in drug use among those who meditated as compared with the controls.
From this Benson concluded that meditation was not acceptable to a
high school age population as a nonchemical alternative to drug use. He
felt this study did not refute the basic usefulness of transcendental
meditation in the treatment of drug abuse, but suggested instead that this
was an inappropriate population in which to use it.

It appears that where individuals are motivated to use meditation
drug use does decline. The key issue, however, is not whether
meditation is effective, but how you induce drug users to be motivated
to use this approach. Benson was able to persuade only 1.3 per cent of his
high school group to use meditation regularly. It also appears that
meditation may offer little in preventing drug abuse where the
overwhelming desire to experiment easily transcends the effects of
meditation. In those who are already using drugs regularly, one is
dealing with a completely different physiological and psychological
phenomenon, and it appears that meditation when used can alter those
forces in such a way as to reduce the desire to continue using drugs. How
such meditation induces specific biochemical changes in the brain or is
purely a psychological phenomenon is hard to tell. However, it remains
a reasonable possibility.

ELECTROSLEEP

Electrosleep or cerebral electrotherapy (CET), neurotherapy and transcranial electrotherapy (TCE) as it is also known is an approach to treatment for a variety of ailments that has been used in the USSR since 1947, and continues to be studied extensively by Soviet researchers (Wesson, 1975).

The period of treatment lasts 30–45 minutes in duration and is usually given in a series of five to ten sessions. The patient reclines in a quiet, semi-darkened room. Four metal electrodes covered by saline-soaked pads are employed in the following manner. An electrode is placed on the forehead just above each eye and the remaining two are placed behind each ear over the mastoid processes. The electrical current is regulated so that the patient feels a slight but not uncomfortable tingling, stinging or pressure sensation at the site of one or more of the electrodes. The effective treatment current is in the range of 0.5 to 1.5 milliamperes.

Most research with this modality has been done in the Soviet Union, Japan or China, and those few studies that have been published in English have serious methodological flaws.

Hood (1972) in California has suggested that with alcoholics 'it has a great deal more effect than just suggestibility, on the ability to aid insomniacs and alcoholics, . . . and has indeed been helpful in assisting relaxation, and in the learning of relaxation by the alcoholic'. Rosenthal and Briones (1972) have demonstrated in their pilot studies that hormonal changes occur with electrosleep.

Although the use of this modality has to date been limited particularly the treatment of drug abuse, Gomez and Mikhail (1974) have ۱onstrated in hospitalized heroin addicts withdrawing from meth- ﹍uone that it produces reduced anxiety and reduced need for methadone. Glen (1974) of the Veterans Administration Hospital in Dallas, Texas used electrosleep therapy for six months on 60 patients in the methadone withdrawal program and reported that 30 per cent improved moderately, and 30 per cent remained unchanged. Ten per cent became worse.

Bearing some similarity to the electrostimulated acupuncture technique of Wen, there is reason to believe that electrosleep may induce certain physiological changes that alleviate withdrawal symptoms.

There is reason to believe also on the basis of Soviet studies that electrosleep may be useful in reducing the anxiety and depression that underlie much of chronic drug-using behavior.

OTHER NON-PHARMACOLOGICAL INNOVATIVE TREATMENT TECHNIQUES

There are now a variety of other new approaches to treatment being tried in the United States. Many of these lack any scientific basis, are in too early a stage of development to warrant any assessment, or represent largely different emphases in rehabilitation rather than being really new treatment techniques. Nutrition therapy with restoration of physical health and well-being as a central focus of treatment has considerable following (Williams *et al.*, 1972, Holan, 1975). There are also a variety of behavior modification programs which use highly structured environments to induce behavioral change. Court diversion programs which suspend jail or other sentences for arrested addicts provided they remain in treatment have also received considerable attention. There are also a wide variety of new treatment programs being established to meet the needs of certain specialized groups such as women, addicted neonates, homosexuals, youth, and psychotic addicts.

NEW PHARMACOLOGICAL APPROACHES TO IMPROVEMENT

Dissatisfaction with methadone and with other traditional pharmacological approaches to treatment has led in the last few years to a search for alternative substances. While many have been tested only a few have shown any significant promise.

PROPOXYPHENE NAPSYLATE

Propoxyphene napsylate (Darvon-N) is a drug whose popularity in the treatment of opiate addiction appears to be in large part due to the timing with which it was first used. Coinciding with increasing disenchantment with methadone, it has been promoted as a substance which retains the beneficial effects of methadone while remaining free of many of its undesirable characteristics. Of interest also is the fact that it has enjoyed its greatest popularity in California where state regulations were the strictest in limiting the use of methadone, particularly in the area of outpatient detoxification.

The pioneer work in the use of propoxyphene napsylate in the treatment of addiction has been done by Tennant and his coworkers (1974). Beginning in 1973, they began administering the drug to addicts and they have now treated more than 400 patients both detoxifying them and maintaining them. Those who were detoxified were hospitalized for up to 21 days and given Darvon-N in gradually decreasing doses. Tennant reports that the initial 230 patients were successfully withdrawn with complete symptom alleviation, and to date, no significant side effects have been noted. More recently, he has successfully detoxified 50 patients on an outpatient basis. In addition to the use of the drug for detoxification, Tennant has used it in a modified maintenance program with 100 patients for periods ranging from 22 to 240 days with a mean of 85 days. Daily doses range from 400–1600 mg with a mean of 400 mg. Seventy-one per cent of Tennant's patients reported diminished desire to use heroin.

In Sacramento, California, Bergin as reported by Gay (1973) had similar results in a brief four-month study. He provided a five-day inpatient detoxification program for 178 patients administering 100–200 mg four to six times daily, a significantly smaller dose than that used by Tennant, but with similar success.

In San Francisco, Inaga, *et al.*, (1974) have established a program using Darvon-N at the Haight-Ashbury Free Medical Clinic. Thirty-two subjects were selected who had demonstrated continued refractiveness to other available treatment.

The duration of therapy was 1 to 66 days with the majority of clients (69 per cent) taking the drug for 5 to 30 days. Propoxyphene napsylate dosages for acute opiate withdrawal symptoms ranged from 600 mg to 1400 mg per day. Success was measured by urine testing and counselor evaluation. In the overall urine picture, the use of Darvon-N appeared to have reduced, by more than one-fourth the proportion of times that the client would be expected to submit dirty urines. Counselors rated 6 per cent as successful or relatively successful.

List, *et al.*, (1973) in Baltimore has used propoxyphene napsylate with apparent success in detoxifying patients on methadone maintenance.

The disadvantages of Darvon-N relate primarily to its potential toxicity particularly in high doses. Five out of 100 maintenance patients and 30 detoxification outpatients in Tennant's study reported a 'seizure-like' event within six hours after taking heroin at a time when 800 mg initial doses were being used. Although there have been reports of hepatic toxicity and bone marrow suppression as well as possible neural, cardiac and endocrine effects, toxicological monitoring for adverse effects of propoxyphene by Tennant showed no adverse effects during short-term detoxification. However, as he points out, considerably more study is needed to determine the possibility of chronic toxicity if patients are to be maintained on the drug for any length of time.

There are problems with Darvon-N which patients are willing to tolerate while enthusiasm for the drug is at high level. However, dizziness, being 'high', having a dry mouth and other somatic sensations might become much less tolerable to the addicts once the Darvon-N was no longer viewed as a potentially 'magical cure' and when there was no longer social pressure to help prove the drug's success.

To date there have been no controlled studies to compare the effectiveness of Darvon-N with methadone although Gay, *et al*., (1973) did select patients who had been unsuccessfully treated previously in methadone programs. Further studies are required to determine whether Darvon-N offers any additional advantages from a scientific standpoint over and above what currently is being derived from the favorable publicity, enthusiasm, and general acceptability.

APOMORPHINE

The use of apomorphine has to date found little application in the United States although in Europe and particularly in Scandinavia several workers are using it on an experimental basis for the treatment of addiction. Historically, apomorphine has been used extensively for the treatment of alcoholism, particularly in aversive conditioning (Liberman, 1968), and also to prevent craving for alcohol. The author William S. Burroughs attributes his recovery from addiction to aversive conditioning with apomorphine and describes his experiences in his book 'The Naked Lunch' (1967).

Recently, several workers in Europe including Martenson-Larsen (1974) who did much of the pioneer work with Antabuse, and Beil (1974a) and Halvorsen (1974) have used apomorphine on a continuing basis as a way of reducing the craving for opiates. According to Halvorsen, apomorphine is a dopamine antagonist causing a reduction in its synthesis. This has also been reported by Hornykiewicz (1966) and Persson (1970). Recently it has been demonstrated in experiments with mice that apomorphine inhibits the locomotory stimulation induced by ethanol.

Beil (1974b) has described his treatment of 38 addicts with apomorphine since 1972. His approach has been similar to that used by Halvorsen although he used no oral administration of the drug and continued the entire period of treatment for only one month. He used 'scattered' small doses of apomorphine at irregular intervals rather than the fixed schedule described by Halvorsen. Beil, unfortunately, has done no follow-up with his patients.

He warns against side effects such as salivation, yawning, nausea, diaphoresis, mild circulatory disturbances, dizziness, feelings of depersonalization and fatigue all of which he believes can be avoided by using the small scattered doses. Apomorphine is not addicting itself and apart from reducing craving apparently also relieves anxiety and creates a general sensation of relaxation.

It is theorized that through their effect in reducing the synthesis of neurotransmitter substances, apomorphine and other similar drugs may significantly reduce the craving of the addict. The similarity in effect of apomorphine in reducing the craving for alcohol and opiates lends support to the suggestion by Davis and Walsh (1970) that alcohol may be broken down with the formation of morphine-like, pathological metabolites.

In March of 1973, Halvorsen (1974) began treating patients with apomorphine after two addicts who had read William Burroughs' autobiography approached him eager to receive the same treatment. His approach is to determine the maximum sub-emetic dose of the drug that each patient can tolerate and then to administer it by subcutaneous injection every two hours. Over a five-day period, the patient gradually tapers off his drug of abuse and then continues taking the injected apomorphine for five additional days. Subsequently, the patient takes apomorphine sublingually in tablet form for a period of approximately two months. According to Halvorsen, this is the period needed for 'normalization of cerebral protein metabolism'. While its value in aversive conditioning and particularly in the treatment of alcoholism is well established, the work so far using apomorphine for the treatment of addiction is limited. Certainly the scientific rationale offered by Halvorsen is plausible but the limited number of patients, the poor follow-up, and the less than encouraging outcome of those he did locate does not suggest widespread acceptance of apomorphine in the future. It is likely, however, that this drug will receive significant additional trials in the next year or so, and once a more substantial body of data is available it should be easier to evaluate its potential efficacy.

PROPANALOL

The application of propanalol, a β-adrenergic blocking agent previously used in the treatment of cardiac arrhythmias, to the treatment of addiction has been largely the result of the work of one man—Dr. Hanus Grosz. Beginning in 1971, he has treated a series of patients with this drug and feels it is a safe, non-addicting, and effective method for dealing with the problem.

Propanalol is generally administered in 10 mg. doses three times a day. In the original case report by Grosz (1972) he noted a reduction in the craving for heroin, relaxation, less nervousness, and better sleep patterns. The patient was able to stop using heroin and after three months was also able to terminate the propanalol. The patient was functioning well and drug free several months later. Since his original report on the initial patient, Grosz has treated more than 50 patients with similar success.

The effects of propanalol described by Grosz are in some ways similar to that described with apomorphine. Specifically he feels that (a) it prevented heroin induced euphoria, (b) caused the use of heroin to precipitate protracted withdrawal symptoms and (c) abolished or greatly altered the residual craving for narcotics which ex-addicts commonly experience in the abstinent state. In studies using rats conditioned to various stimuli, suppression of their response by morphine could be alternated if they were premedicated with propanalol. This suggested, according to Grosz, functional evidence of interaction between morphine and propanalol.

Although the studies by Grosz are persuasive, a paper recently presented by Resnick, *et al.*, (1974) strongly challenges his findings. A series of controlled studies were conducted to evaluate the efficacy of propanalol in blocking the effects of experimentally administered opiates and the effects of propanalol on the signs and symptoms of the opiate abstinence syndrome.

Resnick and his coworkers found that the results of their studies indicated no significant differences between propanalol and placebo on either the time of onset withdrawal, the intensity of withdrawal, or the subjects' responses to acutely or chronically administered opiates. These findings in a well controlled scientifically designed setting certainly contradict the empirical findings reported by Grosz (1973). The problem of unscreened patients, relatively high motivation, the implied demand for success because a new and experimental approach was being used; all such extraneous factors may have contributed to Grosz's success. Also it should be pointed out that Resnick's work does not refute the original contention that propanalol may have an effect in ameliorating the craving for narcotics.

What is clearly needed is substantially larger clinical trials with the drug in the hands of a number of other investigators. There is considerable interest being generated in propanalol in Germany and Scandinavia and perhaps additional clinical trials will be conducted there in the next year. One major problem common to studies with propanalol, Darvon-N and apomorphine is that they tend to presume the utility of a primarily medical model for addiction and tend to ignore the effects of social and psychological determinants of addiction. Even the issue of 'craving' can be strongly psychologically determined and is completely subjective in nature. The importance of controlled studies such as those by Resnick (1974) then become critical in evaluating any of these procedures.

L-ALPHA ACETYL METHADOL (LAAM)

The early work conducted with LAAM by Jaffe *et al.*, (1972) showed that it was a potentially useful tool in the treatment of addiction. It appeared not to differ from methadone in safety or subjective effects, and yet provided considerably greater flexibility for the patients by allowing them to reduce the number of their visits to the clinic. Subsequent work

by Goldstein and Judson (1974) showed that the outcome of treatment with LAAM compared favorably with methadone in terms of
survivorship in the program, attendance record, and cessation of other
drug use. These findings are similar to those reported by Zaks *et al.*,
(1972).

In 1973, a large scale collaborative study of LAAM was initiated by
the Veterans Administration (VA) involving a number of their facilities
around the country. New patients were placed on LAAM and their
progress was compared with patients put on methadone. Although the
study is still in progress, it appears that the only significant difference in
the two groups is that the LAAM patients drop out of treatment with a
slightly higher frequency.

In addition, another collaborative study coordinated by NIDA and
involving 17 non-VA clinics using a variety of different protocols, has
been initiated with the clinics beginning their intake in September, 1974.
Several of the protocols call for the placing of patients on LAAM who
were previously being maintained on methadone as opposed to the VA
study in which all patients were new to treatment.

These two collaborative studies should, during the next year, provide
some important definitive information about the efficacy and safety of
LAAM. At a time when, particularly in New York City, major concern
about methadone diversion is being raised, the availability of a safe,
long-acting substitute that can be administered without ever being
provided as a 'take home' dose, becomes extremely important. The one
disadvantage with LAAM to date appears to be that when it is
administered to new patients who have not previously been stabilized on
methadone, the drop-out rate goes up significantly. This appears to be
due to the fact that when a patient does not have to come to the
treatment facility every day, his emotional ties with the clinic staff are
correspondingly diminished and he becomes much more susceptible to
sudden impulses to return to drug use. It is becoming increasingly clear
that the close relationship with the clinic staff and the daily reinforcement of interpersonal relationships is the critical element in enabling
methadone maintenance patients to achieve an effective degree of
rehabilitation. It is beginning to emerge that LAAM has its greatest
utility during the latter stages of treatment when patients have become
well stabilized and are generally on the road to full rehabilitation with
successful employment and relatively little chance of backsliding.

THE ANTAGONISTS

Antagonist drugs have been available for some time and early interest centered primarily around Naloxone and Cyclazocine. The former had the disadvantage of being short acting and requiring repeated administration and the latter caused side effects in a relatively large number of patients. Although Cyclazocine seems to be virtually discarded at this point a few programs are continuing to use Naloxone, in particular, Kleber at Yale (1974) and Kurland *et al.*, (1973) at the Maryland Psychiatric Research Center.

A number of researchers however, began to look for other antagonists that might be longer lasting and have fewer side effects. Naltrexone (EN-1639A) began to be used on a small scale by a few programs in 1973. Schecter and Grossman (1974), and Resnick, *et al.*, (1974) have treated a small number of patients with the drug with apparently good results.

In order to insure the most appropriate valid testing of this and other antagonist compounds, the federal government decided in December, 1972 to contract with the National Academy of Sciences to develop an overall research design for the development of these drugs. All future federal funding for the clinical testing of antagonists will now be a part of this overall cooperative study coordinated by the Academy.

Naltrexone remains the drug with the greatest promise and five clinics with three different protocols are about to initiate phase II studies. Naltrexone taken orally lasts for approximately 24 hours and to date appears to be virtually free of side effects. A number of other drugs are under investigation but are at an earlier stage of development. Substances identified as M-5050, BC-2605, and BC-2910 are in phase I testing at present. None of these drugs appear to have particular advantage over Naltrexone, although BC-2605 has mildly agonistic properties which may result in making it slightly more reinforcing, although presumably would also give it some dependence liability.

Although the antagonists' blockade against the effect of heroin, they do not suppress narcotic hunger as effectively as methadone and as a result it takes a more motivated patient for this technique to be effective.

CONCLUSIONS

While the range of new and innovative techniques both pharmacological and nonpharmacological is large and intriguing, we should keep in
mind that most as yet are unproven and require considerable additional
scientific research. Also we should remember that there is no magical
cure for drug abuse and that better, more dedicated application of the
techniques we already have is perhaps the best way to increase our
success in rehabilitation, not by looking only for something completely
new. In particular, no matter how effective a new pharmacological
approach may be, addiction remains primarily a social phenomenon and
effective social rehabilitation will still be the critical element in the
restoring of the addict to a happy and meaningful existence.

Perhaps most intriguing in the study of these new techniques is the
finding of the effects of acupuncture, meditation, electrosleep and
biofeedback that suggest that we may be opening the door to a better
understanding of the basic physiological mechanisms in drug abuse, and
to developing a treatment that is nonpharmacological but still based on
inducing specific physiological and biochemical changes in the brain.

REFERENCES

Beil, H. (1974a). Apomorphine in the Treatment of Alcoholism and Multiple
    Drug Use. Presented at the 20th International Institute on the Prevention and
    Treatment of Alcoholism, Manchester
Beil, H. (1974b). Apomorphine in the Treatment of Opiate Addiction and
    Other Drug Dependencies: A General Practitioner's Injection Treatment of
    Out-Patients. Presented at the 20th International Institute on the Prevention
    and Treatment of Alcoholism, Manchester
Benson, H. (1969). Yoga for Drug Abuse. *New England J. Med.* **281**, 1133
Benson, H. (1975). A Non-Pharmacological Approach to Drug Abuse
    Treatment: The Relaxation Response as Elicited by Transcendental Med-
    itation and Other Related Techniques. In 'A Survey of New Treatment
    Techniques for the Treatment of Drug Abuse'. Bourne, P. G., Homiller, J.,
    Smith, D. and Wesson, D. (eds) (National Clearinghouse for Drug Abuse
    Information: Washington, DC)
Benson, H. and Wallace, R. K. (1972). Decreased Drug Abuse with Transcen-
    dental Meditation—A Study of 1862 Subjects. *Proc. Int. Symp. Drug Abuse.*
    (Lea and Febinger: Philadelphia)
Benson, H., Shelley, M. W., Kotch, J. B. and Greenwood, M. M. (1974).
    Unpublished data.

Brautigan, E. (1974). Unpublished data

Burroughs, W. S. (1967). Kicking Drugs: A Very Personal Story. *Harper's*, **235**, 39–42

Bourne, P. G. (1974). The Treatment of Opiate with Acupuncture–A Review. Publication pending

Gay, G. (1973). I got a Yen for That Darvon-N. A Pilot Study of the Use of Propoxyphene Napsylate in the Treatment of Heroin Addiction. Presented at the Eli Lilly and Company Symposium on Propoxyphene Napsylate Treatment of Opiate Dependence, Washington, DC

Glen, R. (1974). Unpublished report

Goldstein, A. and Judson, A. (1974). Three Critical Issues in the Management of Methadone Programs. *In* 'Addiction'

Gomez, E. and Mikhail, A. (1974). Treatment of Methadone Withdrawal with Cerebral Electrotherapy (Electrosleep). Paper presented at the Annual Meeting of the American Psychiatric Association, Detroit, Michigan

Grosz, H. J. (1972). Successful Treatment of a Heroin Addict with Propanalol. Implications for Opiate Addiction, Treatment and Research. *J. Indiana State med. Ass.*, **65**, 505–509

Grosz, H. J. (1973). Effect of Propanalol on Active Users of Heroin. *Lancet* **ii**, 612

Halvorsen, K. A. L. (1974). Apomorphine in the Treatment of Drug Dependence: Psychopharmacological Aspects. Presented at the 20th International Institute for the Prevention and Treatment of Alcoholism, Manchester

Holan, R. (1975). Nutritional Approaches to the Treatment of Drug Abuse. *In* 'A Survey of New Treatment Techniques for the Treatment of Drug Abuse.' Bourne, P. G., Homiller, J., Smith, D. and Wesson, D. (eds.) (National Clearinghouse for Drug Abuse Information: Washington, DC)

Hood, A., Jr. (1972). Alcohol Withdrawal in Electrosleep. (Manuscript.) Program Director, Alcoholic Rehabilitation Program; Napa State Hospital; Imola, California

Jaffe, J. H., Senay, E. C., Schuster, C. R., Renault, P. R., Smith, B. and Dimemza, S. (1972). Methadyl Acetate Vs. Methadone. *J. Amer. med. Assoc.*, **222**, 437–443.

Kamiya, J. (1975). Biofeedback Training as a Modality in the Treatment of Drug Abuse. *In* 'A Survey of New Techniques for the Treatment of Drug Abuse'. Bourne, P. G., Homiller, J., Smith, D. and Wesson, D. (eds.) (National Clearinghouse for Drug Abuse Information: Washington, DC)

Kamiya, J., Barber, T., DiCara, L., Miller, N., Shapiro, D. and Stoyva, J. (1971). Biofeedback and Self Control: Reader. (Aldine-Atherton Inc: Chicago)

Kleber, H. D. (1974). Clinical Experiences with Narcotic Antagonists. *In* 'Opiate Addiction: Origins and Treatment'. Fisher, Seymour and Freedman (eds.) (V. H. Winston and Sons: Washington DC)

Kurland, A. A., Krantz, J. C., Jr., Henderson, J. M. and Kerman, F. (1973). Naloxone and the Narcotic Abuser: A Low-Dose Maintenance Program. *Intern. J. Addict.* **8**, 127–141

Kuska, H. D. (1975). Medical Hypnosis as a Modality in Drug Abuse Treatment. In 'A Survey of New Treatment Techniques for the Treatment of Drug Abuse'. Bourne, P. G., Homiller, J., Smith, D. and Wesson, D. (eds.) (National Clearinghouse for Drug Abuse Information: Washington, DC)

Liberman, R. (1968). Aversive Conditioning of Drug Addicts: A Pilot Study. *Behav. Res. Ther.*, **6**, 229–231

List, D. (1973). Methadone Detoxification Using Propoxyphene Napsylate (Darvon-N). Presented at the Eli Lilly Company Symposium on Propoxyphene Napsylate Treatment of Opiate Dependence, Washington, DC

Martenson-Larsen, D. (1974). Apomorphine or Disulfirm in the Treatment of the Alcoholic. Presented at the 31st International Conference on Drug Abuse and Treatment. Copenhagen, Denmark

Ng, L. K. (1974). Unpublished report

Rajah, S. G. M. (1974). Acupuncture: An Adjunct to Treatment of Drug Addicts. Presented at the African Conference on Drug Abuse, Nairobi, Kenya

Resnick, R. B. (1974). Studies of Propanalol in Opiate Addictions. Presented at the American Psychiatric Association Meeting, Detroit

Resnick, R. B., Volvaka, J., Freedman, A. M., Jones, T. and Thomas, M. (1974). Studies of EN-1639A (Naltrexone)—A New Narcotic Antagonist. *Amer. J. Psychiat.*, **131**, 646–650

Rosenthal, S. H. and Briones, D. F. (1972). Hormonal Studies in Cerebral Electrotherapy. Presented at The Third International Symposium on Electrosleep and Electro-anaesthesia at Varna, Bulgaria

Sacks, L. (1974). Acupuncture: 'Staple-Puncture.' In 'Drug Addiction'. Unpublished manuscript. (Medical Clinic of Torrance, Torrance, California)

Schecter, A. J. and Grossman, D. J. (1974). Natrexone in a Clinical Setting: Preliminary Observations. Presented to the Committee on Problems of Drug Dependence, National Academy of Sciences, National Research Council

Schwartz, G. E. (1974). Unpublished report

Shapiro, D. H. (1974). The Effects of a Zen Meditation—Behavioral Self-Management Training Package in Treating Methadone Addiction: A Formative Study. *Dissertation Abst. Int. (Ann Arbor, Mich.)* Universal M-Films, Nos. 73–70, 474

Shafii, M., Lavely, R. and Jaffe, R. (1974). Meditation and Marijuana. *Amer. J. Psychiat.*, **131**, 60–65

Smith, M. (1973). Unpublished report

Tennant, F. S., Jr., Russell, B. A., McMarna, A. and Cassas, M. (1974). Propoxyphene Napsylate Treatment of Heroin and Methadone Dependence: One Year's Experience. *J. Psychedelic Drugs*, **6**, 201–212

Wen, H. L. and Cheung, S. Y. (1973). Treatment of Drug Addiction by Acupuncture and Electrical Stimulation. *Amer. J. Acupunct.*, 1, 71–75

Wesson, D. R. (1975). Electrosleep (Cerebral Electrotherapy) as a Drug Abuse Treatment Technique. *In* 'A Survey of New Treatment Techniques for the Treatment of Drug Abuse'. Bourne, P. G., Homiller, J., Smith, D. and Wesson, D. (eds.) (National Clearinghouse for Drug Abuse Information: Washington, DC)

Williams, E. Y., Rickman, E. E. and Elder, Z. B. (1972). The Quest of Therapy for Heroin Addiction. Experience with Calcium Gluconate. *J. nat. med. Ass.*, **64**, 205–210

Zaks, A., Fink, M. and Freedman, A. M. (1972). L-Alpha-Acethyl Methadol in Maintenance Treatment of Opiate Dependence. *In* Proceedings of the 4th National Conference of the National Association for the Prevention of Addiction to Narcotics (NAPAN) on Methadone Treatment. (NAPAN: New York)

CHAPTER 9

A therapeutic community for dependent individuals ('addicts') in prison

M. M. GLATT

INTRODUCTION

Dependence on alcohol or 'other drugs' is of course a socio-medical and not primarily a penal problem (Glatt, 1968). Handling offenders with drug or alcohol problems in the past by a predominantly penal approach (involving, for example, repeated court appearances, fines, prison sentences, etc.) has largely led to a 'revolving door' system with no lasting benefit for the individual concerned or society. Every attempt should therefore be made to evolve constructive though realistic (and not merely utopian) alternatives to prison for such offenders—such as, for example, the closest collaboration between voluntary agencies and the probation and aftercare services, ample, suitable hostel accommodation, day training and treatment centres, etc. It is certainly true that people can be better educated for a life of freedom whilst living within the community itself than whilst kept within the confines of prison, with all its accompanying dangers and disadvantages of 'institutionalisation', (Martin et al., 1954) its loss of initiative and feeling of responsibility, and its dependence on prison staff.

The present article is therefore by no means a recommendation to send drug addicts and alcoholics to prison. In the required overall and comprehensive (multidisciplinary) preventive, therapeutic and aftercare programme that should cater for 'addicts' of all types and all phases of their dependence and wherever they may find themselves, prison treatment is no more than a side issue and certainly not the central core of the approach. To mention just one illustration from our own experience, Figure 1 depicts the interrelated chain of (therapeutic, aftercare, educational and training) facilities and connections as they

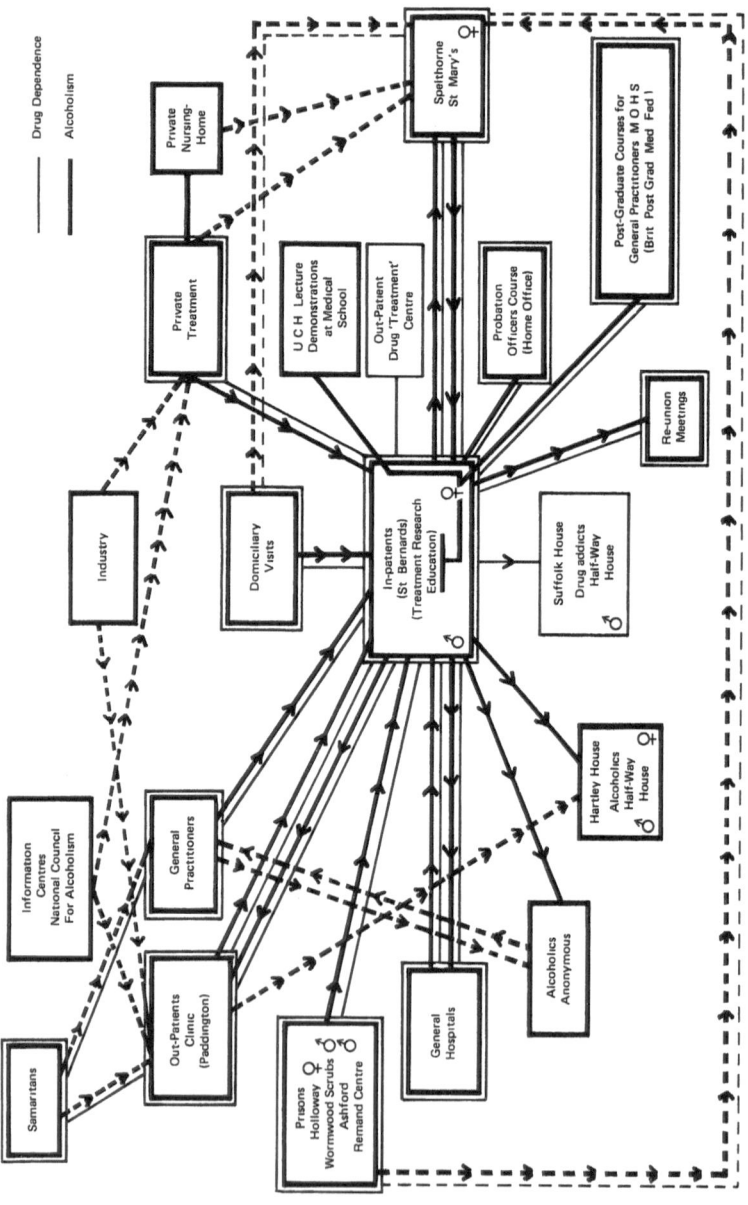

Drug Dependence
Alcoholism

Private Nursing-Home

Spelthorne St Mary's ♀+

Post-Graduate Courses for General Practitioners M O H S (Brit Post Grad Med Fed)

Private Treatment

U C H Lecture Demonstrations at Medical School

Out-Patient Drug 'Treatment' Centre

Probation Officers Course (Home Office)

Re-union Meetings

Industry

Domiciliary Visits

In-patients (St Bernards) (Treatment Research Education) ♀+ ♂+

Suffolk House Drug addicts Half-Way House ♂+

Information Centres National Council For Alcoholism

General Practitioners

Hartley House Alcoholics Half-Way House ♂+ ♀+

Samaritans

Out-Patients Clinic (Paddington)

Prisons Holloway Wormwood Scrubs Ashford Remand Centre ♀+ ♂+

General Hospitals

Alcoholics Anonymous

Figure 1

gradually developed in association with the inpatient facility established at St. Bernard's Hospital in Middlesex in 1958. A glance at the chart indicates that almost all these facilities are primarily concerned with patients who come for help 'of their own free will'.

In general, patients who come for treatment voluntarily stand a better chance than those who are treated compulsorily. However, in our experience the great majority of alcoholic or drug dependent patients who come for treatment 'voluntarily', do so frequently in name only. But for a certain amount of 'back pressure' applied by anxious spouses, well meaning or far-sighted employers, sympathetic friends or understanding courts or Probation Officers, many so called 'voluntary' patients would in fact never have agreed that they were in need of treatment. In practice, however, the question whether such patients originally came for treatment more or less voluntarily, may not be of overriding importance, as it should be the function of any therapeutic set-up wherever it may be situated to induce the initially so often missing motivation in such patients (Glatt, 1974a, 1975).

There are probably many who would reject all compulsory treatment methods as useless and not worth trying in the first instance. On the other hand, from a very recent study carried out in a Californian State Hospital two American workers came to quite different conclusions (Aron and Daily, 1976). According to their findings the 'preferential policy' of many therapeutic commitments '...discriminates against those individuals who are most likely to succeed in completing their treatment'. The authors therefore 'strongly recommend a re-evaluation of that policy'. Their research work compared drug addicts who completed treatment in a therapeutic community with others who terminated their treatment without completing it. They found that abusers with fewer years and milder usage of drugs who entered the therapeutic programme 'under outside pressure from the legal system' tended to complete the programme, whereas abusers 'with more previous years of drug usage and jail time' who had come to the programme voluntarily, tended to leave it before their treatment had been completed. This is in line with our own earlier findings at the St. Bernard's Dependence Unit that 'young addicts admitted under Section 4... with a Condition of Residence stay in hospital longer, thus giving themselves a better opportunity to acquire insight and establish relationships. They are therefore likely to do better than the 'voluntary' patients admitted from treatment centres...' (Glatt, 1972).

As regards imprisonment, everyone would probably agree that in itself it does not constitute treatment for addicts. On the other hand, there will always be alcoholics and addicts who find themselves in prison for some offence or other, which may be more or less directly connected with their compulsion to take drugs at any cost and at any price: for example, those relapsing again and again into alcohol or drug misuse and committing serious offences in a drunken or drugged state. Many emotionally and socially unstable alcoholics and drug addicts may find it very difficult or impossible to co-operate with treatment whilst living in an environment where 'their' special drug, or possibly even any addictive drug, is freely available, and where moreover tradition and culture (in the case of alcohol) or certain subcultures (in the case of 'other drugs') encourage and propagate drug use.

A person cannot be regarded as a free man—free, for example, to co-operate fully in a therapeutic programme—as long as he is enslaved by an overpowering psychological and/or physical dependence on alcohol or other drugs, or a severe psychological dependence on gambling, etc. (Glatt, 1974a). To expect addicts, after release, to maintain the abstinence previously enforced in prison where there had been a purely custodial approach, is futile. Yet 'offender patients, for the period they are in custody, are there to be treated', and in view of 'the assumption by the Prison Medical Service of a positive therapeutic rather than custodial role in the handling of the mentally abnormal offender' (Brit. med. J., 1973), the question arises whether it is possible to approach the addict's enforced sojourn in prison as a challenge and an opportunity to build up a drug-free therapeutic community in which the addict can obtain the initially lacking motivation and insight to keep off drugs. The therapeutic community within the prison would thus have to take care to avoid the dangers of institutionalisation and aim at giving such patients the chance to learn to look at themselves and their problems in a more objective, rational light; and serve as the initial step in a prolonged, comprehensive rehabilitation service.

PREVIOUS RELEVANT EXPERIENCES WITH ADDICTS IN HOSPITAL AND PRISON

There is no such person as the typical alcohol or drug addict (Glatt 1974a, 1975). The wide divergence of personalities among alcoholics, for example, was clearly illustrated by the great differences between samples of patients referred in the early 1950's to the Alcoholic Unit at Warlingham Park Hospital (WPH) by General Practitioners, Alcoholics Anonymous, Probation Officers, etc. (Glatt, 1961a). Similarly a marked difference was later noted to exist among addicts between the middle-aged 'therapeutic' and 'professional' addicts (as they were occasionally admitted to the WPH Unit in the 1950's) on the one hand, and the young, non-therapeutic addicts who in the 1960's were admitted to the Alcoholism and Drug Dependence Unit of St. Bernard's Hospital (Glatt *et al.*, 1968).

One interesting outcome of the great differences between the older, therapeutic and the younger non-therapeutic addicts was seen when attempts were made to include such drug addicts in therapeutic groups and therapeutic communities formed in the main by alcoholics, at WPH in the 1950's and St. Bernard's in the 1960's. Middle-aged (opiate, barbiturate or amphetamine) drug addicts by-and-large fitted in well with the groups consisting predominantly of (middle-aged) alcoholics. Not so successful were our attempts in the sixties at St. Bernard's to include young addicts, or habitual misusers, of heroin, cocaine, barbiturates, amphetamines, in predominantly alcoholic groups. Difficulties arose probably mainly because of the generation gap and the resulting differences in life styles and outlook Nevertheless there were so many resemblances between alcoholics and drug addicts that attempts at St. Bernard's Hospital to treat alcoholics and other drug dependents 'under the same umbrella' (Glatt, 1970a) and in the same therapeutic community were by-and-large regarded by the staff as working quite satisfactorily (Glatt, 1974a). Alcoholics and drug addicts could live and work well together in one therapeutic community although it was later preferable to form separate psychotherapeutic groups for alcoholics and the middle-aged barbiturate addicts on the one hand, and the young addicts to narcotics and polydrug misusers, on the other hand. Aftercare hostels—separate for alcoholics and addicts—were established (Glatt, 1974a, 1975) also running on the principle of therapeutic communities. The in-patient treatment was regarded as no more than the initial step in the long drawn-out rehabilitation programme; the whole constellation of in-patient and community services (see Figure 10.1)—and not merely the in-patient facility—was seen as constituting the 'Unit' (Glatt 1967, 1974a), providing also excellent opportunities for professional training, education and research.

Of some interest as regards certain aspects of our main theme—the possibility of establishing a therapeutic community in prison formed by both alcoholics and addicts on other drugs—were certain impressions gained from lengthy discussions in 1960 with Dr. Leong Hon Koon, who at the time was Medical Officer at the Opium Treatment Centres in Singapore. The latter had been set up to look after Chinese opium addicts who, after arrest, had been compulsorily sent to a prison addiction unit. As described in a joint paper (Glatt and Leong Hon Koon, 1961), initially it seemed to us farfetched to compare English, mainly middle-class alcoholics, treated as voluntary patients in a very permissive English hospital (WPH), with forcibly detained Chinese opium addicts, usually from a poor background, treated in an opium treatment centre under prison conditions in faraway Singapore. Initially we both had expected very considerable differences between these two groups and set-ups, in view of the differences in the 'agent' used (alcohol and opium respectively), in the type of addict, the sociocultural aspects, etc. 'However, after a number of informal exchanges of personal experiences and impressions, gained quite independently of each other (in England and Singapore respectively), . . . there emerged more than a few aspects in which the problems closely resembled each other: . . . such as the indifferent attitude of doctors, the layman and the State towards the addicts, and the latter's ready response to an understanding, accepting attitude within a therapeutic community . . . . Addicts to drugs and alcohol are in general considered to be unco-operative and difficult patients. It seems however that with the background of a therapeutic community, formed by sufferers from the same disorder, and with an understanding, sympathetic staff, such people as a rule become very co-operative and very anxious to work towards recovery . . .'. Dr. Leong's experiences with the Eastern opium smokers certainly indicated that even forcibly detained addicts under certain conditions could co-operate with treatment.

PRELIMINARY EXPERIENCES WITH ADDICTS IN PRISON

During their long drawn-out drinking or drug taking careers many alcoholics and drug addicts will land in prison. For example, out of 200 male alcoholics seen at Warlingham Park Hospital in the early 1950's 20 per cent had at some time or other been in prison; a further 23.5 per cent had been before the courts for an (alleged) offence. (Glatt, 1961a) At WPH all these patients co-operated well with treatment (mainly therapeutic community and group psychotherapy). Had their alcoholism improved at all as a result of their previous prison experience? They all stated that prison had had no lasting effect on their drinking but after all, they claimed, 'we received no treatment for alcoholism at all whilst in prison'. (In all fairness it should be pointed out however, that similar statements were made at the time (the 1950's) by those previously admitted to hospitals because of their alcoholism: they had just been 'dried out' and discharged).

Our early experiences with alcoholics at WPH had shown them—when treated in a therapeutic community—to be much more co-operative patients than generally assumed (Glatt, 1955). Could something be done for alcoholics whilst they are in prison? The Advisory Council on the Treatment of Offenders (Lancet, 1957) was not very hopeful, regarding prison in the case of 'chronic alcoholics' as '... *prima facie* unsuitable and useless'. However it could not see any alternative at the time to imprisonment, 'though occasionally probation and residential treatment methods might be tried'. The Council reported that very few of the alcohol addicts seen in prison were of suitable character and intelligence for psychotherapy. By-and-large, in our experience at the time, alcoholics who had been in prison were likely to be emotionally and socially more unstable than the alcoholic 'non-offenders', and this factor, combined with unfavourable environmental conditions after discharge, would tend to make their prognosis more problematic than that of their factors. Nevertheless in our view, as expressed at the time (Glatt, 1957) '... occasionally a more intelligent type of alcoholic responding to psychotherapy, must turn up in prisons as is evident from the fact that a fifth of the Warlingham Park Hospital alcoholics had been in prison ... . Anyhow, facilities for the residential treatment of alcoholics outside prisons are very scarce, and, where present, their permissiveness makes them not very suitable for the treatment of aggressive psychopathic alcoholics. As the Council did not suggest any alternative to imprisonment, the question arises whether more could not be done for these people whilst in prison. The Council reports that prisoners are allowed to make contacts with Alcoholics

Anonymous (AA) but (in contrast to the United States) there are as yet apparently no AA prison groups in this country (fortunately, in subsequent years, such groups were established in most British prisons, including one at Wormwood Scrubs in the mid-1960's). A great number of the prison alcoholics must be psychopaths who may easily disrupt such a group though it might be expected that the group would be able to 'carry' a few psychopaths. It might therefore be more advisable to have the alcoholic prisoners screened by a psychiatrist and to create separate (and perhaps psychotherapeutic) groups for non-psychopathic and psychopathic alcoholics. Prison treatment would possess at least one advantage in that these alcoholics could be approached while sober, for sobriety is harder to obtain and maintain in a very permissive atmosphere. The result from such an approach might not be overwhelmingly good but some improvement could at least be expected in the non-psychopathic offender of average intelligence' (Glatt, 1957). Clearly like hospital therapy, such prison treatment had no chance of being successful without planned aftercare so that the establishment was also suggested of '... a few experimental special hostels for alcoholics, for example, ... for the down-and-out, ex-prisoners or chronic drunkenness offenders' (Glatt, 1961b). It was also realised that the special services suggested—in hospitals, hostels, prisons—could not be provided 'without the help of medical and ancillary staff with special training and experience in handling the alcoholic and with an understanding of his special problems' (Glatt, 1961b).

With such views and notions arrived at on the basis of my experiences with alcoholics and addicts in hospitals, out-patient clinics, etc. (of the addicts too quite a few had previously been in prison) I started working at the out-patient clinic in Wormwood Scrubs Prison in 1963. The initial idea was to treat both alcoholics and addicts to other drugs, and my bias, in the light of previous experience in hospitals, was treatment by group therapy. As it turned out, the majority referred for treatment in subsequent years were mainly young drug addicts of all types—narcotic addicts, individuals dependent on amphetamines and (in later years) barbiturates, and habitual users of cannabis and LSD; a minority were alcoholics and there were a few compulsive gamblers. As most patients were also heavy cigarette smokers (and very occasionally there was also a very excessive eater among them), the opportunity was explored whether all such patients in spite of their different types of dependence could be treated in the same group. It soon became evident that although the 'agent' differed a great deal (alcohol, other drugs) and although in the case of compulsive gamblers there was no pharmacological 'agent' involved at all, these men had so many experiences in common in view of the common denominator 'dependence', that they were able more or less readily to identify with each other and to evince a lively and constructive interest in each other's problems.

It soon became obvious that in spite of the prevailing custodial atmosphere it was quite feasible to have group-psychotherapeutic sessions with addicts. It soon became equally clear that there were considerable difficulties which made real progress unlikely in spite of the interest shown by quite a few addicts in the group-therapeutic approach.

The group was an 'open' one in the sense that all the time prisoners were discharged and new ones took their place in these group sessions. The aim of the group therapy was to assist these patients to gain some insight into the nature of their problems etc. by freely discussing their personal difficulties. Apart from the fact that sessions were too infrequent anyway (as I attended only once a week), further difficulties arose because as a rule newcomers to the group, understandably enough, kept setting off with complaints about the unfair, unjust and imperfect society in general and the shortcomings of prison and its staff in particular. Therefore it always took some time before discussions moved away from the subject of faults of society and started to concentrate on questions such as to what the individual could possibly do about his own problem—in spite of the admittedly difficult situation in which he found himself, having to accept prison as an unfortunate reality for the time being. Progress was very slow if there was any at all, although even under such difficult circumstances there were those who came to understand that there was no point in bashing their heads against immovable brickwalls, and who began to use uncomfortable reality as a challenge and opportunity to grow in emotional maturity.

At any rate these prisoner-patients living in ordinary prison wings returned after the 'treatment' sessions of one to two hours per week to their cells, and both they and the therapist felt frustrated because the little that might possibly be attempted in these infrequent individual or group therapy sessions seemed only too likely to get 'lost' during the rest of the 24 hour day, or, as Dr. Murray Cox, Consultant Psychotherapist at

Broadmoor Hospital, put it, the 'other 166¾ hours' in the week's stay in a custodial, non-therapeutic atmosphere, in contact with other prisoners not involved in this type of therapy, not suffering from similar problems, and supervised by Prison Officers who had no interest in, or experience with, working with addicted patients.

The majority of these patients were youngsters in their late teens or early twenties—emotionally by-and-large much more unstable and immature than the somewhat older alcoholics and the few gamblers. Most of these were probably basically asocial and antisocial people who later became addicts ('addicted criminals') rather than alcoholics or addicts whose anti-social behaviour was largely the outcome of their fundamental underlying dependence—a difference which probably has an important bearing on the final prognosis and ability to tolerate frustration and to co-operate with psychotherapy under trying conditions (Glatt, 1968). Such patients usually complained bitterly, and in my view with complete justification, that these infrequent sessions in such an unsuitable environment could not really be described as treatment. They felt that their states of tension, frustration, depression, hostility, irritability, etc., were largely reactions to their environment. Although by the time they were referred for this long-term treatment they had been in prison long enough to have passed beyond the initial phase of physical dependence, and though they knew that they would on no account be prescribed their former drugs of addiction, many maintained that they could not overcome their immediate problems without the help of tranquillizers, antidepressants or hypnotics—for which there was a continual demand. Again, discussions arising from refusal to prescribe such drugs took up an inordinate proportion of the little time available for individual and group discussions. Under such circumstances many patients argued that they could not possibly be expected to think of ways and means to keep off drugs after discharge. Quite a number of these prisoner-patients however evinced interest in the approach, as reflected in their active participation in the group sessions and the gradual shift in emphasis away from criticising society, prison and staff towards the development of a more self-critical attitude. Moreover, these sessions also indicated that, in spite of differences of personality, age groups, sociocultural factors and the pharmacological nature of the dependence-producing 'agent', it was possible for compulsive drug users, drinkers, smokers and gamblers to identify with each other, to share their experiences and to enter into meaningful and mutually helpful discussions with each other.

The situation therefore was basically not very different from the one that had existed at Warlingham Park Hospital in 1951/2 prior to the establishment of the first group exclusively formed by alcoholics; living initially in different wards, the formation of an alcoholic group led to their move from different wards into the same ward, and later to the establishment of an Alcoholic Unit (Glatt, 1955).

The preliminary experiences with group sessions at Wormwood Scrubs thus seemed to make it worthwhile to further explore the possibility of the formation of a therapeutic community in prison comprising all types of addicts to be followed up by a planned aftercare programme. As pointed out in a talk at the World Health Session of the Royal Society of Health Congress in Eastbourne in 1969,

'It is an interesting finding that, in our experience, addicts co-operate much better in group therapy sessions held in hospital, and even more so in prison, than in the outpatient treatment centres,* where all too often they insist that they are "not yet ready" to contemplate giving up drugs—and that "it is all the fault of society anyway", and that "there is nothing to come off drugs for anyway". Addicts seen in prison—without any chance for the time being to get hold of drugs—seem much more prepared to consider and to discuss ways and means in which they could help themselves rather than waiting for society to do it all for them.

Under these circumstances, and keeping (the) American experiences in mind, apart from rehabilitation schemes for "volunteers" one might well consider setting up an experimental scheme for the rehabilitation of criminal addicts. Such people could first be treated whilst in prison, and from our own experience of treating prison addicts it should be possible to provide a "therapeutic community"

---

* Whereas until 1968 any British medical practitioner was allowed to prescribe heroin (and cocaine) to addicts, since 1968 only doctors at such official treatment centres have been permitted to do so These centres were established on the advice of the Interdepartmental Committee on Drug Addiction (1965) in order to put an end to the overprescribing of these drugs by a handful of London doctors (Glatt et al., 1968). Officially the centres (the great majority in London) were started in 1968, but two (at the Westminster Hospital and at University College Hospital (UCH)) had opened already in 1967. The later described impressions concerning such centres were gained by the present writer at the UCH Drug Treatment Centre since its inception in 1967 (Glatt, 1974a).

atmosphere for such people there—even if some addicts after discharge from prison state that all they thought about whilst in prison was how to return to drugs immediately the opportunity arose. Such treatment should be combined with attempts at vocational guidance, job training, evening school, etc. Those who co-operate could possibly be transferred to a half-way hostel (if situated within or near the prison precincts, difficulties arising from neighbours' objections, as in the case of half-way houses for addicts discharged from hospital, would not arise) from where they could go out to work; in time some addicts might be well enough to go out on parole whilst still remaining under regular supervision, perhaps working with employers with whom the prison social worker may have established contact. Should there be any return to drugs or any other misdemeanour, the addict would have to return to prison. The knowledge of such a possibility—in the views of a number of prison addicts with whom such a scheme was discussed—would act as a deterrent and as a motivating factor towards keeping off drugs. In the hostel, group therapy and the "therapeutic community" atmosphere would continue; the presence of staff well versed in treating addicts and understanding their special problems would be an essential prerequisite. The whole scheme would be experimental, flexible, and subject to modifications on the basis of experience gained; possibly methods such as Nalline testing might also be applied. The help of voluntary organisations, community agencies and recovered addicts could also be enlisted (possibly for some addict-prisoners part of the prison sentence might experimentally be spent on such a hostel-parole scheme). Such a scheme might mean—in view of the present lack of suitable voluntary rehabilitation facilities—that the addict getting himself into such trouble as to receive longer sentences would be given a better chance of rehabilitation than the one staying out of trouble with the Law, or the one receiving a short sentence only. However, the latter could, of course, volunteer to participate.

The low staying-power and frustration tolerance of many young drug abusers, their passivity on the one hand, their impulsive acting-out on the other (coupled with the desire to achieve a "high" without any effort, and the ready availability of drugs) make it difficult for them to co-operate for long in a permissive atmosphere. At St. Bernard's, for example, addicts admitted informally from treatment centres, frequently discharged themselves after a few days, whereas those admitted from prison or remand home under some order often stayed the course and co-operated fairly well. This ability of many addicts to co-operate with treatment and rehabilitation schemes only if there is some form of compulsion, surely could be better harnessed to a constructive rehabilitation effort than it is at present. Should addicts not in trouble with the Law want to avail themselves of the facilities created originally for those in prison only, this should not create any insuperable problems; and likewise lessons could be learned from such an experimental scheme which could be made use of to improve community, out-patient, in-patient, and rehabilitation facilities for the addict not landing himself in trouble . . .' (Glatt, 1969).

Another important reason for the desire to establish a therapeutic community for those addicts who were in prison was our experience that in those cases where the same patient in the past had been seen in hospital, in an out-patient treatment centre and in prison, he often seemed to co-operate best with group therapy when seen in prison. As described during a talk at the International Conference on Drug Addiction in Quebec in 1968,

'In general, like alcoholics, so also do drug addicts theoretically seem suitable for the group approach. Like alcoholics, . . . they have a common overriding problem and share many experiences; thus there is a natural common bond between them and they identify readily with each other—factors, which, of course, outside hospital contribute to the ease of forming a special subculture. We have found the group approach with drug addicts helpful in a variety of settings, such as a special hospital unit, in prison, in a semi-private nursing home run by a religious organisation, and in a new out-patient treatment centre. "Treatment in a therapeutic group can renew the capacity for social relationships and improve it" (Foulkes), a factor which obviously is of great importance in drug addicts (who, so far, have been able to communicate and to establish relationships only whilst, and by, using drugs) provided the group therapy takes place in a drug-free environment. This is difficult, or almost impossible to achieve in an open ward (such as the Alcoholism and Addiction· Unit at St. Bernard's) where drugs may easily be smuggled in and where even the best motivated addict can readily fall by the wayside, for example by a conditioned reflex type of response when watching another addict "fixing" himself with drugs which he has smuggled in. From the aspect of providing a drug-free atmosphere, of course prison provides an advantage and in our experience group therapy is quite feasible in prison. Here, naturally enough, addicts often complain about prison conditions.... By itself, imprisonment would tend to increase the addict's feeling of "defiant rage" (Rado, 1963) and of impotent embittered resentment, but with psychotherapy he may nevertheless become motivated into wanting help; and under an enlightened, not too restrictive regime he may learn the value of self-discipline, with gradual restoration of self-respect and self-confidence, based on a more realistic appreciation of his abilities, rather than on fantasy-based grandiose and often nebulous notions derived from over-compensation of inadequacy feelings.

... The therapist's tasks would be made much easier by providing institutions with conditions and rules midway between those of hospitals and prison, making the atmosphere within the prison as permissive as possible—by filling the prisoner's day with meaningful occupations, and by trying to establish a therapeutic community within the prison.

... Group therapy, in our experience, so far, seems also a promising tool under the system of the new English out-patient treatment centres. (But) addicts (there) come along in the main because of their need to obtain drugs which are usually prescribed in decreasing dosages, so that they are still taking drugs whilst attending therapy sessions, and a great deal of resistance is expressed, for example by "nodding" (after having drugs shortly before the session) as well as by missing sessions, coming late, and complaining about the therapist's lack of understanding in not giving the addict the amount of drugs which he want and which (in the addict's opinion) is the amount he needs. The same addict has occasionally been seen successively in the permissive hospital set-up, the out-patient centre and in prison, and often such an individual seemed to be to an outside observer (i.e., the same therapist) at his best, and to co-operate best in the drug-free prison atmosphere...' (Glatt, 1970a)

After a great deal of discussion the opportunity for such a therapeutic community for addicts to be set up at Wormwood Scrubs came in 1972.

Preliminary discussions with the addicts in group discussions had shown that what they would have liked would have been to have such a unit exclusively for people dependent on drugs, alcohol, etc.; but when this proved impossible to obtain, the great majority nonetheless voted for starting the "Unit". The Addiction Unit, owing to the administrative and housing problems, thus forms part of a large wing that also contains other psychiatric patient-offenders. Certain problems arose after the unit had been running for about one year, and the section now following is based on two talks given by the author in 1973/4.

A THERAPEUTIC COMMUNITY IN A LONDON PRISON:

PRELIMINARY OBSERVATIONS* (1973/4)

PATIENTS, STAFF AND METHODS

The Annexe in Wormwood Scrubs Prison started to function in December 1972. It forms part of a large wing in the prison, and has four landings, with single cell accommodation for each inmate. Apart from those with problems of dependence the Annexe also provides for the treatment of certain other types of personality disorders. The latter are looked after by other psychiatrists but by the same Hospital Prison Officers as the dependent patients. The great majority of the Annexe inmates partake in the ordinary employment in the main prison, a few working as cleaners in the Annexe (with the standard of cleanliness being remarkably high). Indoor recreation includes such games as table tennis, darts, etc., a library, television, etc.

Admission criteria to the Annexe have remained flexible throughout but were devised so as to exclude those unlikely to benefit from the treatment offered, or highly likely to prove disruptive. Among those

* Based on a talk during a Symposium given at the Prison Medical Officers' South East Regional Conference, London, October 1973 (Three members of the Staff of the unit participated in the Symposium Hospital Principal Officer, M. J. W. Denyer, Hospital Officer, J Brady; and Disciplinary Officer, A L Giddings)· and on a lecture at a plenary session of the 5th International Institute on the Prevention and Treatment of Drug Dependence, Copenhagen, July, 1974 (Glatt 1974a).

who were therefore excluded from admission were, for example, violent patients, aggressive psychopaths, suicidal patients and those with below average intelligence. Among addicts the usual admission procedure as it gradually emerged consisted in their being initially interviewed by the hospital officers working in the Annexe and invited to attend a few out-patient groups. Those considered suitable for the Annexe were subsequently interviewed by the writer. The average length of stay in the Annexe's Addiction Unit varies a great deal but is in the main about six months. Only in very few cases was it found necessary because of lack of co-operation to discharge inmates back into the main prison—a step usually taken only after full discussion with the other inmates.

Between the opening date on 1 December 1972 and 4 September 1973, the highest number of all patients in this wing at one and the same time was 27, and of the addicts among them, 20. Altogether during this initial phase of nine months the number of dependent patients was 34, among them 25 polydrug misusers (aged 21–30 years), seven alcoholics (aged 21–47 years) and two compulsive gamblers. Their personalities—in particular in the case of the younger drug misusers—were often emotionally unstable, immature and inadequate. Their offences covered a wide range (such as forgery, theft, burglary, arson, etc.); their sentences averaged one to three years.

The staff comprised seven Prison Hospital Officers (i.e., Officers who had undergone three months training followed by an examination) who had volunteered for the work in the unit, and who immediately before its opening had spent a special training period of several weeks in Grendon Prison and at the St. Bernard's Alcoholism and Drug Dependence Unit; and two Disciplinary Officers who had been detailed to the unit. The only other staff members were one Assistant Governor, a Welfare Worker, and the writer who attended once or twice a week. The therapeutic programme was essentially in the hands of the Prison Officers and centred on daily group therapy sessions, each Prison Officer looking after his own special group of patients. The atmosphere was therapeutic and non-custodial, with stress being laid on the encouragement of patients' own initiative, responsibility and motivation. A continuing dialogue between staff and patients in time helped to break down initial mistrust and the barrier between 'us and them'. Patients chose their own 'group leader' and published their own magazine.

CRISIS

Things were proceeding smoothly and plans were well in hand to proceed beyond the initial to the second, rehabilitation phase (e.g., giving selected patients the chance to move to a hostel, finding places outside the prison where the Prison Officers could see 'their' patients after discharge, etc.) when a sudden overtime ban for the whole of the prison by the Prison Officers' Organisation led to a crisis in the unit. The necessity to withdraw a number of Officers from the unit to work elsewhere, temporarily brought the work in the Unit to a standstill. At a meeting of the Prison Medical Officers' Regional Conference in October 1973 three of the Hospital Prison Officers who had taken a leading part in the work of the unit clearly expressed their disappoint-ment and frustration, but apart from indicating their sympathy there was little that the meeting could do to help.

When the present writer after a six months' absence due to illness first returned to the unit again—in June 1974—he had expected to find little left in the nature of constructive treatment or a positive 'atmosphere'. However, though still frustrated, staff and patients—though depleted in numbers—showed quite a good morale; two regular group meetings a week (apart from an occasional group for out-patients, i.e. prisoners in other wings who had been referred and were being assessed for admission to the unit) had been kept going, as had been the journal of the unit. Some former patients had been discharged; there were now 19 patients in the wing of whom by now a minority—nine—were addicts: six drug misusers, two alcoholics, one compulsive gambler. Prison Officers' staff now numbered at most six but usually no more than four. Of the former unit inmates who had left the prison quite a few had been reconvicted and were back in prison, but some others had either revisited the unit (permission for this had been obtained some months earlier) or had kept in touch by correspondence or telephone.

RESULTS

The obvious question as to 'results' cannot be answered because a prison unit, like a hospital unit (Glatt, 1967), is quite incomplete by itself, unless it forms part and parcel of an integrated comprehensive service with adequate aftercare and community services (Glatt, 1974a, 1975). Return to old haunts, drug using friends, the addict's former 'subculture' in the absence of strong counteracting supportive rehabilitation facilities makes a return to drugs almost a certainty. The unexpected 'crisis' for the time being interrupted the plans for establishing the aftercare service.

An assessment of preliminary results in a much more modest way—i.e., in its effect on attitudes of staff and patients—would seem to indicate great possibilities inherent in this type of unit, in spite of all the unfortunate unforeseen circumstances. Altered staff attitudes were expressed in such statements as made at the Prison Medical Officers' conference referred to above. For example, one officer mentioned that he had been initially bewildered by the type of 'sink or swim' directive given to the staff with its unexpected delegation of authority, at the start of the experimental unit; but in common with other officers he found that this in time led to a marked development of initiative and interest and to a much more relaxed atmosphere. At the same meeting a Disciplinary Officer who would have initially preferred not to work in the unit as he 'despised' addicts and alcoholics, described how much he had changed his outlook and attitude after closer contact with them. He had experienced great satisfaction in this type of work and no longer resented the remarks of other officers (who did not work in the unit) who called him 'Nurse!' and asked him how the 'Nutfamily' was getting on. Such remarks illustrate the need to educate prison staff not working in the unit about its functioning and objects just as the staff of other departments in a hospital which has an alcoholic unit, should be educated about the work and functioning of the unit, in order to avoid misunderstandings. Most impressive to the present writer, however, was the way in which the depleted and frustrated Hospital Prison Officers' staff often without any medical help in the group sessions and in spite of great difficulties managed to 'activate' and motivate the patients (despite their personality inadequacy) towards dropping their dependency role and assuming a constructive part in working towards their recovery. The staff felt that the patient-offenders during their first two months in the unit perpetuated their customary, passive prisoners' role, but that it was interesting to note how 'veteran' group members questioned newcomers who complained that nobody had ever helped them, 'What have *you* contributed to help yourself? What part did *you* play in all these difficulties?' Of great interest also was the quite unexpected virtual absence of disturbances within the unit and of a demand for tranquilisers, hypnotics or antidepressants.

RECENT DEVELOPMENTS AND PRESENT STATUS
OF THE PRISON DEPENDENCE UNIT

Since the time the report of events described in the previous section had
been written, (Glatt, 1974a), the work of the Annexe has continued, and
in spite of difficulties arising both from staffing and monetary problems,
both the number of staff and patients increased. By now the full number
of patients which could at any one time be admitted to the Annexe is 39,
a figure which is frequently reached. The average number during the
past year was 36. There are three types of patients in the Annexe: sex
offenders, a group of various personality disorders, and the addicts, the
highest number of whom at one and the same time was 26. No inmate in
the Annexe was below the age of 19. Among addicts the great majority
were young addicts, a much smaller proportion were alcoholics and
there were a few compulsive gamblers.

During 1973 24 'dependent' prisoners were discharged from the
Annexe: among them 17 dependent on drugs, six on alcohol, and one
compulsive gambler. Almost all the drug addicts were in their early
twenties, one was 26, one 30 years of age. Of the alcoholics, two were in
their early twenties, one was 27, one 36 and one 47 years of age. The
gambler was aged 25.

During 1974 twenty 'dependents' were discharged from the Annexe:
16 drug addicts, two dependent on alcohol and other drugs, one
alcoholic, and one compulsive gambler. Of the drug takers one was 45
and one 28 years of age, all others were in their early twenties; the two
who were addicted to both alcohol and other drugs were aged 22 and 26
respectively, the alcoholic was 27 and the gambler 29.

During 1975 24 'dependents' were discharged from the Annexe,
among them 16 drug addicts, one dependent on alcohol and drugs, six
alcoholics, and one gambler. Of the drug takers two were aged 29, the
rest 20 to 27; the alcohol and drug dependent was aged 25, the alcoholics
were aged 22, 29, 3–, 41 and 47 respectively, and the gambler 31.

The average age of the addicts was 22 but the Annexe also had one
older junkie aged 45 who had started drug taking in his twenties, had
temporarily abandoned drug taking, only to resume it again after his
family had been killed in a car crash. Most addicts were polydrug users
who took any type of drug coming their way—the prevalent type
among young British drug takers at the present time.

The staff now consists of seven Hospital Prison Officers, but due to the shortage of disciplinary staff the Annexe has no longer any Disciplinary Officers. Closer liaison has been established with the prison welfare staff; two prison Probation Officers regularly participate in the group sessions and the frequent impromptu staff discussion of problems, and they try to arrange for aftercare of discharged prisoners by their local Probation Officers. An Assistant Governor who participates in regular staff meetings maintains liaison between Annexe Staff and the Prison Management.

Most of these offenders had a history of repeated offences, and the great majority stated that in part they had never even considered coming off drugs or drink after receiving a custodial sentence, nor when they had been given a suspended sentence.

Throughout the whole period the same Hospital Principal Officer has remained in charge but for administrative reasons other members of the original staff had to be transferred to other tasks. Most of these would have preferred to stay although this (by losing the opportunity to acquire other experience in other types of prison work) might conceivably have reduced their chances of promotion. On one occasion of such a transfer it was remarkable how strongly the prisoners reacted not only during group discussions, but they also protested against this move in a letter to the Administration signed by all Annexe inmates:

'We have heard, with dismay, that an officer is being transferred from the Annexe to take up other duties in the hospital.

Although we realise it is part of prison routine for officers to be moved from one post of responsibility to another, we feel that, in the case of the hospital Annexe, such transfers have an especially harmful effect.

In the Annexe, the development of officer/inmate personal relationships over a period of time not only results in successful group therapy, but also engenders that indefinable spirit and determination which play such a vital role in the processes of our rehabilitation.

It is our opinion that the systematic transfer of officers from the Annexe is retrograde in the development of what we see as a successful innovation in prison conditions.

We have written this, in the hope that you will take into account these views, whenever you are considering the transfer of officers from the Annexe.'

The remarkable way in which these patients spoke up on behalf of the officers who were leaving the Annexe reflects the extent to which the Staff contributed to the establishment of a good atmosphere, allowing a particular officer's group to develop sufficient trust and confidence in him to approach him with their personal problems. At the same time care is taken to encourage the patient to solve his problems himself and to prevent as far as possible the development of an undue dependence on the staff. In the view of the staff the Annexe now runs much smoother than in the past and the atmosphere has become more relaxed. Two psychologists on the staff of other prisons, after visiting the Annexe, remarked on '... the reality of the community atmosphere, ... the close teamwork and the enthusiasm of the staff running the wing ...' Groups are held daily, with inmates of the Annexe working the rest of the time in the various departments of the prison. The magazine written and published by the Annexe inmates comes out once every three to four months.

As pointed out above, apart from the valiant efforts by the Welfare (Probation) Officers to arrange aftercare, no special follow-up services are at present available. Welfare Officers try to ensure that as far as possible the Probation Officer working on the prisoner's home area is encouraged to visit his client whilst undergoing treatment in the Annexe (in this way he obtains first hand information of the Annexe approach) or when the prisoner has no Probation Officer, to ask the Senior Probation Officer to appoint one. At the same time unless there are special reasons to the contrary, the Welfare Officers also keep the Annexe Staff informed about the prisoner's special home circumstances. All these steps are taken to try as far as possible to provide continuity of care for the prisoner after discharge. Prisoners themselves during their stay in the Annexe often express their concern lest on release they have once more to fend for themselves unaided, and many would welcome a chance to maintain contact with the Annexe staff after release.

For various reasons (see above) unfortunately no results of the outcome of treatment in the Annexe can be given, in terms of statistically significant figures. Keeping the above strictures in mind, some preliminary information is available which might be considered as an indicator of the outcome of treatment—whether the ex-prisoners were convicted after discharge. Details were obtained of reconvictions up to the end of 1975—a period from release of between 2 and 3 years for

1973 discharges and of between 1 and 2 years for 1974 discharges—and are shown in the table below.

Table 1 Discharges from the psychotherapy unit at Wormwood Scrubs in 1973 and 1974, showing whether reconvicted up to the end of 1975

Year of release	*1973*	*1974*
Reconvictions know	13(a)	6
No reconvictions known	6(b)	15
Information not available	2	1
TOTAL	21	22

Lack of known reconvictions does not, of course, necessarily imply that no further offences have been committed, merely that the individual has not been caught and convicted. Nor can the presence or absence of reconvictions imply anything about a return to drug or alcohol misuse, though of the 19 men who were reconvicted, 4 included among their further offences possession of dangerous drugs. Too much can of course not be deduced from these figures: the very brief observation period since discharge, the incompleteness of the information, the fact that not having been caught, of course by no means implies a non-return to drug misuse or criminal behaviour, etc.

Very relevant, in the eyes of the staff, is the noticeable change of attitude as it emerges in the great majority of addicts during their stay in the Annexe. For example, one of the Welfare Officers attached to the annexe stated that 'one cannot but be impressed by the special atmosphere of the Annexe. Nearly 40 men of varied backgrounds, intellectual ability and educational achievement are living in a closely-knit community;' and he remarks... 'From a Social Worker's point of view, the movement observed in a man's attitude, his growth in maturity, and awareness of his difficulties and willingness to face them...' One aspect of such attitude change is reflected in the gradual abandonment of their erstwhile preoccupation with their rights and the theme of how society has failed them; and in place of harping on other people's obligations towards them, they concentrate more and more on a recognition of their own obligations towards family and society.

COMMENTS FROM INMATES

In order to illustrate the typical attitudes of inmates, statements by two addicts in their twenties are presented here:

First addict

Background—A. B. is a 25 year old single, emotionally unstable man, born in London, repeatedly in trouble with the Police since his early teens, with about 10 previous convictions (theft, suspected arson, breaking and entering, possessing dangerous drugs), and now sentenced to three years imprisonment for supplying drugs. He is a polydrug misuser who has taken drugs for four years: starting with cannabis and 'speed' (drinamyl), later 'acid' (LSD) for some time, followed by heroin (mainly 'Chinese H') and methadone. Never registered with any out-patient treatment centre.

Statement—'When coming to the Annexe I felt withdrawn as I was taken off stuff and could not mix or talk to people—I had taken H for three years and I could not understand myself.

When I first came into Nick I thought with all the time I had to do (three years), there was no real rush to finish with drugs, as it would be a simple thing to come off in time. So if any drug would come my way I would not say "no" and in here I could not get addicted anyway. But I had not given the subject any real thought whatsoever. . . .

But the Annexe makes you think, and some of the people who were in here before me and spoke to me, made me see myself and things more clearly. I saw that it was no use going back to the same place or to the people I had known before, and I came to realise that it was me who had to do something about my problem if I wanted to; otherwise whom was I kidding, everyone else or rather myself. . . . I felt quite enlightened when I learnt this and I decided that to live a happy and constructive life and to make something of myself in the future, I would not touch another drug. A while later when someone in the . . . shop offered me some gear, my conscious decision was put to the test. At first I thought I had better take it because he would think I was a bit of a plum if I told him what I wanted to do in the future. But I did say "no" and I told him I had to start somewhere. He said he did not believe me and to stop mucking about but I said that I was serious and that I meant it. Later that day he came again up to me and started talking about old times—he was goofing out and nearly asleep at times— and I thought I should feel jealous and feel "sick" that I had not taken anything, but instead I felt much stronger in myself for saying "no" and I felt a bit sorry for the guy when I was thinking how he would end up ... Anyhow since then I really have more conviction when thinking about drugs and I am quite proud of myself for doing this. Though I know it is only a small step along the way and at least I know that I am not kidding myself, and I know what I want to do in the future .... .

When I came into prison I was sure that my girlfriend (with whom I had been living) would split eventually. I thought if my time in Nick would not break us up the pull of the "gear" on either of us would mean that we would not be able to communicate and I was not sure that we would be able to communicate if we went "straight" ... . But I have been telling her in my letters and on her visits what I want to do and what I have been thinking ... and I wanted to hear from her what she wants to do ... I hope she would not want to go back on drugs ... I hope now we can become a normal and happy family and to have kids of our own, some day .... .

Concerning my family I felt I had done them enough harm and it would be best if I would leave them alone completely. But they wrote to me, saying they hoped that I had now learnt from my many mistakes and they still wanted to help me. Now in their visits I am sure they can see (as I do) that I have been far better off here mentally and physically than I would have ever been, had I stayed outside. They said they would do all they can to help my girlfriend till I come out .... .

So I consider myself lucky that in spite of what I have done to others and myself I still have a girl who loves me and a family who stand by me. Though it still seems a long time off, I know it will happen to me some day that I will have a chance again. Meanwhile I am happy to carry on here, as I know that thinking about things and trying to put them into practice could do nothing but good for me ...'

Second addict

Background—C. D. is a 25 year old, single, methadone addict who is in prison because of theft; he claims that he stole things in order to obtain money to buy drugs. He had been registered with a treatment centre for some time: initially he was prescribed seven ampoules of physeptone (methadone) but, according to his account, his dose was increased to 14 ampoules, as he was also buying barbiturates on the black market and the doctor hoped thereby to cut out his taking barbiturates: 'but I nevertheless continued with my barbs'.

Statement—'. . . having been in the Annexe for a year and with my parole coming up soon I have been advised to go into a drug addicts' hostel for "non-users". I would have liked to go to my relatives' house but as they live in an area where one can easily get drugs I have been warned against going there . . . . So I went for a day's sitting in on a group in the half-way house for addicts in . . . . Soon I felt very disappointed because the other addicts, who had not been in Nick and had come from home or somewhere else, were at a stage I was when I had come into the Annexe a year ago . . . . I felt as if I was dragged back to their level, for example, when they talked about the good effects of drugs, . . . how they would be able to smoke Hash outside the hostel . . . . I had been through all this . . . . I also found the place very untidy . . . . I am not very good at talking in groups but I felt ten feet high when they wanted to take me apart in the assessment group at the hostel. I found that I had no difficulty answering their questions . . .

. . . they seemed to waste most of the time talking about having gone to the Dilly (Piccadilly) but not what made them do it . . . .

In the Annexe people come in with the idea of not giving up drugs but in the end they find out that they are only kidding themselves . . . . I got the idea that these chaps only went to the hostel because they did not want to work . . . .

I would think going into the hostel would be taking a step backwards. I have now so much determination and confidence . . . . I told the other chaps in the hostel that I do not want to have anything to do with drugs and to talk about drugs, and they could not understand it: a junkie not wanting to talk about drugs? Some of the chaps in the hostel turn to drink. I do not want to turn to drink. But I have to go there as my parole is coming up next month. I told them I cannot see that I will get any help from you but I hope that with what I have learnt already I may give you some help and guidance . . . and perhaps in this way I may be building myself up.

. . . It would be much different and much better if our whole group in the Annexe could be sent into the hostel. The great majority of our Annexe group want to leave drugs alone.... .

In the Annexe I found that there is much more to it than just giving up drugs... that is me and my whole attitude.... I have grown up quite a bit. I was never my age. I did silly things, the way kids do. Now I would no longer dream of going into a shop, with enough money to pay for things, but steal, just for excitement and kicks.... .

You ask me what helped me most in the Annexe, other inmates, the Staff, the atmosphere, being locked up?, anything else? I learned in time to want to get something from it all.... . I got much more out of it when beginning to talk about myself. First of all I sat in the group, not saying much unless asked and then I gave the easiest reply. Later on I started to take part in the groups and to take the groups and other person's problems very serious. I started thinking over my past and what I was like. I did a lot of thinking after the groups when I was sitting on my bed and what I had said in that group, and I began to solve it all in my brain.... . I realised that I was changing.

If I had been given by the Court the option to go to a hospital instead of prison I would of course have chosen hospital. Probably I would soon have left hospital and gone to score (buy drugs on the black market).... .

Do I think the Annexe would have worked with me the same way if it would not have been within a Prison? With me, outside Prison the Annexe would probably not have worked during the first six months because I would have wanted to fix, but gradually after the six months this might possibly change...'.

Further comments from inmates

One point emerging frequently from the discussions with the Annexe inmates was their conviction that for many of them a purely voluntary service would not be suitable or would not work. Remarks such as: 'I don't think voluntary services is a good thing for people like us—I'd not be able to do it voluntary—at any rate it hasn't worked for any of us' (the members taking part in the particular group who met that morning were all young drug addicts). 'Living at home or just attending a clinic or day centre for treatment was not enough for me—only prison, or possibly also the threat of imprisonment, might be sufficient to work for me'.

It was, however, a feeling shared by the great majority of addicts in various groups that a hostel stay after discharge from prison might be of considerable help. Leaving prison straight for home, it was said, meant the prison would be 'straight at one's doorstep' 'We need rehabilitation which prepares us for work and which helps us to mix in a "straight" society'.

As regards staffing such a special after-care hostel, the great majority felt that if possible the Annexe staff should also look after the hostel: 'You need personal help and relationship. The Annexe Officers know a prisoner's "tricks" and his particular weaknesses. You need help at the time you cannot cope and, someone to rush to and lean on...'.

At the same time, the inmates, in the various groups in which this theme came up, said that the Annexe patient was not permitted—by fellow patients nor by Staff—to run away from responsibility: 'The community puts pressure on everyone of us. Initially one does not want to learn to face the truth about oneself... but gradually you accept it, and soon you do not want to walk out any longer'.

Why did these people opt for coming into the Annexe in the first place? Most stated that they did not really know what to expect. They had only heard different rumours. A few had hoped that it would be more "cushy" than ordinary prison but they all agreed that essentially it was in fact harder, a 'big mental stress' because they were not permitted to forget their problems but brought face to face with them all the time. Why then did they not leave the Annexe?—seeing that they could of course leave the Annexe for the ordinary prison any time. Initially quite a few had indeed considered it but the Hospital Officers who had initially 'screened' them in the out-patients' groups were soon able to establish a relationship with them, and, with the help of inmates who had been in the Annexe for some time, to persuade the newcomers to give it a somewhat longer try before "opting out"—and soon the initial doubters became anxious to stay.

There are of course many alcoholic or drug dependent offenders for whom community-based alternatives to Prison would be expected to work. But for those who landed finally in the Annexe they had failed to do so, for a variety of reasons given by the inmates. Deferred sentence, for example, had 'made no difference', because... 'even being afraid of a prison sentence did not prevent my drug taking',.... 'I did not have the guts to give up drugs, and I was more afraid of giving drugs up than I was of prison', . . . 'unless you are in a very deep crisis, you do not want to stop drug taking', ... 'I could not really see myself ending up in prison in spite of all the warnings and threats till I finally did land there'.

DISCUSSION

The formation of therapeutic communities provides prisons with the opportunity to greatly improve their psychiatric and therapeutic services without necessarily incurring much additional financial expense. Judges and Magistrates often tell the addict when sentencing him that they hope prison will assist him to get over his addiction problems. In the absence of a therapeutic community and group therapy there seems little chance for such a process to take place. The few psychiatrists working in prison certainly cannot give the large number of addicts in need of help the time, the individual attention, and the therapy necessary for them. A minimum of 1260 individuals sent to prison during 1973 were reported to be drug dependent (Home Office Prison Department Report, 1973). The provision of a special unit within a few selected prisons would make use of suitable staff members and fellow patients as helpers to the psychiatrist and would moreover extend the assistance given to patients over the whole of the day and not limit it to the half hour or so which the overloaded psychiatrist would be able to set aside for a given patient.

A certain proportion among addicts and alcoholics finding themselves in prison would possibly derive much help from being treated in hospitals. On the other hand, their antisocial behaviour—to a certain extent connected with their addiction—has landed them in prison. A prison unit enables the same type of treatment as that available in a hospital therapeutic community, to be carried out in prison under conditions of security—a view expressed by those Prison Officers working in the Annexe who, prior to or during their time in the Annexe, also spent a certain time at the St. Bernard's Hospital Alcoholism and Drug Dependence Unit. Ample opportunity should in fact be provided for Prison Officers employed in prison units to work for certain periods in hospital units, hostels and other community facilities. Those Prison Officers working the Annexe with only minimum special training (but as a rule soon becoming very interested in the approach) seemed to find it surprisingly easy to adopt a therapeutic rather than custodially oriented role and to establish a helping relationship with the prisoner-patients.

Clearly the set-up described in the present report is not an ideal one. Reality was dictated frequently by difficulties arising from staffing, money and similar problems. However mutual support and encouragement from other patients as well as from the Staff, development of insight, self respect and initiative, etc. are all regular features of such a unit, which at the same time provides for supervision by the Staff. Educational and occupational vocational facilities should of course be provided just as well as the more strictly therapeutic ones. Again, as stressed throughout the report, specialised aftercare facilities were woefully inadequate. In the case of dependent individuals with the double handicap of personality disorder and dependency it is not too much to say that lack of planned, adequate aftercare is much more than a great danger, it probably amounts in most individuals to a guarantee for a relapse into drinking or drug taking sooner or later.

By itself imprisonment will do nothing to reduce the likelihood of addicts returning to their dependency immediately after release, and mixing with the 'nick' subculture may well further confirm the antisocial tendencies. Removal from such negative subculture and replacement by a quite different 'subculture' as it emerges in a unit with a high proportion of 'motivated' addicts, supported by an understanding staff, may be one of the most important positive factors at work in such a unit. This encourages the shift from at best meekly passive and indifferent, or indeed hostile, rebellious attitudes towards active participation and towards a change of personality functioning and attitudes. 'Here you are not a number, you are known by your name', as one prisoner put it, 'problems are not solved for you, the staff puts them back to you; you have to work them out yourself'. In the ordinary prison the inmate sees himself as a prisoner, and feels and acts accordingly; in the therapeutic community he is treated as a 'patient' and reacts accordingly—but as a patient who has the responsibility and the possibility to help himself with the assistance of his fellow patients and staff.

Experiences in the Annexe have certainly demonstrated that prisons need not be inflexible, and that Prison Officers can quickly develop a therapeutically oriented role and attitude. They confirm P. D. Scott's view (1974) of the therapeutic capacities of prisons which they should develop for those in whom preventive measures have failed and for whom, for some reason or other, community based alternatives were regarded by the judges as not sufficiently protecting society's interest.

As regards types of personality the majority of inmates of the Annexe were certainly not a positively selected sample. Most were individuals with a relatively unfavourable domestic and social background; in most, delinquent behaviour had antedated their drug taking and drinking career: they were thus 'drinking or drug-dependent delinquents' rather than 'delinquent drug takers and alcoholics', in whom the co-operation in such a scheme could have been expected to be better than in the first group (Glatt, 1968). A description recently given by Washbrook (1976) of a group of chronic alcoholic offenders studied by him in another British Prison would seem to fit equally well also to the great majority of the addicts in the Annexe: (they) '. . . rated very high in terms of mental and social defects' (in the case of the Annexe patients 'emotional' rather than 'mental' would seem more appropriate) 'in prison they are a formidable problem and to society similarly their nuisance value is high'. But within the framework of the therapeutic community formed by the Annexe and with an understanding staff they by-and-large could be handled without too much trouble. As they often explained in the groups: here they had to learn to examine their motives, to listen to other people's views 'even if it hurts', to become more tolerant. Even if making allowances for the finding that so often patients lean over backwards to make the therapist feel that his special brand of therapy is best (and these prisoner-patients all knew that the writer is also connected with out-patient clinics, including a 'treatment [i.e. drug prescribing] centre', a hospital unit, etc.), one was often left with the impression that, rightly or wrongly, these addict-offenders themselves felt that alternative non-compulsory approaches not only had not worked but could not work with *them*—whereas the Annexe at least showed them the way.

Last July the Home Secretary gave a prison population of 42 000 as the breaking point of the system. In a recent article in the Observer, Louis Blom-Cooper, Chairman of the Howard League for Penal Reform, discussing penal reform, stated that with a prison population of 41 400—after a continuing prison population explosion during the past two decades—'the breaking point had been practically reached. There is growing uneasiness both about the inhumanity and the cost of locking offenders up. A much higher proportion of offenders than in the past are now being dealt with by fines, probation and the like rather than by imprisonment'. Research and experience have indicated that prisoners' chances of not offending again remain poor after having been 'confined to an institution too large to provide individual attention, too geographically remote to sustain the vital links with his family and the community, and too regimented to foster the self-esteem necessary to make him a law-abiding citizen'. . . prisons do not reform. But for those who for reasons of public safety, cannot be allowed their liberty, the outmoded prison system should be replaced by a few secure institutions, small enough to provide humane conditions'.

One will, of course, sympathise with much of the above sentiments. There is undoubtedly a great need for services for addicts within the community, the more so as the results of institutional treatment by-and-large have not been promising (D'Orban, 1974). Prolonged hospital (and prison) stay carries the risk of 'institutionalisation) (Martin *et al.*, 1954). The frequent lack of stress on self-help in hospitals which '. . . often encourages people in a dependent role' has been rightly criticised by Willis (1972), who emphasises the importance of "activating" drug addicts, 'especially as they are not usually motivated in any way to do anything constructive'. Yet many drug takers and alcoholics land in prison again and again because the unfortunate combination of personality problem, tendency to act out, and their dependence on drugs, more or less easily available, has foiled any past efforts at their rehabilitation within the community. There is thus also a need to find more constructive methods to make the stay of addicts in prison more therapeutic and more meaningful than is usually the case nowadays. There is likewise a need to educate the staff towards the greater adoption of a therapeutic role. In the view of staff and the great majority of patient-offenders involved in the work of the experimental unit at Wormwood Scrubs Prison, despite all problems and shortcomings, the altered attitudes of staff and patients have indicated the feasibility of establishing a therapeutic community within a prison. Incidentally, the formation of specialised therapeutic communities could avoid most of the pitfalls and drawbacks of larger prisons criticised by Blom-Cooper (1976): inmates do receive a large amount of individual attention, not only from the staff but also from their fellow patients with similar problems to their own and undergoing the same treatment, and as emphasised by prisoners under such conditions, where regimentation is avoided as far as possible, they are able to regain self-esteem, self-respect, and the motivation to work towards their own rehabilitation. Links with the family are certainly difficult to establish, (in particular as in such addicts such family ties were often virtually absent by the time they came into prison) but by encouraging family visits and family discussions with Probation Officers and the Annexe staff, such family links could be fostered and the family kept informed of the patient's progress. Progress under such conditions might enable earlier parole from prison, in particular when specialised hostels and other aftercare facilities are available which enable a gradual adjustment to ordinary life.

Of course, there are as yet no objective results to confirm the favourable impressions gained likewise by staff and patients. It seems difficult to set up a controlled trial with random assignments of comparable patients to either the Annexe or the ordinary prison, and to test attitudes and behaviour, not only before and after the observation and treatment period in the Annexe, but also, and much more importantly, after a period of suitable aftercare in the community. For example, there would have to be a control group consisting of a similar population (composed of drug addicts, alcoholics and gamblers, of similar age groups, social and educational backgrounds, past history of 'dependence' and anti-social activities, etc.), who stay (and receive the attention available for their problems) in ordinary prison; after release one section of these inmates would receive the usual aftercare available to ex-prisoners whilst another section (again the two sections would have to be matched in composition as far as possible) would receive special aftercare. Similarly the Annexe population would also, after release, have to be divided into two matched subsections, the one receiving no more than the usual assistance available to ex-prisoners whereas the other section would receive the special aftercare recommended in the foregoing. The results of the four sections would then have to be compared, not only in regard to (fairly easily measured) numbers (and type) of further offences, and relapses into drug taking and drinking but also as far as possible in regard to behaviour at home, work record, general attitudes to society, personal contentment, etc.

Finally, of some interest may be the comments made by the members of the out-patient group at the UCH Drug Treatment Centre with whom the Annexe was discussed, and of whom one or two had in fact previously been in prison. Their critical comments centred in the main on two queries. The main was their doubt (almost amounting to a conviction) that Prison Officers accustomed to look at their function as mainly custodial would never be able to approach addicts in a therapeutic fashion. The second point concerned their strong belief that inmates would enter the unit mainly because of the greater freedom they could expect in there. Both these points have been briefly dealt with in the foregoing, i.e.,

(a) The Prison Officers concerned soon learned to adopt a therapeutic role. When the comments of the UCH Groups were discussed afterwards during a group session in the Annexe, the Annexe inmates commented that they too were initially very surprised at the way the Officers received and related to them, and later came really to know them with their individual weaknesses, problems, etc.

(b) Whilst probably a proportion or perhaps even the majority entered the Unit in the expectation of an easier life, they soon find that the self-discipline required and having to make decisions themselves and being responsible for the consequences is a much harder task than having all the conflicts and worries about such decisions taken on their behalf by the staff; moreover the initially missing motivation seems in the great majority to arise during their stay in the Annexe whatever their initial reasons for entering it in the first place. The Annexe inmates' own comments on the hospital group's doubts referred to the fact that in the Annexe patients were not allowed just 'to sit back. Neither the staff nor your fellow-patients allow you to "get away" as you may elsewhere in the prison; you are forced to take active part in activities and the group sessions and in time you learn to express yourself'. They also pointed in this connection to the virtual absence of disturbances in the Annexe, despite the lack of use of tranquillisers: 'when you felt grieved and hard done by in prison you perhaps just hit the bloke: in the Annexe you talk your grievances out in the group....'.

The widely held notion that 'any offender with a recognisable mental disorder must necessarily be a suitable case for treatment' has probably been dispelled 'for good' (Brit. med. J., 1975) by the 1975 Report of the Committee on Mentally Abnormal Offenders. This conclusion holds good for addicts as well as for other offenders with personality problems but many addict-offenders are in fact amenable to treatment. In the view of the Annexe staff the formation of experimental units in certain other prisons would seem very desirable. The adoption of slightly different regimes by various units might lead to the elucidation of many unanswered questions, such as the best way of training officers for this work, the best stage during their time in prison when addicts should be admitted to the unit (at present the general feeling would be in favour of admission during the last few months before they are due for parole), the most favourable range of length of stay in the unit (possibly about six months), the composition of the multidisciplinary team, the best ratio between numbers of staff and of inmates, etc. Workers in the field of addiction outside prison often frown altogether at sending alcoholics and addicts to prison, but to imagine that all offender-addicts would be able to summon up the necessary degree of self-discipline required to co-operate with treatment whilst living in the community, is very unrealistic. On the other hand, within the Prison Service, quite a different type of criticism put forward against establishing such units concerns the required outlay of manpower and space at a time when prisons are overcrowded by prisoners and undermanned by staff. Naturally there will be extra costing, arising from the higher staff/inmates ratio required in such a unit to enable more individual attention. At the same time, however, the unit enables officers to assume a definite therapeutic role (and it might perhaps be possible to recruit new applicants specially attracted by such work); and inmates themselves, far from being limited to their customary passive role or even hostile attitude, in time assume a therapeutic role themselves vis-a-vis their fellow patients. Such a unit thus enables the realisation of a therapeutic potential (among inmates as well as among staff) which in ordinary prison remains latent and untapped. Nonetheless, research is needed to show the long-term value of this approach, in particular after the necessary follow-up facilities have been established: therefore in spite of all difficulties involved in such an undertaking it is vitally important to devise some adequate method of evaluation.

CONCLUSIONS

(a) The formation of a therapeutic community for 'addicts' in prison is a feasible proposition.

(b) Many prisoner-addicts—whatever their initial notions—will develop positive 'motivation' in such a unit.

(c) Prison (Hospital) Officers—who, because of their close contact with the inmates, are the most important members of the required integrated multidisciplinary team—in such a unit rapidly assume a therapeutic role completely at variance with the custodial role popularly ascribed to prison staff. The understanding, accepting (though by no means uncritical) attitude of these officers to inmates is probably the main factor in producing an atmosphere of general, constructive co-operation and very active participation of the patients.

(d) Like a hospital unit so also a prison addiction-unit is incomplete and cannot be expected to succeed without a planned, prolonged, specialised, multidisciplinary aftercare service. A special halfway house where these patients can spend the last few months of their sentence before full discharge would seem highly desirable. Continuity of staff—not only within the prison unit but possibly also with the same officers working with 'their' expatients also in the aftercare period, would seem highly desirable.

(e) Evaluation of long-term results (after establishing an adequate aftercare service) is obviously needed, in spite of the problems and difficulties involved. Nevertheless, in the view of all staff members who were involved in this work, the findings in the Wormwood Scrubs Addiction Unit would justify the establishment of a few similar experimental units in other prisons.

(f) The prison addiction unit is well suited for the training of Prison Officers and other professional staff in this field, and for research.

(g) Experiences with Prison Officers in the Wormwood Scrubs Addiction Unit strongly suggest their great, largely untapped, potential for adopting a predominantly therapeutic role—a finding which seems to deserve much wider recognition and utilisation.

REFERENCES

Advisory Council on the Treatment of Offenders (1957) Quoted from *Lancet* (1957), **ii**,
Aron, W. S. and Daily, D. W. (1976) Graduates and Splitees from Therapeutic Community Drug Treatment Programs: A Comparison. *Intern. J. Addict.* **II** (1), 1
Blom-Cooper, L. (1976) Quoted from *Observer* 18 April

British Medical Journal (1973) Leading article, Court Sentences in Female Narcotic Addicts, **4**, 438

British Medical Journal (1975) Leading article. Patients or Criminals, **4**, 70

Cox, M. (1976). Group Psychotherapy in a Secure Setting. *Proc. roy. Soc. Med.* **69**, 215

D'Orban, P. T. (1974). Court Sentences in Female Narcotic Addicts. *Brit. J. Addict.*, **69**, 167

Foulkes, S. H. (1948). 'Introduction to Group-Analytic Psychotherapy' (Heineman: London)

Glatt, M. M. (1955). An Alcoholic Unit in a Mental Hospital—Its Establishment and Functioning. *Brit. J. Addict.*, **52**, 55

Glatt, M. M. (1957). Women in Prison on Attempted Suicide Charges, ii, 387

Glatt, M. M. (1961a). Drinking Histories of English (Middle-class) Alcoholics. *Acta Psychiat. Scand.*, **37**, (1), 88

Glatt, M. M. (1961b). Aspects of the Alcoholic Problem in England. *Med. World*, **95**, 111

Glatt, M. M. (1967). Alcoholism in the United Kingdom. *In* 'New Aspects of the Mental Health Services' (H. Freeman and J. Farndale, eds.) (Pergamon: London)

Glatt, M. M. (1968). Alcoholism in Relation to Crime. *In* 'Gradwohl's Legal Medicine' (F. E. Camps, ed.) (John Wright and Sons: Bristol)

Glatt, M. M. (1969). Rehabilitation of the Addict. *Brit. J. Addict.*, **64**, 165

Glatt, M. M. (1970a). Psychotherapy of Drug Dependence: Some Theoretical Considerations, **65**, 51. Reprinted from: Toxicomanies, *Quebec*, **6**, 33

Glatt, M. M. (1970b). Alcoholism and Drug Dependence—Under One Umbrella? *In* 'World Dialogue on Alcohol and Drug Dependence', (E. D. Whitney, ed.) (Beacon Press: Boston)

Glatt, M. M. (1972) Treatment of Drug Dependency in Treatment Centres, In-Patient Units and Prisons in the London Area. *Brit. J. Addict.* **67**, 125

Glatt, M. M. (1974a). An Addicts' Therapeutic Community in a London Prison. Paper presented at the 5th International Institute on the Prevention & Treatment of Drug Dependence, Copenhagen. ICCA Publications, pp. 13–17

Glatt, M. M. (1974b) 'A Guide to Addiction and Its Treatment—Drugs, Society and Man'. (Medical and Technical Publishing Co: Lancaster)

Glatt, M. M. (1975). 'Alcoholism—A Social Disease' (Teach Yourself Books: London)

Glatt, M. M. and Leon Hon Koon (1961) Alcohol Addiction in England and Opium Addiction in Singapore. *Psychiat. Quart.* **35**, 1 ,

Glatt, M. M., Pittman, D. J., Gillespie, D. G. and Hills, D. R. (1968). 'The Drug Scene in Great Britain' (Revised Edition). (Edward Arnold: London)

Home Office Prison Department Report for 1973. HMSO, London (1974).

Interdepartmental Committee (Second) Report: Drug Addiction (1965). HMSO, London

Martin, D. V., Glatt, M. M. and Weeks, K. F. (1954). An Experimental Unit for the Community Treatment of Neurosis. *J. Ment. Sci.*, **100**, 983

Report of the Committee on Mentally Abnormal Offenders (1975). Chairman Lord Butler. HMSO, London

Rado, S. (1963). Fighting Narcotic Bondage and Other Forms of Narcotic Disorders. *Compreh. Psychiat.*, **4**, 160

Scott, P. D. (1974). Solutions to the Problem of the Dangerous Offender. *Brit. med. J.*, **4**, 640

Washbrook, R. A. H. (1976). The Criminology of the Chronic Drunkenness Offender. *J. Alcohol.*, **11**, 9

Willis, J. (1972). Symposium of the Association for the Prevention of Addiction, London. APA Publication, London. p. 14

ACKNOWLEDGMENTS

I should like to thank Dr. I. G. W. Pickering, former Director, Prison Medical Services; Dr. D. O. Topps, Regional Principal Medical Officer, South East Region Prison Department; Dr. J. Lotinga, Principal Medical Officer, Wormwood Scrubs, for many helpful and stimulating discussions on this project; the Prison Welfare (Probation) Officers for their constant help; and in particular the staff of the Annexe, Mr. J. W. Denyer, Hospital Principal Officer, and the Senior Officers and Officers, for their understanding and exemplary manner in which they carried out their demanding task under often very difficult circumstances.

I am also grateful to Miss S. V. Cunliffe, Director of Statistics, Home Office, for compiling the statistics on the reconvictions of released prisoners and for her kind permission to use them here.

The views expressed in this paper are my own and not necessarily those of the Home Office.

PART IV

Prevention

Social policy and the prevention of drug abuse: Perspectives on the unimodal approach

R. G. SMART

The prospects for successful drug abuse prevention appear to be improving slowly. Effective techniques are still doubtful but considerable work has been done on approaches to prevention. The major problem is to frame acceptable social policies which will allow some test of the major preventive approaches. Concern with prevention should flow from our lack of treatment acumen and from a knowledge that almost no large scale public health problems have been eradicated by treating affected cases. Almost all such problems (with the possible exception of tuberculosis) have been conquered with primary prevention. Few would claim that current theoretical or practical approaches can produce the social policy equivalents of vaccines or immunizations for drug abuse. Presently, schools of thought and doctrinaire approaches to prevention tend to predominate. Because none of the major approaches have been adequately tested choices amongst them are largely arbitrary. The preference here will be for an approach based on the need to reduce the frequency of use of alcohol and drugs in the belief that this will eventually reduce drug problems.

In general, two basic approaches to prevention are based either explicitly or implicitly on explanations of etiology. In one approach drug abuse, including alcoholism is seen as the result of psychological or socio-cultural events predisposing to heavy drinking or excessive drug use. However, the unimodal approach argues that the total *per capita* consumption of drugs must be considered and that where this is high alcoholism or drug abuse will also be high. The purposes of this paper are: (i) to explain each preventive approach with preferential treatment to the unimodal approach, and (ii) to suggest which types of social policy considerations and experiments would contribute most to preventive efforts. Efforts will be made to examine data relevant to alcoholism and the abuse of other drugs.

ABUSE OF ALCOHOL

UNIMODAL MODEL OF PREVENTION OF DRINKING PROBLEMS

Unimodal approaches originated in work by Ledermann (1956) but the implications of this model have been best described by DeLint and Schmidt at the Addiction Research Foundation in Toronto. At the time of their first paper in 1968 (de Lint and Schmidt, 1968) Ontario had the rare requirement that all alcoholic beverages be purchased using sales slips containing the purchaser's name and address. This made it possible to determine how many purchases of alcoholic beverages were being made by given individuals. Purchase forms were collected for some 63 009 transactions made in representative areas of Ontario during 1962 and 1964. Analysis of the forms indicated those who buy more usually consume more since purchasers of large numbers of bottles typically made many separate purchases. The frequency of purchases in Ontario describes a logarithmic normal curve according to Ledermann's model. This is a curve in which there are many infrequent purchases, a somewhat smaller number of more frequent purchasers and even fewer very frequent purchasers. The curve is a smooth, unimodal one with no large discontinuities. This research indicates that there is no clear difference between social drinkers, heavy drinkers and alcohol or problem drinkers on consumption. All drinking categories gradually shade into one another and cannot be clearly distinguished. However, this would be contradictory to a commonly held clinical viewpoint that alcohol consumption should be bi-modal, i.e., that alcoholics or problem drinkers should be distinguishable from normal drinkers in their extent of consumption.

Several studies have shown that the log normal fit holds for alcohol consumption in several countries. Ledermann's early work showed that the fit was good for Finland and selected populations of American drivers and French hospital patients. Later surveys using interviewing techniques have established that the log normal distribution describes alcohol consumption in Finland at several points in time (Ekholm, 1972).

Schmidt and de Lint have also studied the levels of consumption associated with the adverse consequences of drinking. For example, the average *per diem* consumption for most (84 per cent) Canadian drinkers is 5 cl per day or less of absolute alcohol, 5 to 10 cl for 10 per cent of drinkers. Fewer than 3 per cent drink 15 cl per day or more. However, 15 cl is the average amount consumed by alcoholics seen at clinics (de Lint, 1968). Amounts in excess of 10 cl per day taken regularly are associated with marked increases in the risk of liver cirrhosis. The use of liver cirrhosis as an alcohol problem indicator rests both on the known effect of alcohol on the liver and on the high rates of liver disease found amongst alcoholics. These arguments have been strengthened by data showing a significant correlation between liver cirrhosis mortality and *per capita* consumption in several countries (de Lint and Schmidt, 1971). These are spatial and time series correlations for a variety of periods in Australia, Belgium, Canada, Finland, France, Holland, Sweden, and the USA. In summary, the distribution approach suggests that: (i) the general character of the distribution of alcohol consumption is similar from place to place; (ii) alcohol consumption relates to liver cirrhosis; and inferentially, (iii) it may be necessary to reduce *per capita* consumption in order to reduce problems from alcohol.

It should be pointed out that several critics of this approach (e.g., O'Neill and Wells, 1971; Skog, 1971; Ekholm, 1972) have disputed the type of mathematical fit which the distribution may have to the log normal expectancy. However, most proponents (Popham, Schmidt and de Lint, 1974, Smart and Whitehead, 1973) would claim that the main point is that the distribution is smooth and unimodal and apparently constant in character from place to place. The exact fit to the log normal curve is seen to be far less important than that mean consumption and heavy consumption are related.

SOCIO–CULTURAL MODELS OF PREVENTION

The socio-cultural approach to prevention attempts to explain the differences between alcoholism rates of ethnic minorities and national groups with reference to different norms about drinking. Drinking was believed to be a problem amongst Irish-Americans because cultural norms allowed 'institutionalized intoxication'. On the other hand, norms among Jewish drinkers emphasize careful use and the avoidance of intoxication. The contrasting rates of alcoholism among Irish-Americans and Jewish-Americans are well known and presumably related to these norms. Analyses of this sort have led to a socio-cultural hypothesis, e.g., 'in any group or society in which drinking customs, values and sanctions . . . are well established, known to and agreed upon by all, consistent with the rest of the culture and are characterized by prescriptions for moderate drinking and proscriptions against excessive drinking, the rate of alcoholism will be low' (Blacker, 1966).

The socio-cultural model suggests that social and cultural factors are most important and that a set of proscriptive and prescriptive norms allowing controlled, integrated drinking should be established. Essentially, this approach has generally ignored research on the distribution model: its proponents usually assume that the total volume of drinking *per capita* consumption matters little in preventing alcohol problems. Whitehead (1972) has argued that these two positions are not so far apart as has seemed since they emphasize different aspects of alcohol problems, i.e., drunkenness in the socio-cultural and liver cirrhosis in the unimodel. Unfortunately, most approaches taken in the socio-cultural model (e.g., improving the acceptability of bars and taverns as social centres and fostering wine-drinking with meals) would probably increase overall *per capita* consumption.

SOCIAL POLICY CHANGES AND THE PREVENTION ALCOHOL PROBLEMS

Opportunities to experimentally test the implications of either preventive model experimentally have been rare. Few governments change laws on alcohol consumption with either preventive model clearly in view. It is recognized that prohibition did result in remarkable reductions in liver cirrhosis death rates in the USA (de Lint and Schmidt, 1971) but this is an 'experiment' unlikely to be repeated. However there are social experiments which could be based on the two models presented. Some of these are in progress or could easily be suggested.

An interesting social experiment occurred in Finland (Makela, 1972) with regard to alcohol policy. According to some socio-cultural theories one might expect that less drunkenness would result from creating a shift to low alcohol beverages, e.g., beer and wine. By promoting the use of such beverages it may be argued that moderate, drinking habits, e.g., drinking with meals would be generated. However, the uni-modal model would predict that unless *per capita* alcohol consumption (from all sources) decreased there would not be fewer problems from alcohol.

In Finland in 1969 laws were changed to allow the sale of beer in 'unrestricted retail distribution—previously it could be purchased only in stores maintained by the State Monopoly' (Makela, 1972). Unfortunately for clear analysis of causes retail liquor stores were established in rural areas at the same time. The aims were to make low alcohol beverages more readily available through grocery stores etc. and hopefully to moderate drinking practices. Surveys done in 1969 and 1971 showed a 48 per cent increase in overall consumption. Beer accounted for much of the increase but the consumption of liquor occurred at the same rate as earlier. The distribution of consumption described a log normal function both before and after the change (Ekholm, 1972) but with a shift toward much higher *per capita* consumption. The numbers of drinkers reaching consumption levels involving health hazards also rose. In general, it appears that the 'liberalization' merely encouraged people to add a new drinking habit to those already held, without getting them to relinquish any of the older ones. This suggests that changing drinking habits by encouraging new ones may be more difficult than formerly imagined. It also suggests that volume of consumption and *per capita* use has to be reduced or held constant before socio-cultural or normative changes will reduce the hazards of consumption.

There are substantial problems in utilizing the distribution data for alcohol in prevention. One research problem is that no situation has been found where *per capita* consumption is falling so that the effect on the distribution and rate of hazardous drinking can be studied. Consumption seems to be going up everywhere. More generally, to try to reduce or maintain present *per capita* consumption appears to be against most contemporary philosophy and practice in alcohol control. Most such ideologies in Western countries seem to demand more availability of alcohol, e.g., decreasing age limits, increasing numbers and types of outlets, allowing more advertising and promotion, etc.

With regard to policy changes Whitehead suggested that social experiments be made by increasing the cost of alcohol, increasing legal purchase age, elimination of beverage advertising, decreasing bottle sizes and the like. Many of these are at least worth a trial but there is little empirical evidence to suggest that any would be effective, except for increasing the cost of alcoholic beverages.

Popham, de Lint and Schmidt (1974) have masterfully reviewed the known effects of 'legal restraints' on drinking and drinking problems. It is not proposed to duplicate their review here, only to indicate their conclusions and a few relevant papers which have appeared since that review was written. The major conclusions appear to be that:

(i)   numbers of stores or taverns selling alcoholic beverages do not relate well to alcohol consumption or drunkenness except perhaps where the number of outlets was drastically reduced.

(ii) restrictions in hours of sale appear to decrease drinking and drunkenness.

(iii) reductions in drinking age from 21 to 18 result in more drinking and more alcohol-involved accidents for persons 18 to 20.

(iv) conclusions about the effects of monopoly distribution systems are difficult to make.

(v)   increases in the relative price of alcoholic beverages based on alcohol content would be the method most likely to result in decreased consumption.

(vi) differential taxation favouring beer consumption would probably not have more than a small effect on total consumption or on the prevalence of alcoholism.

Two studies done since the Popham *et al.*, review are also of interest. In one study (Smart, 1974a) an examination was made of the effects of the restrictions on hours of sale, numbers and types of outlets, beverage strength imposed during the 1914–18 war in Britain. Conclusions are difficult because of the large number of other events occurring at the same time, however, the restrictions temporarily reduced drunkenness and liver cirrhosis death rates. Part of the reduction also continued after the war when the laws on hours of sale were retained. The other study (Smart, 1974c) showed that self-service stores for alcohol sales generate more impulse buying than do clerk-service stores and that impulse buyers drink more than more planful buyers.

It is clearly the case that the best methods of alcohol control may be rather unpalatable socially and politically. Research suggests controls on availability by not decreasing legal age levels and by substantial increases in price. It has been argued (Addiction Research Foundation (ARF), 1973) that very great increases in relative price of alcohol would be required as a preventive health measure. It has been shown that the relative price of beer and spirits has actually decreased since World War II. In 1949 in Ontario it took 7.2 per cent of the average weekly income to buy 12 bottles of beer but by 1969 only 3.6 per cent. Similar but less striking decreases occurred for spirits. As relative prices of alcoholic beverages have declined in Ontario there has been an increasing prevalence of problems due to alcoholism and heavy drinking. At present, it is not known what acceptance such measures as increasing prices or legal ages would have amongst politicians or the general public. Large scale surveys are underway in Ontario to help determine which measures might be most palatable and in what circumstances. It appears probable, however, that neither politicians nor people in general will be heavily in favour of preventive measures requiring that they modify their own 'safe' drinking in order to reduce the problem in others.

Some gripping and persuasive educational programs will be necessary in order to gain acceptance for social policy measures which restrict alcohol consumption. A survey of 707 adults in 5 Ontario communities (ARF, 1974) indicated that 48 per cent wanted no change in alcohol laws. However, of those who do about twice as many want stricter controls rather than weaker. Attempts to make laws more strict would apparently receive support from less than ⅓ of adults, unless they could be persuaded otherwise. As for alcohol causing problems very few people said that it did (3 per cent) and drugs such as marijuana, LSD, heroin and speed were ranked far ahead of it in causing problems. There was a strong tendency for people to feel that they themselves had sufficient information about alcohol and drugs but that other people needed far more information. There was also a strong tendency for people to believe that although alcohol and drugs are a problem in their community certainly they were never a problem in their neighbourhood. These results suggest the need for alcohol education but also indicate the types of opposition and lack of interest that such education will encounter, at least initially.

ABUSE OF OTHER DRUGS

UNI-MODAL MODEL OF PREVENTION OF DRUG PROBLEMS

The use of the unimodal model for alcohol has created an interest in the possibility that the same relationships might hold for many psychoactive and hallucinogenic drugs. Fortunately, the major implications of the distribution model may not be so difficult to accept for 'drugs' as for alcohol. The author has argued elsewhere (Smart, 1973) that most legal and social policy related to drug control assumes that drug use and not mere 'abuse' or heavy or 'addictive' use is to be controlled. However, control measures are not explicitly based on arguments from epidemiological theory but more on the supposition that all drug use is 'abuse'. Nevertheless, there are dissenting views (e.g., Le Dain, 1972) which maintain that increasing the frequency of drug use would not necessarily increase the number of users who are harmed.

The unimodal model and its implications are less well understood for drug problems than for alcohol. One problem is that the concepts addiction, habituation, dependence and abuse have no clear and agreed meaning (Smart, 1974b; Christie and Brunn, 1969). Individual definitions usually do not include enough sufficiently clear statements to be useful to epidemiological research; terms such as psychic dependence, overpowering desire could rarely be useful. Unlike the field of alcohol studies, clear indicators of pathological consumption have been difficult to determine and have not been related to drug use. Perhaps the exception would be withdrawal symptoms and increased tolerance in the case of narcotics and some other drugs. However, these symptoms are of little use in the study of hallucinogenic drugs such as MDA, Cannabis, LSD, etc. In general, there is no symptom of excessive use such as liver cirrhosis which is a useful indicator of problem drug use.

Also, drug use among adolescents typically involves multi-drug use so that the volume of use of any particular drug may be too small to create any special organic effect. Multi-drug use, of course, also makes it difficult to associate any consequence with the use of a single type of drug. Insufficient attention has been given so far as to how drug problems can be identified in epidemiological work and how their occurrence is associated with the frequency of drug use.

With regard to multi-drug use the most likely problem indicators may be social and psychological and may involve bad trips, dropout from school or other social and familial institutions, personality changes, long-term psychotic reactions, suicide, spontaneous recurrences or treatment for a variety of drug related problems.

Considerable research relevant to the unimodal model has been done for non-alcoholic drugs. Smart *et al.*, (1971) collected data on drug use frequency for five samples of high school students. These samples involved students in Toronto (in 1968 and 1970), in Niagara Counties (in 1970), Montreal (in 1969) and Halifax (in 1969). A variety of sampling methods and sample sizes were employed but all studies utilized adequately chosen samples. The total number of students involved was 27 022. A drug use score was computed for each student indicating the number and frequency of drug use. The drugs used were alcohol, tobacco, glue, marijuana, LSD, other hallucinogens, opiates, tranquillizers, stimulants and barbiturates—10 drugs in all. All five studies enquired about the use of all 10 drugs and depending on the frequency of use drug scores could vary from 1.5 to 75.0. It was found that in all five studies the distributions were smooth and unimodal and that they roughly approximated a log normal distribution. This occurred even in Toronto where *per capita* drug use increased substantially between 1968 and 1970 but the basic character of the distribution remained the same. Similar distributions were found (Smart and Whitehead, 1972) for drugs when considered separately, i.e. in three studies in Canada. The distributions of the frequency of marijuana, LSD, speed, solvents, stimulants, tranquillizers and barbiturates among high school students were continuous and most were approximately log normal (with a few exceptions). For high school students both multi-drug use and use of individual drugs are similarly distributed. This is the case even though some of the drugs are legal and some illegal and they have a wide variety of effects.

A study by Smart and Whitehead (1973) has shown that there is some cross-national generality for these findings. They found that data from a group of British University students also described continuous roughly log normal distributions. Data for a large sample of Canadian adults did not fit the log normal expectancy well (statistically speaking) but the distribution of scores was continuous, unimodal and somewhat similar to the expectancy.

A recent paper by Paton (1974) has taken a different approach to the problem of the mathematical character of drug use distributions. He employed probit analysis which plots per cent using a drug at a given rate or higher, such that if the distribution is normal a straight line is formed. He recast alcohol consumption data from Ledermann and drug use data from Smart and Whitehead as well as drinking and drug use data from a study of US Servicemen by Fisher. It was found that all data fit a log normal distribution well with alcohol having a lower standard deviation than illicit drugs.

Too little work is being done on how drug problems relate to *per capita* drug consumption. A survey of drug use among high school students in Toronto (in 1970) involved some 15 districts. These are units comprising a high school and the several feeder schools associated with it. It was found that the 15 districts varied enormously in rates of drug use—some were low in all types of use, some high, and some varied with the type of drug. The average 'drug use score' was examined for ten drugs as in the earlier study.

Each user's score could vary from 1.5 to 75.0 for the 10 drugs. The average score and the proportion of students receiving scores of 30 or more were computed for each district. However, the mean scores were computed with the 30 or more scores removed so there was no forced correlation between the two. The score of 30 or more was selected somewhat arbitrarily but also because this seemed to be the minimal score held by persons seeking treatment for drug problems. A Spearman rank correlation between the two was 0.75 ($p < 0.001$). This indicates that within a given population where average drug consumption is high, heavy use is also high, even when the heaviest users have been excluded. Essentially, this is the same sort of analysis as has been made for alcohol consumption and liver cirrhosis. However, the data for the latter comparison are far more extensive in that they cover a variety of years and are broadly cross-national in scope.

Unimodal data provided by Whitehead and Aharan (1972) are relevant to the educational and attitude change problems inherent in some preventive efforts. They studied attitudes toward the desirability of intoxication with drugs other than alcohol and have found scores to be a log normally distributed and positively correlated with drug use frequency. This suggests that efforts to reduce favourable attitudes to intoxication may be accompanied by a reduction in drug use. It also

With regard to multi-drug use the most likely problem indicators may be social and psychological and may involve bad trips, dropout from school or other social and familial institutions, personality changes, long-term psychotic reactions, suicide, spontaneous recurrences or treatment for a variety of drug related problems.

Considerable research relevant to the unimodal model has been done for non-alcoholic drugs. Smart *et al.*, (1971) collected data on drug use frequency for five samples of high school students. These samples involved students in Toronto (in 1968 and 1970), in Niagara Counties (in 1970), Montreal (in 1969) and Halifax (in 1969). A variety of sampling methods and sample sizes were employed but all studies utilized adequately chosen samples. The total number of students involved was 27 022. A drug use score was computed for each student indicating the number and frequency of drug use. The drugs used were alcohol, tobacco, glue, marijuana, LSD, other hallucinogens, opiates, tranquillizers, stimulants and barbiturates—10 drugs in all. All five studies enquired about the use of all 10 drugs and depending on the frequency of use drug scores could vary from 1.5 to 75.0. It was found that in all five studies the distributions were smooth and unimodal and that they roughly approximated a log normal distribution. This occurred even in Toronto where *per capita* drug use increased substantially between 1968 and 1970 but the basic character of the distribution remained the same. Similar distributions were found (Smart and Whitehead, 1972) for drugs when considered separately, i.e. in three studies in Canada. The distributions of the frequency of marijuana, LSD, speed, solvents, stimulants, tranquillizers and barbiturates among high school students were continuous and most were approximately log normal (with a few exceptions). For high school students both multi-drug use and use of individual drugs are similarly distributed. This is the case even though some of the drugs are legal and some illegal and they have a wide variety of effects.

A study by Smart and Whitehead (1973) has shown that there is some cross-national generality for these findings. They found that data from a group of British University students also described continuous roughly log normal distributions. Data for a large sample of Canadian adults did not fit the log normal expectancy well (statistically speaking) but the distribution of scores was continuous, unimodal and somewhat similar to the expectancy.

prescription drugs exists e.g., on age of purchasers, number of outlets, numbers of products, hours of sale, than for alcohol. The purpose here is to examine a few studies relevant to the prevention of drug abuse problems.

With regard to illicit drugs such as heroin and cannabis, successful prevention cannot be described. Numerous social policies concerning illicit drugs have been pursued in various countries including different maintenance systems, penalties for users and traffickers, attempts at suppression by educational means and the like. It appears to the present author that no clear statement can be made about the best social policy to follow with regard to illicit drugs such as heroin and cannabis. We appear not to know how to prevent illicit drug use. A few speculations can be made but most current social policy on heroin and cannabis can follow no known successful paths.

A current vogue in many areas, especially education is for drug education programmes. Chiefly these are short term programmes for high school or grade school students. Their aims vary enormously but most seek to change attitudes about drugs in a favourable direction and decrease drug use among students. The author has argued elsewhere (Smart, 1973) that drug education programmes may 'educate' but they do not appear to reduce drug use. At present, numerous drug education programmes have been evaluated (for a review see Goodstadt, 1974). Most such programmes increase knowledge about drugs, a few change attitudes in desirable directions but virtually none reliably reduce drug usage. Unfortunately, at least one programme (e.g., Stuart, 1974) has been shown to actually increase drug use. It will probably be some time before effective drug education programmes will be developed to the point that they could prevent drug abuse on a large scale. Unfortunately, drug education, broadly conceived, represents the only current preventive effort to reduce the demand for drugs in the population.

Most current social policies on illicit drugs attempt to decrease the supply side of the supply and demand function for drugs. These policies essentially provide legal and administrative controls on the production, sale and distribution of illicit drugs. There is a belief that better or bigger repressive policies are decreasing, at least in North America. A long history of severe penalties for possession and trafficking in narcotics and cannabis has not held either use or abuse down to acceptable levels.

Further, it appears unlikely that repressive measures on any drug for which there is a strong, unique demand can succeed. Several economists (Koch and Grupp, 1971; Little, 1967, 1971) have argued that increased enforcement has undesirable side-effects. Heavier enforcement decreases the market supplies and if demand is not totally elastic the price is driven upwards. Unfortunately for prevention by price control, it has estimated that elasticity of demand for heroin is only about 10 per cent (Little, 1967). Thus, small decreases in supply would lead to large increases in price and probably therefore to drug-related crime on the part of addicts.

Other programs of control such as crop-substitution and curtailing illegal diversions of drugs from ethical drug companies have also been suggested. Such solutions are rejected by many (e.g., Lind, 1974) because (i) substitute crops cannot be more profitable than illicit drugs as long as there is a demand for them and (ii) when legal diversions are stopped an illegal manufactured supply of lower quality is likely to appear.

There is little to recommend enforcement without demand reductions as an effective measure. Simmons and Gold (1973) recently pointed out the tremendous difficulties in preventing opium production. They have estimated that the 100 000 to 200 000 pounds of opium used yearly in the USA could be grown in an area between 11.2 to 23.2 square miles. They also refer to a report by the Drug Abuse Council which states that capital intensive cultivation could reduce this to only 5.4 square miles. Surveillance of such a small growing area on a world-wide basis is, of course, almost impossible. Given the large numbers of ships, planes and cars entering the USA each year detection of small amounts of opium is unlikely to be complete.

Not much attention has been given to broad social policy for reducing the use and abuse of prescription drugs. Marketing and distribution has typically been the province of medical associations and pharmaceutical consortium although all western governments screen and licence drugs for sale. The creation of a UN Single Convention on psychoactive drugs is completed but not all countries have signed and it is too early to see its effects. Currently, there is a growing recognition that prescription drugs are frequently abused and that many are addictive (Lennard *et al.*, 1972). There is also growing recognition that much prescription drug use may be unnecessary or essentially the medication of everyday problems, common to anyone and everyone. Seidenberg (1971) has pointed out how often psychoactive advertisements in medical journals and direct mail to physicians recommend drugs for the anxieties and worries of everyday life. That society is over-medicated has been suggested or implied by various authors (e.g. Lennard *et al.*, 1972) but probably not all would agree (Mellinger *et al.*, 1973).

Some maintain that psychoactive drugs are carefully prescribed for real symptoms, given the intent of the physician. However, considerable research on the way in which prescribing is done suggests that the equation between symptoms and a prescribed psychoactive is far more complex than expected. For example, Fejer and Smart (1974) attempted to determine the proportion of 'normal' or 'well' persons among tranquillizer users. Among adults surveyed in Toronto 26.3 per cent of those who had been prescribed tranquillizers reported good or excellent health, had not had a serious health problem in the past 12 months, reported no serious illness in their family in the last year, had not consulted a doctor or psychiatrist for a psychological problem in the past year and in fact had never consulted a mental health professional for psychological problems. One would not claim that these people had absolutely no need for tranquillizers but they do look surprisingly 'well', certainly well enough not to require treatment. Questions are naturally raised about how much of their tranquillizer use is for the minor symptoms of modern life.

The tendency of physicians to prescribe psychoactives appears to depend on many things other than the patients' symptoms. Klerman (1960) found that older physicians, those with administrative duties and nurses more often favoured drug therapy. Prescribing varies with the physician's age and specialty (Cooperstock, 1971), his own drug use (Blum and Wolfe, 1972), and with his experience (Appleton, 1965). Certainly enough data exist to suggest, as has Blum (1974), that 'one might wish to introduce greater rationality into the distribution of drugs that are under control'. Clear action steps are difficult to suggest since it is known that many patients, especially of the lower classes, want and expect medication. However, some efforts in medical education could be made to emphasize the need for controls on psychoactive prescribing where no pressing need exists. Indeed, the whole problem of 'need' for psychoactives for minor anxieties and depressions probably requires re-examination.

CONCLUSIONS

Social policy concerning alcohol and drug abuse is in need of experimental trials. It is likely that *per capita* consumption will have to be decreased before hazardous consumption. In the case of alcohol control many policy changes are being made e.g., with age limits, types of outlets, types of licencing. However, too few are being made with an experimental approach involving comparison areas, before and after measurements and the other experimental deseridata. The best choice for an experiment in social policy concerning alcohol would be one involving striking increases in price. It is likely, however, that public and government acceptance for this will be slow in coming. This makes necessary educational and influence compaigns for legislators and the public.

Social policy concerning illicit and prescription drugs is more difficult to frame. It appears likely however that reductions in the use of drugs will be necessary before heavy use can be reduced. Demand for the narcotics is far less price elastic than for alcohol. This makes it necessary to reduce demand functions rather than merely hoping to reduce supply as in past efforts of control. Elasticity of demand for prescription drugs is probably high since many have a low addictive liability although this has apparently not been studied. The most promising approaches with both illicit and prescription drugs would appear to involve educational efforts. Currently, research on these efforts is underway but effective programs have not been created yet. With regard to prescription drugs research and educational efforts should be directed to attempts to reduce the occasions on which prescription drugs are prescribed. Reductions in demand for illicit drugs probably depends on the educational efforts made for young people and their parents.

REFERENCES

Addiction Research Foundation. (1973). Proposal for a Comprehensive Health-Oriented Alcohol Control Policy in Ontario, Toronto
Addiction Research Foundation. (1974). Public Drug Education and Information Needs in Five Ontario Communities, Toronto. (Unpublished)
Appleton, W. S. (1965). Now Phenomenon. *Psychiatry,* **28**, 88
Blacker, E. (1966). Socio-cultural Factors in Alcoholism. *International Psychiatry Clinics*; **3**, 51

Blum, R. H. and Wolfe, J. (1972). *In* 'The Dream Sellers: Perspectives on Drug Dealers' (R. H. Blum, ed.) (San Francisco: Jossey-Bass)

Blum, R. H. (1974). *Studies on Natural Groups in Controlling Drugs.* (R. H. Blum, ed.) (San Francisco: Jossey-Bass)

Christie, N. and Brunn, K. (1969). Alcohol Problems: The Conceptual Framework. *Proceedings of the 28th International Congress on Alcohol and Alcoholism,* Vol. 2. (Hillhouse Press: Rutgers)

Cooperstock, R. (1971). Sex Differences in the Use of Mood-modifying Drugs: An Explanatory Model. *J. Health Hum. Behav.,* **12**, 238

de Lint, J. and Schmidt, W. (1968). The Distribution of Alcohol Consumption in Ontario. *Q. J. Stud. Alcoh.,* **29**, 968

de Lint, J. (1968). Alcohol Use in Canadian Society. *Addictions,* 14

de Lint, J. and Schmidt, W. (1971). Consumption Averages and Alcoholism Prevalence: A Brief Review of Epidemiological Investigations. *Brit. J. Addict.,* **66**, 97

Ekholm, A. (1972). The Lognormal Distribution of Blood Alcohol Concentrations in Drivers. *Q. J. Stud. Alcoh.,* **33**, 508

Fejer, D. and Smart, R. G. (1974). *Tranquillizer Users: How Many are Without Physical or Psychological Problems.* (ARF Substudy)

Goodstadt, M. (1974). *Myths and Methodology in Drug Education: A Critical Review of the Research Evidence.* (ARF Substudy No. 588)

Klerman, G. (1960). Staff Attitudes, Decision Making and Use of Drug Therapy in the Mental Hospital. *In* 'Research Conference on the Therapeutic Community' (H. C. Denber, ed.) (Springfield: C. C. Thomas)

Koch, J. V. and Grupp, S. E. (1971). The Economics of Drug Control Policies. *Int. J. Addict.,* **6**, 571

Le Dain, G. (1972). *Cannabis: A Report of the Commission of Inquiry into the Non-Medical Use of Drugs.* (Ottawa: Information Canada)

Lederman, S. (1956). *Alcool, Alcoolisme, Alcoolisation.* Donnees Scientifiques De Caractere Physiologiques, Economique Et Social (Institut National d'Etudes Demographiques, Travaux et Documents, Cahier (No. 29). (Paris: Presses Universitaires de France)

Lennard, H. L. and Associates. (1972). *Mystification and Drug Misuse.* (New York: Harper & Row)

Lind, R. C. (1974). Benefit—Cost Approach to Evaluation of Programs. *In* 'Controlling Drugs'. (R. H. Blum, D. Bovet, J. Moore eds.) (San Francisco: Jossey-Bass)

Little, A. D. (1967). *Drug Abuse and Law Enforcement.* (Cambridge: Presidents' Commission on Law Enforcement and the Administration of Justice)

Little, A. D. (1971). *A Study of International Control of Narcotics and Dangerous Drugs.* (Bureau of Narcotics and Dangerous Drugs)

Makela, K. (1972). Consumption Level and Cultural Drinking Patterns as Determinants of Alcohol Problems. *Proceedings of 30th International Congress on Alcoholism and Drug Dependence.* (Amsterdam)

Mellinger, G. D., Balter, M. B., Parry, H. J., Manheimer, D. I. and Cisin, I. H.

(1973). *An Overview of Psychotherapeutic Drug Use in the United States.* Paper prepared for Epidemiology of Drug Abuse Conference, Puerto Rico

O'Neill, B. and Wells, W. T. (1971). Blood Alcohol Levels in Drivers Not Involved in Accidents and the Log Normal Distribution. *Q. J. Stud. Alcoh.*, **32**, 798

Paton, W. D. M. (1974). The Uses and Implications of the Log Normal Distribution of Drug Use. *Proceedings of 3rd Cannabis Conference* (London)

Popham, R. E., De Lint, J. and Schmidt, W. (1974). The Effects of Legal Restraint on Drinking. (ARF Substudy 581, 1973). *In* 'Biology of Alcoholism' (B. Kissin and H. Begleiter, ed.) (Plenum Press: New York)

Seidenberg, R. (1971). Drug Advertising and Perception of Mental Illness. *Mental Hygiene*, **55**, 21

Simmons, L. R. S. and Gold, M. B. (1973). The Myth of International Control: American Foreign Policy and Heroin Traffic. *Int. J. Addict.*, **8**, 779

Skog, O. J. (1971). *Alkohalkonsumets Fordeling i Befolkningen.* (Statens Institutt For Alkohol-Forskning, Oslo)

Smart, R. G., Whitehead, P. and Laforest, L. (1971). The Prevention of Drug Abuse by Young People: An Argument Based on the Distribution of Drug Use. *U.N. Bul. Narc.*, **XXIII**, 11

Smart, R. G. and Whitehead, P. C. (1972). The Consumption Patterns of Illicit Drugs and Their Implications for Prevention of Abuse. *U.N. Bul. Narc.*, **XXIV**, 39

Smart, R. G. (1973). The Ethics and Efficacy of the Prevention of Drug Dependence. *Report on WHO Conference on Epidemiology of Drug Use*, Euro 5436IV (Regional Office for Europe)

Smart, R. G. and Whitehead, P. C. (1973). The Prevention of Drug Abuse by Lowering Per Capita Consumption Distributions of Consumption from Canadian Adults and British University Students. *U.N. Bul. Narc.*, **XXV**, 49

Smart, R. G. (1973). *Factors in the Effectiveness of Drug Education.* Paper Presented at the Conference on Drug Education, Montreux

Smart, R. G. (1974a). The Effect of Licencing Restrictions During 1914–1918 on Drunkenness and Liver Cirrhosis Deaths in Britain. (ARF Substudy 578, 1973). *Br. J. Addict.* In Press

Smart, R. G. (1974b). Addiction, Dependency, Abuse or Use: Which Are We Studying with Epidemiology. *In* 'Epidemiology of Drug Use' (E. Josephson, ed.) (New York: R. H. Winston and Co.)

Smart, R. G. (1974c). *The Effect of Self-Service Stores on the Purchase of Alcoholic Beverages.* (ARF Substudy No. 595)

Stuart, R. B. (1974). Teaching Facts About Drugs: Pushing or Preventing. *J. Educ. Psyc.*

Whitehead, P. C. and Aharan, C. H. (1972). *Drug Using Behaviours and Attitudes: Their Distributions and Implications.* (Addiction Research Foundation: London)

Whitehead, P. (1972). *The Prevention of Alcoholism: An Analysis of Two Approaches.* (Addiction Research Foundation: London)

CHAPTER 11

An enforcement—Prevention perspective on drug abuse

J. H. LANGER

The complex phenomenon of abuse of natural and synthetic chemical substances is not new. Nor are efforts by social and political institutions to attempt to regulate or control it. Every society, large or small, seeks to preserve and perpetuate itself. When a threat to its viability arises, defense mechanisms are brought into play. This Toynbeean concept cannot have eluded the serious observer of the present crisis in drug and alcohol abuse.

Recent developments in the United States and elsewhere have complicated any analysis of drug trends. Yet some things have been learned and may prove to be useful to those who must continue to operate the social mechanisms which control, or try to regulate, consumption of potentially harmful substances. At present (mid-1975) a reassessment of both the supply (enforcement) and demand (treatment/prevention/education) sides of the drug problem is underway in the US, by the Federal government. However, the fifty states and hundreds of local governments are continuing to carry on programs of drug abuse prevention, treatment, and law enforcement. Evolving from this broad spectrum of activity are common experiences which have utility for future planning.

The basic themes of this paper are the need for a coherent strategy and the definition of the roles of institutions, with emphasis on the role of law enforcement and the criminal justice system. It is not the contention here that enforcement and extrinsic control are the most effective means of handling drug abuse. Rather, it is asserted that the society itself must recognize the inter-relationships among the roles of the many agents of control and education which influence the drug problem.

A BASIC DRUG STRATEGY

The 1974 Federal Response to drug abuse has been published by the White House Special Action Office for Drug Abuse Prevention (SAODAP). Its major themes emphasize the balance needed between treatment, rehabilitation and education on the one hand, and the criminal justice system on the other. Even more significant is the explicit focus on the role of the criminal justice system in outreach, and cooperation with the drug treatment system. The major themes of Federal Strategy II are:

1. Continued support for heroin treatment programs.
2. Expand treatment emphasis on poly-drug abuse.
3. Outreach through the criminal justice system and other mechanisms to bring into treatment those drug abusers who would not seek it of their own volition.
4. New rehabilitation and vocational training efforts.
5. Nationwide school-based early intervention programs.
6. Increased cooperation among Federal, state and local law enforcement programs.
7. Expand programs to strengthen the interrelationship between the criminal justice system and the drug treatment system.
8. Increased enforcement efforts directed at all levels of illicit drug traffic.

A key part of the making of Federal Strategy II was the process of reaching out to all parts of the country for comments, criticisms and new concepts. SAODAP took inventory of the first strategy statement, and synthesized private sector input to strengthen this effort.

A great many US Federal agencies have been active in dealing with the multiple facets of drug abuse, in treatment, education, and rehabilitation. Over the past five years the Drug Enforcement Administration (DEA) and its predecessor agency have worked quietly to promote the concept of law enforcement-criminal justice-community cooperation. Before it was popular, DEA proposed that the police and treatment and rehabilitation people sit down and discuss their differences and establish mutual goals in the field of drug abuse prevention—as well as ways of handling the various types of drug offender. Publications were produced that really lived up the 'factual, accurate, no-exaggeration' dictum. Reaching the grass-roots level and finding out the needs of people was basic to DEA's prevention program.

Although control, prevention, and treatment measures taken earlier were sometimes criticized, in 1973 there was less heroin on the street than for a number of years, and the purity was lower. In effect, some addicts were detoxified by the low potency of the heroin supplied by their dealers. The number of addicts had dropped, and estimates range to 300 000 in 1973 from a high of 600 000 three years earlier. The recent decision by Turkey to resume poppy-growing may have an adverse effect on the supply of heroin, as will increased smuggling from Mexico. How much is difficult to predict. Developments in 1975 reveal that addiction in the US is increasing, though it is still below the levels of 5 years ago.

The drug problem is far from solved. Poly-drug abuse, and alcohol abuse has increased, though total drug abuse statistics seem to be levelling off. Nevertheless, DEA's DAWN (Drug Abuse Warning Network) finds that drugs—hypnotic, barbiturate, opiate, cannabis—in combination with alcohol is the most frequent cause of drug-related medical incidents such as overdose, death, and hospital admissions.

Examination of the relationship between treatment and the criminal justice system can be instructive should another drug problem occur such as the one we are experiencing. Today, the major source of addicts and other persons in treatment is the criminal justice system—and far from objecting, treatment programs are eager to obtain such clients. Other easy sources of addicts have dried up, and obtaining clients is a matter of survival for many treatment programs.

There is no delusion that a sudden change of heart has occurred among the critics of the police. (It should be recognized that some of the criticized practices were those of prosecution and adjudication and are erroneously attributed to the police.) There is a good deal of self-interest in much of the criticism, but recently greater cooperation has developed between enforcement and treatment programs in many places, and penalties for possession have been reduced in some places.

A recent meeting in the Netherlands, of persons working in pre-vention and treatment, indicated that in Europe, too, with some exceptions, penalties have been made less severe for drug abusers, and more severe for dealers. In Germany, where even penalties for possession have increased, the courts have still been given, and are exercising, greater discretion in sentencing. As a point of interest for the treatment establishment, in Austria the chronic cannabis abuser can be certified and required to undergo treatment.

It is desirable that we learn from experience. But Bismarck once said, that 'Only a fool says he learns through his own experience; I have always contrived to learn from the experience of others'. As oversimplified as that may be, there is an undeniable element of truth in it. Society cannot afford to permit the lessons regarding cooperation between the criminal justice system and the rest of the community in drug abuse prevention and treatment to be forgotten. Both the justice system and the community need a great deal more education in the process of communication, and mechanisms must be made more flexible and responsive to emerging needs.

ROLE DEFINITION IN PREVENTION OF ABUSE

In the US there are 50 states laws on drugs, as well as the Federal law, and hundreds of local ordinances—all different in some way, and all enforced by different police and regulatory agencies. Laws act as deterrent to the majority of the public, even today, despite mass media distortions to the contrary. Problems with the law have risen because of inconsistent enforcement, and even more inconsistent prosecution and judicial disposition—e.g., differing sentencing, dismissals, arbitrary action by judges, and a number of other technical issues. Yet the great majority of the public believes that drug laws are necessary and should be reasonably and rationally administered. It is the application of them by some jurisdictions that creates controversy—they may be too severe, too lenient, or irrelevant to the local problem.

Penalties for some drug-related activities may have been unreasonable, but this is being remedied by many states. The issue of drug abuse as a 'victimless crime' is still being raised in some places—but the public generally does not accept this concept completely, nor should it. Perhaps the victims are once or twice removed from drug dealers' transactions, but a look at our drug abuse statistics and the actual drug casualties refutes the idea that drug dealing is a victimless crime.

The issue of 'social harm' must be faced. How many people who are unproductive or dependent can the society support? Drug abuse challenges the basic desire of a society to be in control of itself, to be able to call upon itself—on all of its members when necessary, and have them respond. Most communities cannot afford the luxury of a large unproductive or dependent population.

Very slowly a recognition of the distinction between the criminal who is incidentally an addict, and the addict who is not otherwise a dangerous criminal is becoming clearer. Still more difficult to sort out, however, is the distinction between the addict who sells drugs only to support his habit, and the criminal who is in business to make a profit who may incidentally use drugs. Where treatment is available and the addict may choose between treatment or continued criminal conduct, the addict-criminal merits imprisonment, not for his addiction, but for his illegal trafficking. In the US treatment is available for any addict who wants it, thus negating the argument that the addict was 'forced' to resort to crime to obtain drugs.

Continuing pressure of law enforcement, along with treatment availability, has brought many addicts into treatment. The majority of addicts in treatment were identified by enforcement and some form of coercion into treatment was involved. There is a 'Partnership' of sorts developing between the criminal justice system and some treatment agencies. Treatment of persons dependent on drugs other than opiates also is an emerging option available to police and the courts, but there are fewer treatment programs for non-opiate users.

Another unsolved issue is the varying levels of effectiveness of state regulations and voluntary self-regulation of physicians and pharmacists who handle legal drugs. State regulatory boards and associations of registrants have both legal and professional responsibilities. If the public will identify and require controls from regulatory agencies and the health professions, the need for drug enforcement by police could be greatly reduced. The prescriber and seller of legal drugs, the physician and pharmacist, and their licensing boards and associations must be educated to meet their obligations to control drugs and their patients' use of them.

It is important to distinguish the role of the police from the roles of courts, corrections and prosecutions. Courts decide upon punishment, control, and rehabilitation of offenders. They still are not able to distinguish well between the hardened criminal who should be imprisoned for a long period to protect the community, and the petty criminal who might, with training, become rehabilitated. Prison-conducted rehabilitation has not been successful. Some consistent legal distinctions are needed between:

—the hardened criminal who incidentally uses drugs
—the drug abuser who has committed only crimes involving drug possession
—the non-user who sells to the user for profit
—the trafficker who sells only to dealers
—the maker of illicit drugs
—the diverter of legally-produced drugs
—the seller of legally-produced drugs to drug abusers
—the physician who prescribes unneeded drugs
—the physician who supplies drugs to addicts illegally

A new court diversion approach to deal with the non-criminal addict who is arrested for drug possession is the TASC, or Treatment Alternatives to Street Crime program, funded by the Law Enforcement Assistance Administration. It will be in over 30 US cities by 1975.

Diversion programs of this and other kinds generally remove the drug-dependent person from the criminal justice system without sending him to jail first. Such programs for first offenders, and in some cases others, may function at the arrest level, the pre-trial hearing level, and the hearing-pre-plea level. Diversion post-plea is really a kind of probation. Unfortunately, judges are often uneducated in distinguishing between the defendant who needs treatment and the one who should be imprisoned. Staff capable of assisting the court are not generally available.

DEA's 1973 study of the sentencing practices of Federal Courts reveals that twenty-five per cent of kilo-amount heroin dealers never go to jail. Many others are free on bond for periods of a year or more. And often continue their drug dealing. State statistics on this are unknown, but thought to be as high or higher. Of course the role of the prosecutor in drug cases is critical. The prosecutor is the single most powerful and frequently inaccessible element in the criminal justice system. His decision on whether or not to prosecute is the least public. Reform of prosecutor and court practices especially at the local level is long overdue.

THE ROLE OF LAW ENFORCEMENT

The task of law enforcement agencies is made very difficult when society has passed laws which it may not want consistently enforced, but does not wish to say so. This basic problem is a continuing issue in the US, although drug laws and judicial decisions are slowly becoming more consistent. It is clear from recent experience that effective law enforcement depends upon public support as well as upon efficient enforcement techniques and judicial consistency.

In the field of prevention, some large-city police forces have instituted the position of 'Crime Prevention Specialist' which is not primarily drug abuse prevention, but which includes such responsibilities. The Community Relations Officer on a city police force also has many functions that deal with drug abuse and community programs for prevention, and even treatment.

Unfortunately, local law enforcement in some communities has become isolated from the public. This loss of two-way communication has made it difficult for the police to ask for cooperation in drug traffic prevention. Some communities, recognizing this need, have established programs to 'Turn in the Pusher' or TIP programs. Although they have had limited success, TIP programs do bring the community into closer cooperation and communication with the police. A critical need in police-community relations is to give the citizen a safe, easy and effective way of reporting criminal activity—and to guarantee anonymity or protection if needed. It is essential, in high-crime, high drug abuse areas, to obtain the cooperation of the community, to allay fear of reprisal—police cannot expect citizens all to be heroes. In some communities, however, especially large cities with minority populations, vigilante groups have threatened to find and themselves execute or expel drug dealers. This occurs when the authorities do not seem to be communicating with these groups or are not cutting down on drug traffic in that community.

A basic aspect of drug abuse prevention by the police is gaining the trust and confidence of the public that drug law enforcement can be effective, and is in fact working. This requires meeting and working with community groups, professional organizations, etc. If the police can work effectively with youth, in and out of school, and cooperate with those who work with youth, in the long range drug abuse prevention will be effective—but such a program requires trained officers, and long-range planning, something most communities do not have. Small towns and rural areas are most deficient, because of lack of resources. A study conducted by the White House Special Action Office for Drug Abuse Prevention, in 1974 warned of the increase in drug abuse, and even heroin addiction, in small communities in the US. DEA's Community/Justice System program provides technical assistance on this problem to community and state officials.

A prognosis of what may occur in the next few years can serve as a sort of summary of these observations. Drug abuse in various forms will remain part of our culture at an undetermined level for a number of reasons:

1. Society really does not seem to believe itself capable of eliminating drug abuse of all kinds, but wishes to minimize it. So many psychoactive drugs are being produced that it is impossible to control all of them—especially the legally produced ones. The poly-drug abuse phenomenon is likely to increase. Combinations of drugs, and drugs with alcohol are now becoming popular, and such abuse is almost impossible to completely eliminate.

2. A reduction in drug abuse can occur if the public and special interest groups will agree on certain basic measures of prevention, education and control.

3. Fluctuations in heroin availability in the US (now again on the increase due to an influx of brown heroin through Mexico) shows that it is possible to control and reduce the traffic in illicit substances such as heroin and cocaine, LSD, and cannabis, if sufficient resources are provided, but constant enforcement, control and deterrent pressure is necessary.

4. Enforcement agencies are becoming more skillful in identifying dealers and traffickers, and discriminating between them and their victims.

5. The public is now recognizing important distinctions between some drug abuse as a stage through which a minority of youth go, and drug trafficking, conducted by ruthless dealers who victimize the ignorant. Well-planned, permanent education about drugs integrated into the school curriculum at all grade levels including the primary grades, can reduce the number of

experimenters. Parents and teachers also require training and education.

6. Courts, it is hoped, will become capable of making more intelligent judgments about various types of offenders, and utilize community resources for diversion to appropriate control facilities.

7. The public has slowly become aware of the socially destructive nature of drug abuse—regardless of which drug—when it affects large numbers of people. This may result in the most effective type of controls—family, peer group, and social-cultural.

8. The cost of maintaining large numbers of unproductive people in costly programs that are not very effective is becoming more burdensome. The US is coming to believe it can no longer afford them. There are nations which cannot and will not tolerate addicts who are unproductive, hence, some, like China, and Japan take positive action to deal appropriately with both trafficker and user.

9. The dealer in illicit drugs who does so for profit and in large quantities must be dealt with effectively. Long prison terms are the only protection a society has against the hardened criminal. When penalties are inconsistent or minimal, when the profits are large, and when the public is not willing to assist law enforcement in controlling illicit selling, control is not likely to be effective.

10. Mass media and its excessive reporting of insignificant or obviously anti-social views was a basic reason for the problem in the US, for example, Timothy Leary and LSD and the present cannabis decriminalization controversy. Greater social responsibility is needed in press and other media, otherwise the next drug fad will, like the present one, attract large numbers of youth.

11. If, to repeat, *if* schools and parents continue effectively to teach very young children about drugs and to counsel them on the dangers and the constructive alternatives, drug abuse is likely to level off and perhaps decline—as it shows signs of doing in some areas of the US.

The most important concept in the drug demand-and-supply equation is that the level of drug abuse in a community is a function of the *total availability* of drugs of all kinds. This idea focuses our attention on the inter-relationships of law enforcement, community education programs, and the treatment needs of a community. If, to repeat if, total drug supplies are controlled by the police, physicians, and pharmacists, manufacturers and wholesalers, and parents, less will be available to the actual and potential user; therefore, the level of abuse will decrease. But cooperation by all who are responsible for control is necessary, otherwise drug abusers will do what they do now in many places—use the drug that is available, whatever it is.

The immediate problem faced by those responsible for drug abuse prevention is to keep the numbers of people who use drugs as a kind of self-medication to minimum:

(a) If they use drugs to cope, other ways for them to cope must be found.
(b) If they use drugs to escape, other ways to rescue them are needed.
(c) If they use drugs for recreation, alternatives must be provided, and especially taught to the young.
(d) If they use drugs to defy society, they will have to be controlled insofar as they become antisocial.
(e) If they use drugs because others do so, they need counseling, or new friends or environments.

Whatever the reason, an alternative to drugs as a solution must be found.

The inter-relationships of social institutions are so complex that accurate prediction of the next drug fad is impossible. Nevertheless, unless reasonable and consistent controls, acceptable to and accepted by the public, are developed, inevitably the next drug fad will come and with it more people will be affected or destroyed.

Ultimately, it is self-control rather than extrinsic control which will be a final solution to any drug crisis. The basic issue is whether the people in our society recognize the inherent dangers of chemical dependence and manipulation of consciousness, or whether, as individuals, they understand the value and necessity of being in command of themselves.

BIBLIOGRAPHY

BNDD (Drug Enforcement Administration) (1973). Proceedings of the Second Alternatives to Drug Abuse Conference (Airlie, Virginia)
Drug Abuse Council (1974). Recent Spread of Heroin Use in the United States: Unanswered Questions (Washington, D.C.)

Drug Enforcement Administration (1974). Drug Abuse and the Criminal Justice System (Washington, D.C.)

International Union for Child Welfare (1974). Summary Report Second Extra-Ordinary Session of the IVCW Consultative Group in Social Problems of Children and Youth (Amusfoort, Netherlands)

Langer, J. H. (1973). Drug Information, Drug Education, and Law Enforcement. Report of the International Conference on Alcoholism and Drug Abuse (ICAA) p. 400 (San Juan, Puerto Rico)

White House Special Action Office for Drug Abuse Prevention (1974). Federal Strategy for Drug Abuse and Drug Traffic Prevention (Washington, D.C.)

PART V

The Laboratory's Contribution

Detection and measurement of drugs in biological fluids: Their relevance to the problem of drug abuse

V. MARKS AND D. E. FRY

INTRODUCTION

The large increase in drug abuse, especially during the 1960's, resulted in a demand for laboratory methods suitable for detecting drugs in biological fluids under routine clinical conditions. Many methods have been published and are the subject of a number of reviews (Kaistha, 1972; Mulé, 1972).

It is first necessary to consider the technical and analytical requirements of a drug screening programme. The best methods will depend on circumstances. Firstly; what drugs are being sought—and why? In the United Kingdom, where multiple drug abuse is the main problem, a wide spectrum of drugs must be included and the reason is usually clinical rather than forensic. Secondly, the sensitivity of the testing procedure must be considered. Increasing the sensitivity of the method usually involves more difficult laboratory procedures, which decreases the number of samples that can be handled and increases the cost. Thirdly, the accuracy of the procedure must be taken into account. The elimination of false positives is especially important when the method is used for follow up of drug addicts that are being rehabilitated.

Other factors which must be taken into account include the number of specimens requiring analysis, the time taken to produce a result and the instrumentation available. In general, rapid qualitative screening is best carried out using a thin-layer chromatography (TLC) system or immunochemical procedure (Mulé, et al., 1974a, 1974b) but the latter is only useful when a limited number of known drugs are being sought. Quantitative measurement of drugs requires the use of more sophisticated equipment and is of questionable value in the management of drug addiction.

For most procedures, drugs must first be extracted from the sample by solvent extraction, ion exchange, or an adsorption method. The extracted drugs are then further purified, if necessary, by a chromatographic procedure and finally measured either qualitatively or quantitatively. For immunochemical identification prior purification is seldom necessary but specificity is generally low.

This article will first consider the commonly used methods for extracting drugs from urine and their detection using thin-layer chromatography (TLC) as nearly all screening programmes depend upon this technique. The most commonly used drugs will then be considered in detail and the methods for their identification and measurement discussed.

GENERAL ANALYTICAL CONSIDERATIONS

SOLVENT EXTRACTION

Direct extraction of the commonly abused drugs from urine by organic solvents, is simple and widely used. Provided the pH and salt concentration of the aqueous phase is optimal and a suitable organic solvent is chosen, most drugs can be extracted, in good yield, from biological fluids. Acidic and neutral drugs can be extracted from an acidified solution into chloroform or ether whilst the basic drugs, such as amphetamine, can be extracted into ether from an alkaline solution.

The extraction of morphine from urine requires more critical adjustment of pH and the use of a more polar solvent system such as chloroform-isopropanol. Attempts to extract both basic and acidic drugs in one step have resulted in diminished recovery of drugs. More recently a procedure has been proposed by Stoner and Parker (1974) which is quicker than multiple extraction procedures, especially when large numbers of urines are processed. The method employs bromo-cresol purple which reacts with basic drugs at pH 6.0 to form organic salts which are extractable into an organic solvent. The acidic drugs are also extracted at this pH. The solvent is evaporated and the dried down residue can then be used for TLC detection of both basic and acidic drugs.

ION EXCHANGE RESIN

Ion exchange procedures give a cleaner extract than direct extraction—but only at the expense of recovery. This can, however, generally be compensated for by use of a larger urine volume.

Dole *et al.*, (1966) suggested the use of Reeve Angel SA2 cation-exchange paper to remove and concentrate drugs from the urine. The various drugs could subsequently be eluted from the paper with three consecutive extractions at pH 2.2, 9.3, and 11.0 respectively. The main advantage of this technique was that drugs could be extracted onto the paper at the clinic and the paper sent to a distant laboratory for analysis.

This procedure has found little application in the United Kingdom where the distances between clinics and laboratories are smaller and the transport of urine specimens presents few problems.

The Dole extraction procedure has the additional advantage that pigments and other interfering substances present in urine are not absorbed onto the paper so that subsequent TLC analysis is subject to less interference. However, the method has been criticised by Heaton and Blumburg (1969) and by Mulé (1969) because of the poor recovery of barbiturates and amphetamines. Mulé (1969), using radioisotope markers, obtained only a 2.4 per cent recovery of pentobarbitone and a 21 per cent recovery of amphetamine. Marks and Fry (1968) had overcome these difficulties by using a preliminary extraction of the urine with ether, at pH 2.0, to remove barbiturates. The urine was then made alkaline with sodium hydroxide (NaOH) and again extracted with ether to remove amphetamines. The pH was finally adjusted to pH 5.0–6.0 and the morphine extracted with SA2 ion exchange paper. This procedure, though more complicated than that described by Dole *et al.*, (1966) was found to be more suitable for the urine specimens received in the United Kingdom where multiple drug abuse is prevalent.

Zeocarb 225 resin could be used for the extraction of morphine from urine instead of SA2 paper (Marks and Fry, 1968). However, the paper is easier to handle than the resin, especially when large numbers of urines are being examined.

Kaistha and Jaffe (1971) reported a modification of the method of Dole *et al.*, (1966) in which 40–50 ml of urine was used. The sedative-hypnotics were eluted at pH 1.0, and the opiates and amphetamines at pH 10.1, using an ammonium chloride/ammonium hydroxide buffer. The decreased extraction efficiency of the ion exchange paper was overcome by the use of a much larger volume of urine. For urine volumes under 40 ml Kaistha and Jaffe (1971) recommended direct extraction but in our experience the volume of urine submitted for analysis is frequently less than this and so presents difficulties.

NON-IONIC RESIN (AMBERLITE XAD-2)

Amberlite XAD-2 resin is an insoluble synthetic cross-linked, poly-styrene polymer. The adsorption forces involved are primarily of the Van der Waals' type, hence by changing the hydrophobic/hydrophilic balance of the molecule to be adsorbed the extent of its adsorption can be altered. In the case of ionic drugs the hydrophilic/hydrophobic balance of the molecule can be altered by changing the pH. Mulé *et al.*, (1971) studied the use of XAD-2 resin for the routine identification of drugs of abuse in urine. They found that recovery of amphetamine was only 49 per cent but that of other drugs of abuse was more complete. Weissman *et al.*, (1971) on the other hand, obtained 90–100 per cent recovery from urine for all of the major drugs of abuse. More recently Kullberg and Gorodetzky (1974), in a detailed study of the factors involved, reported 80–90 per cent recoveries of drugs in the organic eluates from Amberlite XAD-2 columns.

Adsorption of drugs onto resin in a column depends on pH, flow rate and urine/resin ratio; elution from the resin is dependent on solvent polarity, flow rate of the solvent and the degree of contact between the solvent and the resin beads. Because of the large number of factors capable of affecting the overall recovery of drugs from the urine using Amberlite XAD-2 resin, it is difficult to maintain consistent results. One of the most difficult factors to control, when dealing with large numbers of specimens, is the flow rate of urine and/or solvent through the column. Mulé *et al.*, (1971) used a hydraulic flow control apparatus while Kullberg and Gorodetzky (1974) used a Technicon two speed Proportioning Pump II to maintain satisfactory flow rates but both modifications tend to make the method too cumbersome for routine use.

THIN-LAYER CHROMATOGRAPHY (TLC) IDENTIFICATION

Numerous thin-layer chromatographic techniques have been described for the separation and identification of the extracted drugs. The two commonest are those of Dole *et al.*, (1966) and of Davidow *et al.*, (1968). Both methods use the same solvent system, namely ethyl acetate: methanol: NH$_4$OH (85:10:5). The detection systems differ in so far as Dole *et al.*, (1966) ran three separate plates—one each for barbiturates, narcotics and amphetamines respectively, whereas Davidow *et al.*, (1968) ran only one plate but applied a sequence of various spray reagents to it to detect the different drugs.

Kaistha and Jaffe (1972a) have described a modification of the development system which they claim gives better differentiation of drugs of abuse from drugs used for treatment.

Variations in the conditions of running TLC plates can produce marked differences in the Rf values, and the separation, of individual drugs. The size of the tank, the temperature and other factors can all affect the degree of solvent saturation and hence the Rf. The type of silica gel—and what additional additives and hardeners are present—also has an effect. Each laboratory must, therefore, determine its own best solvent system and running conditions. Standards must also be spotted on each plate to correct for variations in running conditions.

The spotting of urine extract onto a TLC plate is tedious and accounts for much of the time taken to screen a urine sample for drugs. Various automatic devices are available which help to overcome the tedium but they generally are slow in use. Considerable time saving can, however, be achieved by using a new type of TLC plate which is available commercially from a number of manufacturers, although the cost is somewhat greater than conventional plates.

Visualisation systems are even more numerous than solvent systems bearing testimony to the unsatisfactory nature of many of the spray reagents. Amphetamine is usually detected using a ninhydrin spray followed by exposure to UV light; or by using a Fast Blue B salt spray but neither spray reagent is specific. Barbiturates are usually detected by spraying sequentially with mercuric sulphate solution followed by diphenylcarbazone; but compounds other than barbiturates also react. Narcotics are detected by spraying the TLC plate with iodoplatinate, but this visualises many different compounds including several widely used psychotropic drugs, e.g., the phenothiazines.

Davidow *et al.*, (1968) recommended sequential spraying of a single TLC plate for the detection of amphetamines, barbiturates and narcotics respectively. The ammonia and volatile solvents were removed, after development, by heating the TLC plates in an oven at 75°C. The hot TLC plate was then sprayed with ninhydrin; put under a UV lamp for 2 minutes and any pink spots, due to amphetamine, noted. The plate was then sprayed with diphenylcarbazone followed by mercuric sulphate and dried. Barbiturates and glutethimide appeared as blue to pink spots. The plate was then heated to 75°C for 2 minutes when the phenothiazine drugs showed up as violet to orange-red spots. Finally, the plate was sprayed with iodoplatinate followed by Dragendoff reagent, to detect the narcotics. In practice considerable care is needed with the Davidow spraying sequence as overspraying with ninhydrin affects the sensitivity of the subsequent morphine detection.

Further details relating to the detection of individual drugs in urine will be given later. Sufficient has been said, however, to show the non-specificity of these crude TLC identification procedures. It cannot be emphasised too strongly that they are *screening* procedures only and that positive drug *identification* cannot be made on the basis of a single Rf value and one or two colour reactions. For positive identification of a specific drug independent analytical methods must be used. These will be further discussed under specific drugs.

Providing the limitations of the method are remembered, however, TLC procedures can be very useful for rapid screening of large numbers of urine samples. The reliability of the method depends, to a large extent, on the experience of the personnel and their skill in interpreting the colours and Rf values of the spots seen on the final sprayed chromatogram.

GAS-LIQUID CHROMATOGRAPHY (GLC)

The main use for gas-liquid chromatography, in the present context, is in the confirmation of drugs detected by TLC. GLC is too slow for routine screening of large numbers of urines but used in conjunction with TLC doubtful results can be confirmed with a high degree of reliability.

The simplest method of confirming the identity of a drug is by comparison of the retention time of the unknown substance with that of an authentic sample of the drug. Additional confirmation can be obtained by derivative formation of the authentic and putative substances and comparing their retention times. Examples of these techniques are given under individual drugs.

Considerable increase in specificity can be obtained by using a nitrogen detector instead of the conventional flame ionization detector. This type of detector is particularly sensitive to nitrogen-containing compounds and is useful for the GLC of plasma specimens when interference from lipids can be a problem (Toseland *et al.*, 1975).

IMMUNOCHEMICAL METHODS

This type of method can be used in the routine screening of urine specimens for drugs. In general, sensitivity is greater than that of TLC procedures. The specificity is often not as good but is tremendously dependent on the nature of the antibody. The reagent cost is generally high in comparison with TLC. Immunoassay methods are usually not suitable where multiple drug abuse is suspected as the procedure then becomes very time consuming. Furthermore, the numbers of different drugs that can be tested for is limited by the availability of antisera. However, Sulkowski *et al.*, (1975) used a semi-automated immunoassay method for the mass screening of urine for morphine, barbiturates and amphetamine.

Immunoassay methods are of greatest value in the detection and measurement of drugs that are present in biological fluids in exceedingly small amounts and which can only be detected with great difficulty—or not at all—by other methods. The quantitative measurement of morphine in blood (Aherne *et al.*, 1975), for example, and the detection and measurement of cannabinoids in blood and urine (Teale *et al.*, 1974; 1975) is relatively easily performed by radioimmunoassay, but is extremely difficult by other methods. In these and similar instances where the sensitivity of existing methods is insufficient for clinical use, immunoassay techniques have great advantages. They enable drugs to be detected and quantitated routinely in cases in which this was previously not possible.

HIGH-PRESSURE LIQUID CHROMATOGRAPHY (HPLC)

Recent progress in the development of high-pressure liquid chromatography has resulted in this technique being used for the detection and quantitation of drugs of abuse (Jane, 1975). HPLC has some advantages over GLC in that high molecular weight compounds can be separated at room temperature without the formation of volatile derivatives. Decomposition of thermal labile compounds is also avoided. Drugs are usually detected by their ultra-violet absorption at 254 nm or at the wave length of maximum absorption if a variable wave length detector is used. The fluorescence detector is more sensitive and was used by Jane and Taylor (1975) to measure morphine in urine down to levels of 0.01 $\mu g/ml$.

INDIVIDUAL DRUGS

DIAMORPHINE AND MORPHINE

Extraction

Diamorphine (heroin) is excreted in the urine principally as morphine and its derivatives. Subjects receiving diamorphine by injection excrete only a very small amount of the unchanged drug in their urine but this can, if necessary, be detected and measured by sensitive GLC methods. Codeine is also partially hydrolysed to morphine in the body, and is excreted as morphine and its conjugates as well as native codeine.

About 90 per cent of both diamorphine and morphine are excreted in the urine as water-soluble morphine glucuronide. Most of the remainder is excreted unconjugated, and is commonly referred to as 'free' morphine. Most screening methods for morphine detect only the 'free' drug. This avoids the technical difficulties associated with hydrolysis of morphine glucuronide, including the time taken to achieve complete hydrolysis. It also reduces interference from other substances in the urine in the final detection system.

Hydrolysis may be necessary, however, to increase the sensitivity of the method if it is required to detect sporadic misuse of diamorphine or morphine in contrast to habitual use. The morphine glucuronide can be hydrolysed by acid or by incubation with an enzyme. Boiling with hydrochloric acid, at atmospheric pressure, does not produce complete hydrolysis. To achieve this it is necessary to autoclave urine with 10 per cent hydrochloric acid at 120°C for 15 minutes. Alternatively, overnight incubation with β-glucuronidase at 37°C and pH 4.7, can be used to achieve complete hydrolysis and production of a cleaner extract than boiling with hot acid. Because urine contains enzyme inhibitors these must be removed before hydrolysis (Fry *et al.*, 1974) if quantitative results are required.

Morphine can be extracted from the urine, either before or after hydrolysis, by solvents, ion exchange resins or by adsorption on XAD-2 resin. Numerous solvent systems have been used but in order to extract the maximum quantity of morphine from urine it is first necessary to adjust the pH to 9.0 and ensure that the salt concentration is high. This can be achieved in a number of ways. The simplest is to make the urine strongly alkaline with sodium hydroxide and to add sufficient solid sodium bicarbonate to restore the pH to 9.0.

Single solvents do not generally give good recoveries of morphine. Better results can be obtained using a mixture of chloroform:isopropanol in the proportions 3:1. Unfortunately, this solvent also removes large quantities of impurities from the urine and these can interfere with subsequent TLC detection. Extraction of ammonium sulphate saturated urine with ether produces a much cleaner extract but only at 54 per cent yield. Ion exchange paper and XAD-2 resin have also been used to extract morphine. These are particularly useful for rapid screening methods. For quantitative work a correction for recovery can be made using ^{14}C labelled morphine (Fry *et al.*, 1974).

Fluorimetry

Morphine can be measured quantitatively in biological fluids by means of spectrophotofluorimetry, gas-liquid chromatography, high-pressure liquid chromatography, or immunoassay.

Kupferberg (1964) described a sensitive and relatively specific fluorimetric method for measuring morphine which employed ferriferrocyanide oxidation of morphine to pseudomorphine. Blackmore *et al.*, (1971) adapted this method to the AutoAnalyzer for the rapid screening of urine. For morphine extracted from urine the limit of detection was said to be 0.2 μg/ml. Jane and Taylor (1975) used this fluorimetric method for the detection of morphine in urine after HPLC and were able to measure down to levels of 0.01 μg/ml. Mulé and Hushin (1971) used the fluorescence formed by heating morphine with sulphuric acid as the basis of a simple method for screening urine for morphine. The method was said to be sensitive to a concentration of morphine in urine in the region of 0.2–0.3 μg/ml.

TLC

Morphine can be detected on the TLC plate by spraying with iodoplatinate reagent. This is a non-specific reagent which reacts with a large number of nitrogen-containing drugs. Consequently other drugs present in the urine can sometimes cause confusion, especially if they have similar Rf values to morphine. In particular the presence of phenothiazine drugs can effectively mask the presence of morphine in some TLC solvent systems. Confirmation of morphine can be obtained by overspraying with ammoniacal silver nitrate solution and heating the plate (Dole *et al.*, 1966).

Kupferberg *et al.*, (1964) described a fluorimetric method for the detection of morphine after TLC, based on the oxidation of morphine to pseudomorphine. They claimed the sensitivity was of the order of 0.1 μg but the application of this method to urine extracts creates problems due to the presence of other fluorescent compounds in the extracts.

GLC

Gas-liquid chromatography (GLC) of morphine is best carried out by forming either the acetates or silyl ethers. Wallace *et al.*, (1972) used a simple acetylation procedure for measuring morphine extracted from the urine of heroin addicts. Wilkinson and Way (1969) prepared the BSTFA [N-o-bis-(trimethylsilyl) (trifluoroacetamide)] derivative of morphine and, in this way, were able to measure as little as 25 ng morphine per sample of plasma or CSF. Wilkinson and Way (1969) used a flame ionization detector but the sensitivity of their technique could undoubtedly have been increased by means of an electron capture detector or mass spectrometer (mass fragmentography).

Fry *et al.*, (1974) used the N-o-bis-(trimethylsilyl) acetamide derivative and a flame ionization detector to measure morphine quantitatively in the urine of patients receiving morphine therapeutically for the relief of pain.

GLC methods are more specific than most other methods but are not sensitive enough to measure morphine in blood accurately or precisely. Moreover, they are slow and not suitable, therefore, for routine detection of morphine in urine from addicts. They may, however, have a place in the confirmation of positive tests from thin-layer chromatography.

Immunochemical

Immunoassay methods are the most sensitive available for the detection and measurement of morphine but they are seldom as specific as GLC. Many different immunoassay methods have been described but all are based on the production of an antibody to morphine. The specificity of the method is generally dependent on the cross-reactivity or specificity of the antibody used. This can vary enormously—not only from animal to animal but even from bleed to bleed.

Most antibodies to morphine that have been produced cross-react with codeine, heroin and morphine glucuronide. The latter is an advantage if the sole object is to detect morphine or heroin misuse as it increases the already excellent sensitivity of the technique without the need to hydrolyse the urine. They do, of course, limit the usefulness of the assay for measuring morphine accurately in blood and, for this purpose, a non-cross-reacting antiserum is required (Aherne *et al.*, 1975).

Morphine antibodies have been used in four different ways for the detection and measurement of morphine in blood and urine. These have recently been described in great detail by Mulé *et al.*, (1974a; 1974b).

Spector (1971) described the first standard-type radioimmunoassay for morphine; and results obtained with it, on urine and blood from drug addicts, were reported by Catlin *et al.*, (1973). The lowest concentration of morphine that could be measured by Spector (1971) was 10 ng/ml. This has recently been reduced to less than 1 ng/ml by Morris *et al.*, (1974).

The second type of morphine 'immunoassay' is the free radical assay technique (FRAT) developed by Leute *et al.*, (1972). FRAT uses a spin-labelled analog of morphine, prepared by introducing a stable nitro-oxide radical at position C-3 of the morphine molecule, instead of the conventional radioisotope label of an RIA. Although it is very sensitive, FRAT requires expensive instrumentation and reagents. Nevertheless, it is capable of giving quick results and can be used for testing specimens whilst patients are still in the clinic.

The third immunochemical method for detecting morphine in biological fluids is the so-called enzyme multiplied immunoassay technique (EMIT) first described by Rubinstein *et al.*, (1972). An enzyme, lysozyme, is labelled with morphine and complexed with a morphine antibody. This lysozyme–morphine–antibody complex has no enzyme activity although the simpler and smaller lyzosyme–

morphine conjugate does. The addition of unlabelled morphine releases some of the enzyme labelled morphine from its binding to morphine antibody. The morphine–lysozyme so liberated is then able to react with an appropriate substrate and its enzyme activity can be measured spectrophotometrically. The enzyme activity observed is proportional to the amount of morphine present in the original sample.

The fourth, and least sensitive type of immunoassay—but easiest to perform—is the haemaglutination method which uses sheep erythrocytes coated with carboxymethyl morphine conjugated to rabbit serum albumin, as the indicator system (Adler et al., 1972). Urine which is believed to contain morphine is mixed with morphine antibody and allowed to react with it before the sensitised red blood cells are added. If morphine was present in the sample it 'neutralises' the antibody which is no longer available to agglutinate the sensitised red cells. As a result they settle as a clear pellet. If the antibody is not neutralised by morphine it reacts with the sensitised red cells causing them to adhere and produce a sediment which can be distinguished by naked eye from the pellet of cells which is characteristic of a positive reaction. This haemaglutination method is sensitive down to about 30 ng/ml of morphine.

An evaluation of the immunoassay methods available for the detection of drugs of abuse in urine has been made by Mulé et al., (1974a; 1974b) who concluded that they are highly sensitive but lack specificity. They are relatively easy to use, as no sample treatment is normally required, but their cost is relatively high.

Summary

Morphine is best detected in the urine of drug addicts by TLC, especially if other drugs are also being looked for. Positive results can be confirmed by GLC. Immunological methods will undoubtedly become increasingly important, particularly for the quantitative measurement of morphine and other opiates in the blood.

AMPHETAMINES

Extraction

Amphetamines and related compounds can readily be extracted from urine by making it alkaline (pH approximately 10) and using an organic solvent such as ether. Blood and plasma can be extracted either directly (Bruce and Maynard, 1969) or after protein precipitation and alkalinisation of the filtrate (Lebish *et al.*, 1970). The latter produces an extract that contains less interfering substances.

Because amphetamine base is volatile it can easily be lost by volatilisation during evaporation of solvent prior to separation by TLC. It is essential, therefore, to convert it to a salt, by the addition of acid, before the evaporation is commenced.

TLC

Most of the methods used to detect amphetamines and related compounds by TLC and subsequent colour development employ chemical reactions associated with the presence of primary, secondary or tertiary amine groups. For this reason they are non-specific and naturally occuring amines may also be detected with the possibility of producing false positive results. Nevertheless, these methods are extremely useful for screening but absolute identification requires confirmation by some other method.

The commonest spray reagent for the detection of amphetamine after TLC is ninhydrin in acetone. This produces a pink spot with primary amines (but not with secondary amines, e.g., methylamphetamine) after irradiation with UV light. Another spray sequence is hexan-2:5 dione followed by *p*-dimethylaminobenzaldehyde (Dickes and Ellis, 1967), which gives a stable red colour after suitable treatment. As little as 1 µg of amphetamine is said to be detected by this means.

Marks and Fry (1968) used a spray containing Fast Blue B salt to detect amphetamine after TLC. Their method is sensitive to both primary and secondary amines and is capable of detecting amphetamine at a concentration of about 1 µg/ml of urine.

A method recently introduced by Bussey and Backer (1974) uses ninhydrin–phenylacetaldehyde and dimethylaminobenzaldehyde in sequence as spray reagents, and is said to be even more sensitive but does not detect secondary amines.

Fluorescamine, a sensitive fluorogenic reagent, has recently been used for the detection of primary amines (Klein *et al.*, 1974) and has the advantage that it does not interfere with subsequent over-spraying with reagents used to detect any other drugs that may be present.

GLC

Beckett *et al.*, (1967) used GLC to detect and measure amphetamine and also provided extensive data on a large number of related drugs. Initial confirmation of amphetamine, detected by TLC, can be achieved by injecting a concentrated ether extract of alkalinised urine directly into the GLC column. By use of the 'peak-shift technique', which involves the formation of a derivative with a slightly different retention time to the parent compound, virtually absolute identification of amphetamine can be achieved. Jain *et al.*, (1975) used GLC for mass screening and confirmation of amphetamine in urine.

Quantitative measurement of amphetamine requires the formation of less volatile derivatives prior to analysis. Toseland and Scott (1969) originally employed the acetate derivatives but latterly the halogenated acyl derivatives have become increasingly popular. These are readily produced, show excellent peak shapes and, with GLC instruments fitted with electron capture detectors, enable much smaller amounts of the drug to be measured. The increased sensitivity is particularly important in the measurement of amphetamine in blood, and permitted Bruce and Maynard (1969) to detect amphetamine in the blood of a subject up to 6 hours after initial injection of a 5 mg dose.

The same procedure enabled them also to measure the concentration of fenfluramine, methylamphetamine and ethamphetamine in blood. Even more sensitive techniques, using perfluorbenzene derivatives, have recently been proposed for measuring this group of compounds (Moffat *et al.*, 1972).

Miscellaneous methods

Immunochemical techniques have been described for the detection of amphetamine in the urine and some are available in kit form. Spectrophotofluorimetric methods (Nix and Hume, 1970; Stewart and Lotti, 1971) have also been used to detect and measure amphetamines in urine. One of them has been adapted for use with the AutoAnalyzer (Hayes, 1973) and is sensitive to about 50 μg of amphetamine per litre of fresh urine. Another automated method for screening uring for amphetamine utilises the reaction between amines and 2, 4, 6-trinitrobenzene sulphonic acid to produce an orange–yellow colour (Rutter, 1972). These methods are not very specific and their clinical usefulness is limited to mass screening for a single drug.

METHADONE

The detection and identification of methadone in urine has assumed importance because of its extensive use in rehabilitation programmes for heroin addicts. Most urines from patients receiving treatment contain a greater or lesser amount of the drug, approximately 60 per cent of which can be recovered in the urine as unchanged methadone or its mono-*N*-demethylated derivative (Beckett *et al.*, 1968).

TLC

Methadone is extracted from alkaline aqueous solution by most organic solvents and can readily be detected by TLC. It runs in the common solvent system ethyl acetate/methanol/ammonia, with an Rf so similar to cocaine that the two drugs cannot be differentiated if an iodo-platinate spray is used. The two drugs can be distinguished, however, by over-spraying with ammoniacal silver nitrate (Kaistha and Jaffe, 1972a) which bleaches the methadone spot and converts the cocaine spot to a yellowish colour.

A methadone metabolite can be identified by spraying the TLC plate with Fast Blue B salt when it shows up as a bright orange–yellow spot, with an Rf slightly less than that of methadone itself. A metabolite can also be detected on the TLC plate used for detection of amphetamine in the system employed by Marks and Fry (1968) where it appears as a spot with an Rf of about 0.3 and shows up when the plate is sprayed with Fast Blue B salt.

GLC

Many methods are available for the detection and measurement of methadone and its metabolites by GLC. For the simultaneous detection of methadone and morphine (Van der Slooten *et al.*, 1971) it is first necessary to hydrolyse the morphine conjugates with β-glucuronidase, extract into chloroform–isopropanol and purify on TLC before proceeding to GLC separation and measurement. The method of Van der Slooten *et al.*, (1971) is said to be sufficiently sensitive to detect methadone in urine after a dose of less than 50 mg per day.

Valentine *et al.*, (1972) described a method for the GLC measurement of methadone in urine which omitted the TLC purification step. This method was sensitive to 3–30 μg of methadone per ml of urine. Inturrisi and Verebely (1972) described a similar method that can be applied to plasma.

Miscellaneous

Immunochemical methods have been used to detect methadone in urine (Mulé *et al.*, 1974b) and a fluorimetric method has also been described (McGonigle, 1971), although it has not been applied directly to biological specimens.

COCAINE

Cocaine is extensively metabolised in the body to yield first benzoylecgonine and finally ecgonine; less than 10 per cent of the dose is excreted unchanged in the urine (Fish and Wilson, 1969a). It is important, therefore, to look for cocaine metabolites, as well as for the unchanged drug, if maximum sensitivity is required.

Cocaine is readily extracted into organic solvents and can be detected by TLC, using an iodoplatinate spray. As has already been noted, however, it runs with a very similar Rf to methadone—from which it can be distinguished by over-spraying with ammoniacal silver nitrate, or by use of a different solvent system that separates the two compounds. Unfortunately, cocaine metabolites are not detected by commonly used procedures for drug detection, though two recently introduced TLC systems (Valanju *et al.*, 1973; Bastos *et al.*, 1974) do permit their identification.

Several GLC methods are available for measuring cocaine and its metabolites. One such method (Fish and Wilson, 1969b) permits determination of both morphine and cocaine on the same urine extract. Benzoylecgonine can be detected and measured by first reconverting it to cocaine, by methylation with diazomethane, and then measuring it by GLC (Fish and Wilson, 1969a). Another simple GLC method for confirming the presence of cocaine and other alkaloids in urine has recently been described by Sine *et al.*, (1973). Jatlow and Bailey (1975) have described a GLC method for cocaine in human plasma, with use of a nitrogen detector to give increased sensitivity.

Benzoylecgonine can also be detected by the EMIT immunochemical system which has an acceptable specificity and is sensitive to the presence of 1 μg of the drug per ml of urine.

BARBITURATES

Probably more methods are available for the detection and measurement of barbiturates in blood and urine than for any other group of drugs.

TLC

Simple screening methods for urine samples generally involve TLC of an organic solvent extract prepared from acidified urine. One of the commonest TLC developing systems uses chloroform–acetone but better separation of the different barbiturates—especially from the non-specific materials often present in urine—can generally be obtained by using an ethyl acetate/methyl alcohol/ammonia mixture. Neither system gives good separation of the individual barbiturates. Better separation can be achieved, however, with the technique described by Curry and Fox (1968) but the conditions for development are critical and this makes it less suitable for routine use. The spray reagent commonly used to detect barbiturates on TLC plates contains mercuric sulphate and diphenylcarbazone and reacts with some other drugs, such as glutethimide and phenytoin, which may also be present in the urine. Despite these drawbacks, TLC is perfectly adequate for rapid screening of urine for barbiturates, though further investigation is necessary for confirmation.

GLC

GLC is now commonly used for confirming the presence of barbiturates in plasma and urine and for identifying them. It can also be used to measure them. For best results, and in order to prevent adsorption of the drug onto the column, and consequently tailing, it is generally necessary to produce a more volatile derivative of the native drug. Several ways of achieving this are available, including the use of diazomethane (Cook *et al.*, 1961) which is, unfortunately, potentially explosive and toxic. Dimethyl sulphate has also been used (Martin and Driscoll, 1966) and is more satisfactory when the reaction mixture is buffered with a borax buffer (Baylis *et al.*, 1970). Dimethyl sulphate is also toxic, however, and consequently not well suited to routine use. Other GLC techniques, such as those employing on-column methylation (MacGee, 1971; Stevenson,

1966) or butylation prior to injection (Greeley 1974), have been developed. These are generally adequate for urine but in order to produce successful chromatograms of barbiturates in plasma it is first necessary partially to purify the plasma extract so as to prevent interference by plasma lipids.

Tailing of barbiturates on the column can be prevented, without the necessity of forming derivatives, by saturating the carrier gas with formic acid. This technique has been applied by Papadopoulus *et al.*, (1973) to the routine measurement of phenobarbitone and other anticonvulsant drugs in plasma. A major advantage of this method is that it is free from interference from lipids and a simple ethyl acetate extract of plasma can be injected directly onto the GLC column.

Miscellaneous methods

Spectrophotometry has been widely used, in the past, for detecting and measuring barbiturates in urine and tissues especially for toxicological purposes. Its insensitivity and relative non-specificity makes it unsuitable for work with drug addicts though Blackmore *et al.*, (1971) have recently described an automated method, with a sensitivity of 2.5 μg barbiturate per ml, which they claim is suitable for this purpose.

Immunoassay methods have been described for the detection of barbiturates in urine (Cleeland *et al.*, 1975; Mulé *et al.*, 1974a) and are sensitive to about 1–2 μg barbiturate per ml. Glutethamide interferes, but only at a concentration about 25 times as great as for barbiturates.

METHAQUALONE

Methaqualone abuse can be detected by means of a routine TLC procedure after extraction from alkaline urine by an organic solvent. Much of the drug is excreted in the urine either as the glucuronide or as a methaqualone metabolite. In our laboratory we use a modification of the method of Allen *et al.*, (1970) in which a metabolite of methaqualone is first extracted from alkaline urine prior to detection by TLC. The metabolite appears as a blue–mauve spot after irradiation under UV light and spraying with Fast Blue B salt, and has an Rf of about 0.35. It can easily be detected in the urine of normal volunteers after the ingestion of as little as 150 mg methaqualone. The TLC method

Probably more methods are available for the detection and measurement of barbiturates in blood and urine than for any other group of drugs.

TLC

Simple screening methods for urine samples generally involve TLC of an organic solvent extract prepared from acidified urine. One of the commonest TLC developing systems uses chloroform–acetone but better separation of the different barbiturates—especially from the non-specific materials often present in urine—can generally be obtained by using an ethyl acetate/methyl alcohol/ammonia mixture. Neither system gives good separation of the individual barbiturates. Better separation can be achieved, however, with the technique described by Curry and Fox (1968) but the conditions for development are critical and this makes it less suitable for routine use. The spray reagent commonly used to detect barbiturates on TLC plates contains mercuric sulphate and diphenylcarbazone and reacts with some other drugs, such as glutethimide and phenytoin, which may also be present in the urine. Despite these drawbacks, TLC is perfectly adequate for rapid screening of urine for barbiturates, though further investigation is necessary for confirmation.

GLC

GLC is now commonly used for confirming the presence of barbiturates in plasma and urine and for identifying them. It can also be used to measure them. For best results, and in order to prevent adsorption of the drug onto the column, and consequently tailing, it is generally necessary to produce a more volatile derivative of the native drug. Several ways of achieving this are available, including the use of diazomethane (Cook *et al.*, 1961) which is, unfortunately, potentially explosive and toxic. Dimethyl sulphate has also been used (Martin and Driscoll, 1966) and is more satisfactory when the reaction mixture is buffered with a borax buffer (Baylis *et al.*, 1970). Dimethyl sulphate is also toxic, however, and consequently not well suited to routine use. Other GLC techniques, such as those employing on-column methylation (MacGee, 1971; Stevenson, column coated with OV-17, and said to be capable of measuring Δ^9-THC in blood at a concentration as low as 1 ng/ml, has been described by Fenimore *et al.*, (1973) but no data are yet available concerning its clinical use. In 1973 Agurell *et al.* used a GC–MS method to measure the concentration of Δ^9-THC in the plasma of three subjects who had recently smoked a cannabis-containing cigarette. They obtained values comparable to those observed in volunteers given similar amounts of Δ^9-THC. Despite its sensitivity and specificity the GC–MS technique is, because of its great expense, impracticable except as a research tool and only one confirmatory study has so far been published (Rosenfeld *et al.*, 1974).

Radioimmunoassay techniques for the measurement of cannabinoids in blood and urine have recently been described by Teale *et al.*, (1974; 1975) and by Gross *et al.*, (1974). Neither technique is absolutely specific for Δ^9-THC because of cross-reactivity between the antibody and other cannabinoids, notably 11OH-Δ^9-THC. The radioimmunoassay described by Teale *et al.*, (1974) is sensitive to approximately 1 ng Δ^9-THC (or 11OH-THC) per ml of urine (or 7.5 ng/ml of plasma) and is sufficiently simple for it to be used as a routine procedure. It is possible, by this means, to detect cannabinoids in the urine of volunteers up to 48 hours after the smoking of a single cigarette containing only 5 mg Δ^9-THC, i.e. about the same as an average 'reefer'. The extremely high group specificity of the antiserum used in this assay makes any risk of false positive results arising from interference by other drugs extremely unlikely and has not been observed in many hundreds of assays carried out in the authors' laboratories (Marks *et al.*, 1975).

LSD

The detection and measurement of LSD in biological fluids is extremely difficult because of the very low concentrations present. A screening test, based on fluorimetry (Faed and McLeod, 1973), has been used to detect LSD and its metabolites in urine after hydrolysis with β-glucuronidase, solvent extraction and purification by paper chromatography. Two commonly used anti-migraine drugs, ergotamine and methysergide, interfere with the method.

A quantitative fluorimetric method, based upon that of Aghajanian and Bing (1964) and said to be capable of detecting LSD after an oral dose, has recently been reported by Upshall and Wailing (1972).

A radioimmunoassay method has been described by Van Vunakis *et al.*, (1971) but so far information relating to its use for detection and measurement of LSD in biological fluids is limited. The RIA procedure used by Taunton–Rigby *et al.*, (1973) was reported to be more specific. This method is claimed to be sensitive to as little as 16 pg of LSD and to be capable of detecting it in the urine of volunteers given 200–400 µg of the drug by mouth.

THE CLINICAL APPLICATION OF DRUG DETECTION METHODS AND INTERPRETATION OF RESULTS

Some of the methods available for the detection and measurement of drugs of abuse in urine and plasma have been reviewed briefly. It is now necessary to consider their usefulness in clinical and forensic practice. In doing so we move from a situation in which there is almost a surfeit of knowledge and information to one of virtual ignorance, surmise and speculation.

GENERAL CONSIDERATIONS

The ability of the laboratory to detect and, if necessary, to measure common drugs of abuse in blood and urine is limited, nowadays, by the time and money available rather than by lack of suitable methods.

Interpretation of the results obtained depends upon a host of factors—not least amongst them being the sensitivity and specificity of the analytical method used. With specific, sensitive and reliable methods it may be possible to say, with almost absolute certainty, that the subject had, at some time in the recent past, taken some of the drug in question. This information may be all that is required by an epidemiologist investigating the prevalence of drug abuse in a community—or by law-enforcement agencies—but is generally not sufficient for the clinician who may want to know how much of the drug the patient has taken and how often. Unfortunately neither of these questions is amenable to satisfactory answer by urine analysis. The first requires a knowledge of the absorption, metabolism and excretion of the drug and even then provides only a minimal figure which cannot be interpreted rationally without knowledge of the time of the last dose, and the previous drug history—neither of which is readily or reliably available.

It is in the investigation of the absorption, metabolism and excretion of drugs that the more sophisticated techniques of analysis are invaluable. Some aspects of the metabolism of individual drugs has already been discussed—especially in so far as it affects their detection. There are, however, other factors to be considered.

NATURE OF THE SPECIMEN

The type of specimen submitted for analysis is important. The interpretation of results obtained with urine and blood, for example, is very different. The blood level of a drug depends on the balance, at the time it was taken, between its rate of entry into the blood from the gut, or site of tissue injection, and its rate of removal by redistribution, metabolism or excretion. The amount of drug in the urine, on the other hand, is an integrated function of drug concentration in the body pool over a finite period.

A low urinary concentration of a drug may indicate that a small dose of the drug was taken recently or that a large dose was taken many hours, or days, beforehand.

One of the many factors that can affect renal excretion of unconjugated basic and acidic drugs is urinary pH. The rate of excretion of acidic drugs, e.g., phenobarbitone, is increased in alkaline and decreased in acid urine. Conversely, and even more profoundly, the excretion of basic drugs, e.g., amphetamine, is increased by acidification and decreased by alkalinisation of the urine. This is due to changes in the ratio of ionised to un-ionised drug in the glomerular filtrate and, consequently, their rate of reabsorption by the tubule—the un-ionised drug being rapidly and almost completely reabsorbed, whilst the ionised compound is barely reabsorbed at all.

AMPHETAMINE

Beckett *et al.*, (1965) studied the effect of urinary pH extensively in relation to the excretion of amphetamine. They showed that 5–30 per cent of a 10–15 mg dose of amphetamine was excreted in the urine, by normal subjects, over a 16-hour period when urinary pH was not controlled, but the proportion was increased to 55 per cent when the urine was acidified to pH5.0 by ingestion of ammonium chloride. On a third occasion, when the same subjects were given sodium bicarbonate so as to produce an alkaline urine of pH 8.0, only 3 per cent of the ingested amphetamine was excreted over 16 hours. The relevance of these observations to the interpretation of urine amphetamine analyses is immediately evident. A negative amphetamine result on a strongly alkaline urine specimen is of doubtful significance in excluding recent amphetamine ingestion as such a small percentage of the dose is excreted under these conditions. Beckett *et al.*, (1965) suggested that doubt could be resolved by giving subjects sufficient ammonium chloride to reduce urinary pH to less than 6.0 before collecting urine specimens for amphetamine analysis. But whilst this may be practicable and, indeed, enforceable in sport it is clearly not so in the average outpatient clinic.

It should perhaps be stressed that whilst the effect of urinary pH on excretion has been demonstrated most clearly for amphetamine, it applies equally to all basic drugs which are excreted largely or wholly as the free base. Moreover, it is apparent that under everyday conditions, in which urinary pH is not controlled, no reasonable correlation can be expected to exist between the dose of amphetamine taken and the amount found, at any one time, in the urine.

MORPHINE

Morphine, though a basic drug, is excreted in the urine largely as the water-soluble glucuronide and consequently is not pH dependent. Fry *et al.*, (1974) measured total 24-hour urine morphine excretion in 37 terminal cancer patients who were receiving either morphine or diamorphine by mouth or by injection. The mean daily excretion was 68 per cent (range 20–112 per cent) of the daily dose but large fluctuations were found in excretion, both from day-to-day and during a single 24-hour period. Extreme caution must, therefore, be exercised in drawing any conclusions about the amount of morphine (or heroin) administered on the basis of quantitative morphine measurements which are made on untimed or isolated urine specimens. However, whilst it is clear that no conclusions can be drawn regarding the dose of morphine or diamorphine that any individual patient has received, there is, as a group, a remarkably good correlation ($r = 0.82$; $P < 0.001$) between urine morphine excretion and the dose of morphine administered (Twycross *et al.*, 1974). Consequently, although valid conclusions cannot be drawn from urine excretion data about the amount of morphine (or heroin) taken by any individual subject, such data can, nevertheless, provide valuable information about drug usage by groups of patients. It is reasonable to believe that such information could be extremely useful as the basis of a method for comparing morphine (or heroin) abuse in different groups of users in both epidemiological and sociological surveys.

CLINICAL VALUE OF QUALITATIVE URINE ANALYSIS

We would now like to consider the interpretation of the results of qualitative analysis of urine for drugs by thin layer chromatography in so far as they affect clinical practice.

Most screening procedures aim at a sensitivity of about 1 μg of drug per ml urine. Sensitivity can be altered by changing the volume of urine extracted, by introducing a hydrolysis stage and by varying the amount of the extract applied to the thin layer plate. The nature of the spray reagent also affects sensitivity. It is, however, important to remember that sensitivity refers to the mass of drug present in the actual urine specimen and not to the dose of drug taken by the patient. A negative result on TLC screening merely means that the specimen contained less than the lowest amount of drug detectable by the method employed. It cannot be construed as proof of complete absence of the drug, though this becomes increasingly likely as the sensitivity of the assay procedure increases. Moreover, a small amount of drug in the urine may signify a small dose of drug taken recently or a much larger dose taken some days previously.

Kaistha and Jaffe (1972b) reported drug excretion data for several commonly abused drugs. A single minimum therapeutic dose of each drug was given orally to a number of staff personnel. Urine was collected at various time intervals thereafter and analysed by a TLC method sensitive to about 1 μg/ml for each of the drugs detected. Most of the drugs investigated could be detected in the urine about 6 hours after the dose and subsequently for the next 24 hours. There were wide individual variations in drug excretion rates and this means, in practice, that in some patients a minimal dose will be detectable for less than 24 hours, whilst in others it will persist for much longer. It is assumed that with drug addicts a much larger dose of drug is normally taken than would be used therapeutically so that the likelihood of detecting drug abuse by urine testing up to 24 hours after the last dose becomes almost a certainty. A negative urine test under these circumstances must throw serious doubt upon the reputed addict's (physical) dependence upon the drug(s) to which he claims to be addicted. When sporadic misuse of drugs is the problem under investigation a negative result may merely mean that some considerable time has elapsed since the last dose. Detection rate under these circumstances is increased by using more sensitive methods, some of which are capable of detecting the presence of drugs taken up to a week beforehand.

The significance of a positive urine test for drugs must be considered in the context of the specificity of the method. We have already emphasised that positive identification of a drug solely by thin layer chromatography is fraught with difficulties and confirmation by another method is essential. However, due to the pressure of work, many laboratories report their results solely on the basis of a TLC analysis. Under these circumstances the possibility of false positive results is very real, especially when the patient is taking other drugs, either legitimately or illegitimately.

The application and general usefulness of urine analysis to the diagnosis and treatment, as opposed to detection, of addicts has received extremely scant attention, especially in view of the vast amount of resources devoted to it. The problems are different in different countries, depending on the laws and social climate prevailing in them. Our experience is necessarily limited to the UK where treatment of heroin and cocaine addiction is available free in Government clinics, and where the abuse of other drugs is strongly disapproved of but, with the exception of cannabis, rarely illegal.

In our opinion urine analysis is an essential first step in the diagnosis of heroin and morphine addiction. Participants in the 'drug-scene' are notoriously unreliable people who may not only refuse to help, but often positively obstruct or mislead clinicians to whom they have gone ostensibly for treatment.

Marks *et al.*, (1969) reviewed the results of urine analysis on specimens

The laboratory's contribution

collected from 107 patients at their first visit to the clinic, who claimed to be addicted to heroin which they had hitherto obtained illicitly. No morphine was detected in the urine of 37 of these patients. Because the results of urine analysis could not be made available immediately 8 of the patients were prescribed either methadone or heroin on the basis of clinical impression. Of the remaining 29 patients who were not prescribed any drugs, only 7 returned to the clinic. Repeated examination of urine from these seven patients revealed a positive result for morphine on only one occasion.

Essentially similar results were obtained by Gardner and Connell (1970). No less than 27 patients (27 per cent) failed to exhibit either morphine or methadone in their urine at their first attendance at the clinic but despite this 10 were prescribed heroin or methadone. Gardner and Connell (1970) considered, in retrospect, that eight of these ten patients were probably sporadic users, of whom two were converted to daily use by the clinic. Because of this danger Gardner and Connell (1970) suggested that three consecutive positive urine samples, collected on different days and over a period of 10 days, could be taken as evidence of daily use. A negative urine result for morphine, whilst not proof that the patient has never taken heroin, is nevertheless evidence that less than 10 mg has been taken in the past 24 hours—and this is less than the amount generally taken by regular users.

The two surveys, by Marks *et al.*, (1969) and Gardner and Connell (1970), suggest that a fair proportion of the patients presenting themselves at the drug treatment clinics, shortly after their inauguration at least, were either sporadic users who were trying to establish a regular habit on free and legitimate drugs or else were seeking to obtain heroin in order to sell it.

Misuse of other drugs is also important. Addicts will often confess to heroin misuse, in order to obtain free supplies of it, but will not admit to using other drugs which are not covered by the Act. Gardner and Connell (1970) found that of the 27 urine samples from patients that were negative for morphine and methadone, 17 contained amphetamine, and in our own laboratory a good proportion of the urine samples received for analysis from drug treatment clinics are found to contain diverse drugs, such as barbiturates, methaqualone and amphetamine analogues. The results for the four main classes of drugs in urine specimens obtained from patients attending two of the Government

Table 1   **Percentage of urine specimens positive for drugs for the years 1970–73**

Year	Morphine	Methadone	Amphetamine	Barbiturates
1970	20	85	4.5	23
1971	18	89	3.5	20
1972	14	93	1.5	16
1973	10	94	2.5	12

Drug Dependency Treatment Units because of opiate addiction during four consecutive years are given in the Table 1. The increasing proportion of specimens positive for methadone undoubtedly reflects the policy of using this drug for 'maintenance' therapy. On the other hand, the percentage of specimens which were positive for morphine, amphetamines and barbiturates has halved over four years. These figures necessarily give an indication of the relative frequency with which different drugs are abused in one, rather localised, area in one country in the world and are not necessarily typical.

Gardner and Connell (1972) reported details of the pattern of drug misuse in non-opiate users in London over several years. Amphetamine and methylamphetamine were the most frequently detected drugs but the misuse of methylamphetamine declined dramatically after it was withdrawn from the market in injectable form in 1968—a finding which conforms to our own experience.

Because of the lack of a suitable detection method no information was available, until recently, regarding the prevalence of cannabis derivatives in the urine of habitual or casual users of drugs. Teale *et al.*, (1974) demonstrated the presence of cannabis derivatives in the urine in 5 out of 7 random urine specimens received from patients attending a drug treatment centre. Subsequently, analysis of 393 urine samples selected at random over a two month period from amongst more than 1000 specimens received in our laboratory with a request for routine analysis for drugs of abuse, revealed 165 (42 per cent) positive for cannabis (Marks *et al.*, 1975). In many of the urine samples the concentration of cannabis derivatives exceeded 1000 ng/ml. None of 82 urine specimens received in the laboratory from hospital in-patients, and in whom a diagnosis of drug abuse was not suspected, gave a positive response (i.e., > 10 ng/ml) for cannabis.

The ability to detect cannabis in the urine raises several questions, not least of them being the ethical one as to whether a laboratory should report the result of a positive test to the clinician when neither he, nor the patient, has specifically requested it.

REFERENCES

Adler, F., Lui, C.-T. and Catlin, D. H. (1972). Immunological studies on heroin addiction, I, Methodology and application of a hemaglutination inhibition test for detection of morphine. *Clin. Immunol. Immunopathol*, **1**, 53

Aghajanian, G. K. and Bing, O. H. L. (1964). Persistence of lysergic acid and diethylamide in the plasma of human subjects. *Clin. Pharmacol. Ther.*, **5**, 611

Agurell, S., Gustafsson, B., Holmestedt, B., Leander, K., Lindgren, J., Nilsson, J., Sandberg, F. and Asberg, M. (1973). Determination of Δ^1 Tetrahydrocannabinol in plasma from cannabis smokers. *J. Pharm. Pharmacol.*, **25**, 554

Aherne, G. W., Piall, E. M., Robinson, J. D., Morris, B. A. and Marks, V. (1975). Two applications of a radioimmunoassay for Morphine. *In* 'Radioimmunoassay and related techniques in Clinical Biochemistry' (C. A. Pesternak, ed.) (London: Heyden)

Akagi, M., Oketani, Y. and Takado, M. (1963). Studies on metabolism of 2-Methyl-3-o-tolyl-4(3H)-quinazolinone, I The estimation of 2-methyl-3-o-tolyl-4(3H)-quinazolinone in biological materials. *Chem. Pharm. Bull. (Japan)*, **11**, 62

Allen, J. T., Fry, D. E. and Marks, V. (1970). Urine spot-test for methaqualone. *Lancet*, **i**, 951

Anderson, J. M., Nielsen, E., Schou, J., Steentoft, A. and Worm, K. (1971). A specific method for the demonstration of cannabis intake by TLC of urine. *Acta Pharmacol. Toxicol.*, **29**, 111

Baylis, E. M., Fry, D. E. and Marks, V. (1970). Micro-determination of serum phenobarbitone and diphenylhydantoin by gas-liquid chromatography. *Clin. Chim. Acta*, **30**, 93

Bastos, M. L., Jukofsky, D. and Mulé, S. J. (1974). Routine identification of cocaine metabolites in human urine. *J. Chromatog.*, **89**, 335

Beckett, A. H., Tucker, G. T. and Moffat, A. C. (1967). Routine detection and identification in urine of stimulants and other drugs, some of which may be used to modify performance in sport. *J. Pharm. Pharmacol.*, **19**, 273

Beckett, A. H., Taylor, J. F., Casy, A. F. and Hassan, M. M. A. (1968). The biotransformation of methadone in man: synthesis and identification of a major metabolite. *J. Pharm. Pharmacol.*, **20**, 754

Beckett, A. H., Rowland, M. and Turner, P. (1965). Influence of urinary pH on excretion of amphetamine. *Lancet*, **i**, 303

Berry, D. J. (1969). Gas chromatographic determination of methaqualone, 2 methyl-3-o-tolyl-4(3H)-quinazolinone, at therapeutic levels in human plasma. *J. Chromatog.*, **42**, 39

Blackmore, D. J., Curry, A. S., Hayes, T. S. and Rutter, E. R. (1971). Automated Analysis for Drugs in Urine. *Clin. Chem.*, **17**, 896

Brown, S. S. and Smart, G. A. (1969). Fluorimetric assay of methaqualone in plasma by reduction to 1, 2, 3, 4-tetrahydro-2-methyl-4-oxo-3-o-tolylquinazoline. *J. Pharm. Pharmacol.*, **21**, 466

Bruce, R. B. and Maynard (Jr.), W. R. (1969). Determination of amphetamine and related amines in blood by gas-chromatography. *Anal. Chem.*, **41**, 976

Bussey, R. J. and Backer, R. C. (1974). Thin-layer chromatographic differentiation of amphetamines from other primary-amine drugs in urine. *Clin. Chem.*, **20**, 302

Catlin, D., Cleeland, R. and Grunberg, E. (1973). A sensitive rapid radioimmunoassay for morphine and immunologically related substances in urine and serum. *Clin. Chem.*, **19**, 216

Cleeland, R., Davis, R., Heveran, J. and Grunberg, E. (1975). A simple, rapid ^{125}I Radioimmunoassay for the detection of barbiturates in Biological Fluids. *J. forensic Sci.*, **20**, 45

Cook, J. G. H., Riley, C., Nunn, R. F. and Budgen, D. E. (1961). Gas chromatography of methyl derivatives of some barbiturates. *J. Chromatog.*, **6**, 182

Curry, A. S. and Fox, R. H. (1968). Thin layer chromatography of the common barbiturates. *Analyst*, **93**, 834

Davidow, B., Petri, N. L. and Quame, B. (1968). A thin-layer chromatographic screening procedure for detecting drug abuse. *Amer. J. clin. Path.*, **50**, 714

Dickes, G. J. and Ellis, A. C. (1967). The detection of amphetamine in urine by thin layer chromatography. *J. Ass. Pub. Anal.*, **5**, 103

Dole, V. P., Kim, W. K. and Eglitis, I. (1966). Detection of narcotic drugs, tranquilizers, amphetamine and barbiturates in urine, *J. Amer. med. Ass.*, **198**, 349

Evenson, M. A. and Lensmeyer, G. L. (1974). Qualitative and quantitative determination of methaqualone in serum by gas chromatography. *Clin. Chem.*, **20**, 249

Faed, E. M. and McLeod, W. R. (1973). Urine-screening test for lysergide (LSD-25). *J. chromat. Sci.*, **11**, 4

Fenimore, D. C., Freeman, R. R. and Loy, P. R. (1973). Determination of Δ^9-tetrahydrocannabinol in blood by electron-capture gas chromatography. *Analyt. Chem.*, **45**, 2331

Fish, F. and Wilson, W. D. C. (1969a). Excretion of Cocaine and its metabolites in man. *J. Pharm. Pharmacol.*, **21**, (Suppl.), 1355

Fish, F. and Wilson, W. D. C. (1969b). Gas chromatography determination of morphine and cocaine in urine. *J. Chromatog.*, **40**, 164

Fry, D. E., Wills, P. D. and Twycross, R. G. (1974). The quantitative determination of morphine in urine by gas-liquid chromatography and variations in excretion. *Clin. Chim. Acta*, **51**, 183

Gardner, R. and Connell, P. H. (1970). One year's experience in a drug-dependence clinic. *Lancet*, **ii**, 455

Gardner, R. and Connell, P. H. (1972). Amphetamine and other non-opioid drug users attending a special drug dependence clinic. *Brit. med. J.*, **2**, 322

Goudie, J. H. and Burnett, D. (1971). A rapid method for the detection of methaqualone metabolites. *Clin. Chim. Acta*, **35**, 133

Greeley, R. H. (1974). New approach to derivatization and gas-chromatographic analysis of barbiturates. *Clin. Chem.*, **20**, 192

Gross, S. J., Soares, J. R., Wong, S.-L. R. and Schuster, R. E. (1974). Marijuana metabolites measured by a radioimmune technique. *Nature (London)*, **252**, 581

Hayes, T. S. (1973). Automated fluorometric determination of amphetamine in urine. *Clin. Chem.*, **19**, 390

Heaton, A. M. and Blumberg, A. C. (1969). Thin-layer chromatographic detection of barbiturates, narcotics and amphetamines in urine of patients receiving psychotrophic drugs. *J. Chromatog.*, **41**, 367

Inturrisi, C. E. and Verebely, K. (1972). Gas-liquid chromatographic determination of methadone in human plasma and urine. *J. Chromatog.*, **65**, 361

Jain, N. C., Budd, R. D. and Sneath, T. C. (1975). Rapid mass screening and confirmation of urinary amphetamine and methamphetamine by Gas Chromatography. *Clin. Toxicol.*, **8**, 211

Jane, I. and Taylor, J. F. (1975). Characterisation and quantitation of Morphine in Urine using high-pressure liquid chromatography with fluorescence detection. *J. Chromatog.*, **109**, 37

Jane, I. (1975). The separation of a wide range of drugs of abuse by high-pressure liquid chromatography. *J. Chromatog.*, **111**, 227

Jatlow, P. I. and Bailey, D. N. (1975). Gas-chromatographic Analysis for Cocaine in Human Plasma, with Use of a Nitrogen Detector. *Clin. Chem.*, **21**, 1918

Kaistha, K. K. (1972). Drug abuse screening programs: Detection procedures, development costs, street-sample analysis and field tests. *J. pharm. Sci.*, **61**, 655

Kaistha, K. K. and Jaffe, J. H. (1972a). TLC techniques for identification of narcotics, barbiturates and CNS stimulants in a drug abuse urine screening programme. *J. pharm. Sci.*, **61**, 679

Kaistha, K. and Jaffe, J. H. (1972b). Reliability of identification techniques for drugs of abuse in a urine screening programme and drug excretion data. *J. pharm. Sci.*, **61**, 305

Kaistha, K. K. and Jaffe, J. H. (1971). Extraction techniques for narcotics, barbiturates and central nervous system stimulants in a drug abuse urine screening programme. *J. Chromatog.*, **60**, 83

Klein, B., Sheehan, J. E. and Grunberg, E. (1974). Use of fluorescamine ('Fluram') to detect amphetamines in urine by thin-layer chromatography. *Clin. Chem.*, **20**, 272

Kullberg, M. P. and Gorodetzky, C. W. (1974). Studies on the use of XAD-2 resin for detection of abused drugs in urine. *Clin. Chem.*, **20**, 177

Kupferberg, H. J., Burkhalter, A. and Way, E. L. (1964). Fluorometric identification of submicrogram amounts of morphine and related compounds on thin-layer chromatographs. *J. Chromatog.*, **16**, 558

Kupferberg, H., Burkhalter, A. and Way, E. L. (1964). A sensitive fluorometric assay for morphine in plasma and brain. *J. Pharm. exp. therap.*, **145**, 247

Lawson, A. A. H. and Brown, S. S. (1967). Acute methaqualone (Mandrax) poisoning. *Scot. Med. J.*, **12**, 63

Lebish, P., Finkle, B. S. and Brackett, J. W. (1970). Determination of amphetamines, methamphetamine and related amines in blood and urine by gas chromatography with hydrogen-flame ionization detector. *Clin. Chem.*, **16**, 195

Leute, R., Ullman, E. F. and Goldstein, A. (1972). Spin immunoassay of opiate narcotics in urine and saliva. *J. Amer. med. Ass.*, **221**, 1231

MacGee, J. (1971). Rapid identification and quantitative determination of barbiturates and glutethamide in blood by gas–liquid chromatography. *Clin. Chem.*, **17**, 587

McGonigle, E. J. (1971). Determination of microgram quantities of methadone by fluorescence. *Anal. Chem.*, **43**, 966

Marks, V. and Fry, D. (1968). Investigation of drug addiction in the routine clinical biochemistry laboratory; detection and identification of amphetamine and morphine in urine. *Proc. Ass. Clin. Biochem.*, **5**, 95

Marks, V., Fry, D., Chapple, P. A. L. and Gray, G. (1969). Application of urine analysis to diagnosis and treatment of heroin addiction. *Br. med. J.*, **2**, 153

Marks, V., Teale, D. and Fry, D. (1975). Detection of Cannabis Products in Urine by Radioimmunoassay. *Brit. med. J.*, **3**, 348

Martin, H. F. and Driscoll, J. L. (1966). Gas chromatographic identification and determination of barbiturates. *Anal. Chem.*, **38**, 345

Mitchard, M. and Williams, M. E. (1972). An improved quantitative gas–liquid chromatographic assay for the estimation of methaqualone in biological materials. *J. Chromatog.*, **72**, 29

Moffat, A. C., Horning, E. C., Martin, S. B. and Rowland, M. (1972). Perfluorobenzene derivatives as derivatising agents for gas chromatography of primary and secondary amines using electron capture detection. *J. Chromatog.*, **66**, 255

Morris, B. A., Robinson, J. D., Piall, E., Aherne, G. W. and Marks, V. (1974). The development of a radioimmunoassay for morphine having minimal cross reactivity with codeine. *J. Endocrin.*, **64**, 6

Mulé, S. J. (1969). Identification of narcotics, barbiturates, amphetamines, tranquilizers and psychotominetics in human urine. *J. Chromatog.*, **39**, 302

Mulé, S. J. (1972). Detection and identification of drugs of dependence. *In* 'Chemical and biological aspects of drug dependence'. (S. J. Mulé and H. Brill, ed.) (Cleveland, Ohio: CRC Press)

Mulé, S. J., Bastos, M. L., Jukofsky, D. and Saffer, E. (1971). Routine identification of drugs of abuse in human urine, II Development and application of the XAD-2 resin column method. *J. Chromatog.*, **63**, 289

Mulé, S. J., Bastos, M. L. and Jukofsky, D. (1974a). Evaluation of immunoassay methods for detection in urine of drugs subject to abuse. *Clin. Chem.*, **20**, 243

Mulé, S. J. and Hushin, P. L. (1971). Semi-automated fluorimetric assay for submicrogram quantities of morphine and quinine in human biological material. *Anal. Chem.*, **43**, 708

Mulé, S. J., Sunshine, J., Braude, M. and Wilbette, R. E. (1974b). *Immunoassays for drugs subject to abuse.* (Cleveland, Ohio: CRC Press)

Nix, C. R. and Hume, A. S. (1970). A spectrophotofluorometric method for the determination of amphetamine. *J. Forensic Sci.*, **15**, 595

Papadopoulos, A. S., Baylis, E. M., Fry, D. E. and Marks, V. (1973). A rapid micro-method for determining four anti-convulsant drugs by gas-liquid chromatography. *Clin. Chim. Acta.*, **48**, 135

Rosenfeld, J. J., Bowins, B., Roberts, J., Perkins, J. and Macpherson, A. S. (1974). Mass fragmentographic assay for Δ^9-tetrahydrocannabinol in plasma. *Anal. Chem.*, **46**, 2232

Rubinstein, K. E., Schneider, R. S. and Ullman, E. F. (1972). Homogeneous enzyme immunoassay: A new technique for the quantitative determination of abused drugs. *Clin. Chem.*, **18**, 714

Rutter, E. R. (1972). Automated method for screening urine for amphetamine and some related primary amines. *Clin. Chem.*, **18**, 616

Sine, H. E., Kubasik, N. P. and Woytash, J. (1973). Simple gas–liquid chromatographic method for confirming the presence of alkaloids in urine. *Clin. Chem.*, **19**, 340

Spector, S. (1971). Quantitative determination of morphine in serum by radioimmunoassay. *J. Pharmacol. exp. ther.*, **178**, 253

Stoner, R. E. and Parker, C. (1974). Single-pH extraction procedure for detecting drugs of abuse. *Clin. Chem.*, **20**, 309

Stevenson, G. W. (1966). On-column methylation of barbituric acid. *Anal. Chem.*, **38**, 1948

Stewart, J. T. and Lotti, D. M. (1971). Fluorometric determination of amphetamines with 3-carboxy-7-hydroxycoumarin. *J. Pharm. Sci.*, **60**, 461

Sulkowski, T. S., Lathrop, G. D., Merritt, J. H., Landez, J. H. and Noe, E. R. (1975). A Semiautomated Radioimmunoassay for Mass Screening of Drugs of Abuse. *J. Forensic Sci.*, **20**, 524

Taunton-Rigby, A., Sher, S. E. and Kelley, P. R. (1973). Lysergic acid diethylamide: radioimmunoassay. *Science (N.Y.)*, **181**, 165

Teale, J. D., Forman, E. J., King, L. J. and Marks, V. (1974). Radioimmunoassay of cannabinoids in blood and urine. *Lancet*, **ii**, 553

Teale, J. D., Forman, J. E., King, L. J., Piall, E. M. and Marks, V. (1975). The development of a radioimmunoassay for cannabinoids in blood and urine. *J. Pharm. Pharmac.*, **27**, 465

Toseland, P. A., Albani, M. and Gauchel, F. D. (1975). Organic nitrogen-selective detector used in gas-chromatographic determination of some anticonvulsant and barbiturate drugs in plasma and tissue. *Clin. Chem.*, **21**, 98

Toseland, P. A. and Scott, P. H. (1969). Determination of amphetamine as its N-acetyl derivative by gas–liquid chromatography. *Clin. Chim. Acta.*, **25**, 75

Twycross, R. G., Fry, D. E. and Wills, P. D. (1974). The alimentary absorption of diamorphine and morphine in man as indicated by urinary excretion studies. *Brit. J. Clin. Pharmacol.*, **1**, 491

Upshall, D. G. and Wailling, D. G. (1972). The determination of LSD in human plasma following oral administration. *Clin. Chim. Acta.*, **36**, 67

Valentine, J. L., Weigert, P. E. and Charles, R. L. (1972). G.L.C. determination of methadone in human urine. *J. Pharm. Sci.*, **61**, 797

Valanju, N. N., Baden, M. M., Valanju, S. N., Mulligan, D. and Verma, S. K. (1973). Detection of bio-transformed cocaine in urine from drug abusers. *J. Chromatog.*, **81**, 170

Van der Slooten, E. P. J., Van der Helm, H. J. and Geerlings, P. J. (1971). Gas chromatographic detection of methadone and morphine in the urine of drug addicts. *J. Chromatog.*, **60**, 131

Van Vunakis, H., Farrow, J. T., Gjika, H. B. and Levine, L. (1971). Specificity of the antibody receptor site to D-lysergamide: Model of a physiological receptor for lysergic acid diethylamide. *Proc. Nat. Acad. Sci.*, **68**, 1483

Wallace, J. E., Briggs, J. D. and Blum, K. (1972). Gas-liquid and thin-layer chromatographic determination of morphine in biologic specimens. *Clin. Chim. Acta*, **36**, 85

Weissman, N., Lowe, M. L., Beattie, J. M. and Demetriou, J. A. (1971). Screening method for detection of drugs of abuse in human urine. *Clin. Chem.*, **17**, 875

Wilkinson, G. R. and Way, E. L. (1969). Submicrogram estimation of morphine in biological fluids by gas–liquid chromatography. *Biochem. Pharmacol.*, **18**, 1435

Index